# FERTILITY AND ASSISTED REPRODUCTIVE TECHNOLOGY (ART)

**Eleanor L. Stevenson, PhD, RN,** is an assistant professor of nursing at Duke University School of Nursing in the Division of Health for Women, Children, and Families. She received her BS in nursing from Rutgers University College of Nursing–New Brunswick and her MS as a women's health nurse practitioner from Rutgers University College of Nursing–Newark. She received her PhD in nursing research and theory development from New York University College of Nursing. Her area of inquiry focuses on the multidimensional psychological stress women who have conceived pregnancies via in vitro fertilization experience, as well as the adaptive behaviors of men with male-factor infertility. Dr. Stevenson is an active member of Sigma Theta Tau International, Beta Epsilon, the American Society for Reproductive Medicine–Nurse Professional Group, and the Association for Women's Health, Obstetrical and Neonatal Nursing (AWHONN). She has received numerous awards including the New York University Alumni Association Doctoral Achievement Award; the Sigma Theta Tau International Upsilon Research Award; the Rudin Family Award for Doctoral Achievement; the McRae Foundation Award; and the American Society for Reproductive Medicine Nursing Professional Group Prize Paper Award (2011, 2012, and 2014). Dr. Stevenson's clinical career has focused on women's health issues, including clinical practice in various settings such as high-risk labor and delivery, mother–baby, antepartum, family planning, and infertility services. At Duke University, she teaches in the DNP, MSN, and ABSN programs. Dr. Stevenson has also applied her clinical expertise in the research and development of women's health and infertility medications. She enjoys sharing her passion for this patient population with students by mentoring baccalaureate, master's, and doctoral students who focus their inquiry and practice on fertility issues to advance science and clinical care.

**Patricia E. Hershberger, PhD, MSN, RN, FNP-BC,** a registered nurse and board-certified family nurse practitioner, is an associate professor of nursing and an affiliate professor of medicine at the University of Illinois at Chicago (UIC). Dr. Hershberger received her ASN and BSN degrees from Indiana University–Northwest, her MSN from Valparaiso University, and her PhD from UIC. She completed postdoctoral training at the University of Michigan. Dr. Hershberger's multidisciplinary research, which is shaped by her clinical practice experiences, aims to improve the health and health care of individuals, couples, and families with fertility challenges. Her research has been supported by the National Institutes of Health, the International Society of Nurses in Genetics, Sigma Theta Tau International (Alpha Lambda Chapter), and the UIC College of Nursing Internal Research Support Program. Dr. Hershberger is the recipient of numerous awards for her research, including the National Award of Excellence in Research from the Association of Women's Health, Obstetric, and Neonatal Nurses (2013) and the National Institutes of Health Building Interdisciplinary Research Careers in Women's Health (BIRCWH) scholar award (2009). She is among a handful of nurses who received a prestigious BIRCWH award. Dr. Hershberger is a recipient of the American Society for Reproductive Medicine Nursing Professional Group Prize Paper Award (2005, 2014). Committed to advancing research and fostering the next generation of scientists, Dr. Hershberger was elected to the Midwest Nursing Research Society board of directors in 2014. She is also an active member of the American Society for Reproductive Medicine.

# FERTILITY AND ASSISTED REPRODUCTIVE TECHNOLOGY (ART)

Theory, Research, Policy, and Practice
for Health Care Practitioners

Eleanor L. Stevenson, PhD, RN
Patricia E. Hershberger, PhD, MSN, RN, FNP-BC

*Editors*

SPRINGER PUBLISHING COMPANY
NEW YORK

Springer Publishing Company, LLC
11 West 42nd Street
New York, NY 10036
www.springerpub.com

*Acquisitions Editor*: Elizabeth Nieginski
*Composition*: Newgen KnowledgeWorks

*ISBN*: 978-0-8261-7253-2
*e-book ISBN*: 978-0-8261-7254-9

16 17 18 19/ 5 4 3 2 1

The author and the publisher of this Work have made every effort to use sources believed to be reliable to provide information that is accurate and compatible with the standards generally accepted at the time of publication. Because medical science is continually advancing, our knowledge base continues to expand. Therefore, as new information becomes available, changes in procedures become necessary. We recommend that the reader always consult current research and specific institutional policies before performing any clinical procedure. The author and publisher shall not be liable for any special, consequential, or exemplary damages resulting, in whole or in part, from the readers' use of, or reliance on, the information contained in this book. The publisher has no responsibility for the persistence or accuracy of URLs for external or third-party Internet websites referred to in this publication and does not guarantee that any content on such websites is, or will remain, accurate or appropriate.

**Library of Congress Cataloging-in-Publication Data**

Names: Stevenson, Eleanor, editor. | Hershberger, Patricia E., editor.
Title: Fertility and assisted reproductive technology (ART) : theory, research, policy, and practice for health care practitioners / Eleanor Stevenson, Patricia E. Hershberger, editors.
Description: New York, NY : Springer Publishing Company, LLC, [2016] |
    Includes bibliographical references and index.
Identifiers: LCCN 2015037357| ISBN 9780826172532 | ISBN 9780826172549 (e-book)
Subjects: | MESH: Fertility—Nurses' Instruction. | Reproductive Techniques, Assisted—Nurses' Instruction: | Infertility—Nurses' Instruction.
Classification: LCC RG133.5 | NLM WP 565 | DDC 618.1/78—dc23
LC record available at http://lccn.loc.gov/2015037357

Printed in the United States of America by Gasch Printing.

*To the women and men who have fertility challenges*

# CONTENTS

*Contributors* xi
*Foreword* Susan Seenan, HND *xv*
*Foreword* Marcia C. Inhorn, PhD, MPH *xvii*
*Preface* xxi
*Acknowledgments* xxv

## PART I: THEORY: ENGAGING THEORIES AND CONCEPTUAL CONCEPTS IN ART

1. A Template for a Comprehensive Theory of Infertility: A Roy Adaptation Model Perspective *3*
   *Jacqueline Fawcett*

2. Shifting Family Structure: Theoretical Perspectives of Worldwide Population and Family Composition *15*
   *Jennie M. Wagner*

3. A Theoretical Approach to Multidimensional Stress Experienced During Pregnancy by Women Who Conceive Via In Vitro Fertilization *29*
   *Eleanor L. Stevenson and Kristina Cobb*

4. Examining the Unit of Analysis in Assisted Reproduction: Conceptual Insights Into Individual, Couple, and Family Research in Education and Counseling *49*
   *Patricia E. Hershberger and Sooyoung Yeom*

5. *Exemplar*: Using an Egg Donor: Insights Into an Infertile Woman's Experience *59*
   *Patricia E. Hershberger*

## PART II: RESEARCH AND REVIEWS: DELINEATING THE STATE OF THE SCIENCE IN ART

6. Psychological Stress and Fertility *65*
   *Angela K. Lawson*

7. The Illusion of Normal Fertility: Women's Experiences of Pregnancy and Birth After Oocyte Donation *87*
   *Astrid Indekeu and Ken Daniels*

8. Individual and Family Outcomes of First-Time Parents Older Than 40 Years: Implications of Later-Life Parenting *103*
   *Julia T. Woodward and Katherine E. MacDuffie*

9. Understanding the Impact of Delayed Parenting: Gender, Paid Work, and Work–Family Strategies   *121*
   *Tiffany Romain and Robert D. Nachtigall*

10. Young Women's Reasons Regarding Whether to Undergo Fertility Preservation Treatment When Facing a Cancer Diagnosis: A Literature Review   *143*
    *Patricia E. Hershberger*

11. Accommodating Assisted Reproductive Technologies to Rabbinic Law   *153*
    *Tsipy Ivry*

12. "If Some Is Good, More Must Be Better": Diverging Goals Between Patient and Provider About Multifetal Pregnancies in ART   *161*
    *Alexandra Cooper, Kathryn E. Flynn, and Elizabeth A. Duthie*

13. *Exemplar*: Medically High-Risk Conditions Necessitating Utilization of a Gestational Carrier   *183*
    *Eleanor L. Stevenson*

**PART III: POLICY: EXPLORING ACCESS AND CHALLENGES IN ART**

14. Challenges to Infertility Advocacy in the United States: Defining Infertility and Barriers to Access to Care   *191*
    *Barbara Collura and Eleanor L. Stevenson*

15. Utilization of ART Services in Developed Countries and Impact on Cross-Border Reproductive Care   *201*
    *Eleanor L. Stevenson and Jamie Kanehl*

16. Utilization of Fertility Care in Developing Countries: Challenges in Family Building Around the Globe   *211*
    *Nathalie Dhont and Willem Ombelet*

17. Emerging "Cost-Effective" Treatments Including Low-Cost IVF   *223*
    *Willem Ombelet and Nathalie Dhont*

18. Defining Infertility: Global Views on Timing of IVF and the Ability to Access Care   *235*
    *Irma Scholten and Ben W. Mol*

19. Changing Times: How Is Same-Sex Relationship Equality Impacting the Fertility Care Landscape?   *245*
    *Bethany G. Everett, Oluwatitofunmi O. Apatira, and Katharine McCabe*

20. *Exemplar*: A Genetically At-Risk Couple Considers the Use of Preimplantation Genetic Diagnosis in the United States   *257*
    *Patricia E. Hershberger*

**PART IV: PRACTICE: IMPROVING THE DELIVERY OF CARE IN THE ART SETTING**

21. Assisted Reproductive Technology Treatment Options for Couples With Fertility Issues   *263*
    *Eleanor L. Stevenson*

22. Polycystic Ovary Syndrome: Reproductive and Psychological
Implications   277
*Osama S. Abdalmageed, Jennifer L. Eaton, and William W. Hurd*

23. Team Communication: Critical in the Care of the Couple
With Fertility Challenges   295
*Jamie Leonard and Eleanor L. Stevenson*

24. Focusing on Nursing: Emerging Specialty
Practice in the United Kingdom   **311**
*Eilis Moody*

25. Men and Infertility: Their Experience With Challenges
in Family Formation   323
*Kevin McEleny*

26. *Exemplar*: An Adolescent Seeking Fertility Treatment   337
*Anne Derouin*

Epilogue: Family Formation—What Is Ahead?   343
*Eleanor L. Stevenson and Patricia E. Hershberger*

*Index   355*

# CONTRIBUTORS

**Osama S. Abdalmageed, MBBCh**   Research Fellow, Division of Reproductive Endocrinology and Infertility, Department of Obstetrics and Gynecology, Duke University School of Medicine, Duke Fertility Center, Durham, North Carolina

**Oluwatitofunmi O. Apatira, MS, RN**   PhD Student, Department of Health System Sciences, University of Illinois at Chicago, Chicago, Illinois

**Kristina Cobb, BSN, BA, RN, PCCN**   Staff Nurse, Rex University of North Carolina Healthcare, Raleigh, North Carolina

**Barbara Collura, MA**   President/CEO, RESOLVE: The National Infertility Association, McLean, Virginia

**Alexandra Cooper, PhD**   Associate Director for Education, Social Science Research Institute, Duke University, Durham, North Carolina

**Ken Daniels, ONZM, MA (Hons), Dip. Soc. Stu.**   Professor (Adjunct), University of Canterbury, Christchurch, New Zealand

**Anne Derouin, DNP, MSN, CPNP**   Assistant Professor, Duke University School of Nursing, Durham, North Carolina

**Nathalie Dhont, MD, PhD**   Gynecologist, Genk Institute for Fertility Technology, Genk, Belgium

**Elizabeth A. Duthie, PhD**   Instructor and Research Fellow, Department of Medicine, Center for Patient Care and Outcomes Research, Medical College of Wisconsin, Milwaukee, Wisconsin

**Jennifer L. Eaton, MD, MSCI**   Assistant Professor of Obstetrics and Gynecology, Division of Reproductive Endocrinology and Infertility, Department of Obstetrics and Gynecology, Duke University School of Medicine, Duke Fertility Center, Durham, North Carolina

**Bethany G. Everett, PhD**   Assistant Professor, Department of Sociology, University of Utah, Salt Lake City, Utah

**Jacqueline Fawcett, RN, PhD, ScD (Hons), FAAN**   Professor, Department of Nursing, University of Massachusetts Boston, Boston, Massachusetts

**Kathryn E. Flynn, PhD**   Associate Professor, Department of Medicine, Center for Patient Care and Outcomes Research, Medical College of Wisconsin, Milwaukee, Wisconsin

**Patricia E. Hershberger, PhD, MSN, RN, FNP-BC**   Associate Professor, College of Nursing, Department of Health Systems Science; Affiliate Professor, College of Medicine, Department of Obstetrics and Gynecology, University of Illinois at Chicago, Chicago, Illinois

**William W. Hurd, MD, MPH**   Professor of Obstetrics and Gynecology, Division of Reproductive Endocrinology and Infertility, Department of Obstetrics and Gynecology, Duke University School of Medicine, Duke Fertility Center, Durham, North Carolina

**Astrid Indekeu, PhD, L. Psy., M. Sexol.**   Postdoctoral Researcher, Department of Neurobiology, Care Sciences and Society, Karolinska Institutet, Huddinge, Sweden and Fellow, Centre for Sociological Research, University of Leuven, Leuven, Belgium

**Tsipy Ivry, PhD**   Senior Lecturer, Department of Anthropology, University of Haifa, Haifa, Israel

**Jamie Kanehl, BSN, BS, RN**   Staff Nurse, Cone Health, Greensboro, North Carolina

**Angela K. Lawson, PhD**   Assistant Professor, Departments of Obstetrics and Gynecology and Psychiatry, Northwestern University, Chicago, Illinois

**Jamie Leonard, BSN, RN**   Infertility Support Group Facilitator, Bennett Fertility Institute, Oklahoma City, Oklahoma

**Katherine E. MacDuffie, MA**   PhD Student, Department of Psychology and Neuroscience, Duke University, Durham, North Carolina

**Katharine McCabe, MA**   PhD Student, Department of Sociology, University of Illinois at Chicago, Chicago, Illinois

**Kevin McEleny, BSc, BM, PhD, FRCS (Eng.), FRCS (Ed.), FRCS (Urol.)**   Consultant Urologist, Newcastle Fertility Centre, The Newcastle-Upon-Tyne Hospitals National Health Service Foundation Trust, Newcastle-Upon-Tyne, United Kingdom

**Ben W. Mol, MD, PhD**   Professor, Department of Obstetrics and Gynecology, The University of Adelaide, Adelaide, South Australia, Australia

**Eilis Moody, RGN, BA (Hons)**   Senior Nurse, Newcastle Fertility Centre, The Newcastle-Upon-Tyne Hospitals National Health Service Foundation Trust, Newcastle-Upon-Tyne, United Kingdom

**Robert D. Nachtigall, MD** Clinical Professor Emeritus, Departments of Obstetrics and Gynecology and the Institute for Health and Aging, University of California, San Francisco, California

**Willem Ombelet, MD, PhD** Professor, University of Hasselt, Genk Institute for Fertility Technology, Genk, Belgium

**Tiffany Romain, PhD** Advisory Research Anthropologist, Ricoh Innovations Corporation, Cupertino, California

**Irma Scholten, MD** PhD Student, Reproductive Medicine, Department of Obstetrics and Gynecology, Academic Medical Center, Amsterdam, The Netherlands

**Eleanor L. Stevenson, PhD, RN** Assistant Professor, Duke University School of Nursing, Division of Health for Women, Children, and Families, Durham, North Carolina

**Jennie M. Wagner, EdD, RN, MSM, IBCLC** Assistant Professor, University of North Carolina at Chapel Hill, Chapel Hill, North Carolina

**Julia T. Woodward, PhD** Infertility Psychologist, Duke Fertility Center, Duke University Medical Center, Durham, North Carolina

**Sooyoung Yeom, BSN, RN** Graduate Student, College of Nursing, University of Illinois at Chicago, Chicago, Illinois

# FOREWORD

The agony and anguish fertility struggles wreak go right to the heart of what it means to be human. Being able to reproduce and bring forth new life is the basis of human biology; when this ability is damaged, our very existence is threatened. That is why problems with fertility often cut harder and deeper than other issues. Infertility is also far more than just a physical malfunction: It affects individuals profoundly at emotional, social, and cultural levels. It is not uncommon to hear those battling to become parents talking of how life loses all meaning; men describe feeling less of a man and, for women, the empty womb can challenge all notions of womanhood. Considering this, the importance of fertility care is paramount.

It is approaching 40 years since the world's first "test-tube" baby was born in the United Kingdom; since then, assisted reproductive technologies (ARTs) have transformed our world for the better. Those who struggle with fertility challenges experience a very simple story: that of restoring the gift of life. However, as advances in ART, including in vitro fertilization (IVF), continue to improve success rates there is a growing threat for those unable to have children without medical assistance. Across the world, access to fertility treatment is being denied to those who cannot afford it, or those whose medical insurance does not cover it. Although we may applaud developments in ART, it would be a hollow victory indeed if novel fertility therapies were only available for the richest few in society.

I am one of the lucky ones who finally became a mother after struggling with fertility problems. I got the chance to try IVF. I want to see all others in need have the same opportunities. In my office, I have the following patient quote pinned up: "I can accept failure; everyone fails at something. But what I cannot accept is not trying." The real challenge in the years ahead for fertility treatment will be making sure all who want to try to become parents via ART have the chance to do so.

*Fertility and Assisted Reproductive Technology (ART): Theory, Research, Policy, and Practice for Health Care Practitioners* addresses the many facets of infertility and fertility care around the world. Discussion of these topics will help physicians, nurses, and others who care for those with fertility challenges to not only increase awareness of the issues surrounding access and policy, but also highlight some key clinical

care considerations. The wide range of topics provides a wealth of information and
helps to bring awareness of the many struggles and issues for people with fertility
concerns.

*Susan Seenan, HND*
*Chief Executive*
*Infertility Network United Kingdom*
*East Sussex, United Kingdom*

# FOREWORD

Infertility is estimated to affect as many as 186 million people worldwide. On average, 9% of all reproductive-aged couples suffer from this condition. In some regions of the world, the rates of infertility are much higher, affecting as many as 30% of all couples. Infertility thus remains a challenging global reproductive health problem. Yet, in vitro fertilization (IVF)—the nearly 40-year-old assisted reproductive technology (ART) designed to overcome infertility—is still not readily available to those who need it, either in resource-poor settings or in countries such as the United States where lack of public funding of IVF remains a potent barrier to fertility care.

Fertility care is the main theme of this edited volume brought together by two professors of fertility nursing. Their notion of "care" is admirably broad and reflected in diverse and comprehensive chapters on a wide range of subjects. This welcome and much-needed interprofessional volume provides a state-of-the-art, cutting-edge overview of infertility and ART in the 21st century. Indeed, this volume presents a veritable treasure trove of useful information for both clinicians and scholars. Four key themes shine through the chapters.

## CAUSATION

This volume clearly challenges the assertion that the causes of infertility have been completely discovered. Several chapters address both the most proximate (e.g., genetics and stress) and distal (e.g., global demographic shifts and delayed child-bearing) causes of infertility, suggesting that more research is needed on the global epidemiology of infertility. Particularly welcome are chapters devoted to male infertility and polycystic ovary syndrome (PCOS). Both of these conditions are increasing in prevalence around the world, with male infertility contributing to more than half of all cases of childlessness. Both of these conditions also reflect the interaction of genes and environment. For example, most cases of severe male-factor infertility reflect genetic mutations or chromosomal abnormalities. But smoking and various environmental toxins also diminish men's sperm profiles. Similarly, PCOS, which is related to insulin resistance and diabetes, is often triggered by lifestyle changes such as increased sedentarism and weight gain. Indeed, PCOS is a growing cause of women's infertility around the globe, but one that has received insufficient scholarly attention.

Another issue that is particularly well addressed in this volume is the relationship between age and fertility, both maternal and paternal. As several chapters demonstrate, changing norms of marriage and cohabitation, increasing educational and professional opportunities for women, workplace policies that do not support parenting, and concomitant delays in childbearing are serving to increase the age of first pregnancy in many societies around the globe. In the United Kingdom, for example, the average age of first-time mothers is 30 years. In the United States, one out of every five women will become a first-time mother after the age of 35 years, an eightfold increase over the previous generation of women. These shifts toward older childbearing have, in effect, "caused" more infertility, with advanced maternal age (AMA) as one of the primary indications for IVF due to poor ovarian reserve and poor oocyte quality. At last, advanced paternal age is also being questioned for its links to poor fertility and child health outcomes. Like male infertility in general, advanced paternal age—including its effects on parenting and life expectancy—has been relatively neglected and misunderstood. Thus, the attention in this volume to all of these issues is quite laudable, suggesting that much more research, both on the basic science of infertility etiology and on the social science of gender norms and family formation, deserves to be undertaken.

## ACCESS

This volume also prioritizes issues of access—namely, why millions of people worldwide face obstacles to receiving infertility diagnosis and care, including access to ART. ART access varies widely around the globe, due to the lack of IVF clinics in some regions (e.g., sub-Saharan Africa), and due to the lack of public IVF funding (i.e., state subsidization) in the majority of non-Western European countries. As a result, IVF and other ARTs are unaffordable for most people. In the United States, which is the main focus of this volume, the average cost of an IVF cycle exceeds $12,000 and is not covered by most health insurance plans. Furthermore, the few "mandate states" where IVF cycles are publicly financed are paradoxically being challenged by the Affordable Care Act (ACA), which does not cover infertility treatment. In the United States, as elsewhere, infertility is too often viewed as a "luxury" condition, making IVF an "elective" procedure. This view is strongly challenged by the reproductive rights focus forwarded in this volume, in which ART access is a form of reproductive justice for the infertile.

Several chapters in this volume highlight ART activism. Most notably, the low-cost IVF (LCIVF) movement—which is being promoted most forcefully by the Walking Egg nonprofit organization in Belgium—hopes to bring a very low-cost form of IVF to sub-Saharan Africa and other parts of the Global South. LCIVF also has great potential in "developed" countries such as the United States, where the unmet need for IVF among low-income and minority populations represents a potent reproductive health disparity. Eventually, LCIVF may serve to mitigate what has become a worldwide phenomenon of cross-border reproductive care (CBRC), or the reproductive travel of infertile patients across national borders. As shown in this volume, much CBRC is attributable to the search for affordable IVF care.

## CARE

As mentioned earlier, care is the key trope of this volume. What does it mean to deliver high-quality care to those needing help with conception? This volume takes an expansive view of those needing help—not only infertile heterosexual couples in marriages or committed partnerships, but also same-sex couples (i.e., gay men needing gestational surrogates and gay women needing sperm donors), transgender individuals who may desire fertility preservation, adolescents who desire early childbearing, single women seeking oocyte cryopreservation for either medical or elective fertility preservation, and couples facing genetic conditions (e.g., sickle cell disease), where IVF-related preimplantation genetic diagnosis may prevent genetic disease in their offspring. As the remit of (in)fertility services for ever-more-diverse populations grows wider, the need for clinically, psychologically, socially, culturally, and religiously "competent," "patient-centered" (in)fertility care and ART services will continue to expand. Fortunately, this book offers much guidance and advice for those working in the clinical realm. Several chapters are oriented toward psychologists and nurses, demonstrating what a crucial role they play in helping to relieve patient anxiety, in developing effective clinical teamwork, and in introducing patients to helpful adjunct services such as support groups and complementary and alternative medicine (CAM). In addition, patient-centered infertility care involves understanding the lifeworlds of patients themselves—their psychological distress, their social and structural vulnerabilities, and their special needs for support, including those after the birth of their children. For example, as shown in this volume, parenting after oocyte donation may require special clinical skills and psychological reassurance to women who have grieved the loss of their biogenetic reproductive potential. These women deserve to be supported in their mothering roles, so they may form strong and positive attachments to their children through pregnancy, childbirth, and breastfeeding.

## OUTCOMES

In other words, the "aftermath" of ART—the actual outcomes of infertility services, including the successful births and the reproductive failures—requires more scholarly attention and care. As this volume makes abundantly clear, new ARTs are continuously on the horizon. This includes, for example, IVF through uterine transplantation, mitochondrial transfer to overcome inherited mitochondrial disease, ovarian tissue freezing, and ovarian tissue transplant. How will these new technologies change the face of fertility care as well as the families created by them? This volume suggests that much research will need to be undertaken, not only on the "new" reproductive technologies, but also on the ART outcomes already in our midst. This includes the high rates of excess embryo transfer and iatrogenic multifetal pregnancies in many parts of the world. Moreover, with egg donation already firmly in place, and with egg freezing increasingly being undertaken by women in their late 30s and 40s, more research on age, ART outcomes, and "peri-menopausal parenting" will need to be conducted.

Overall, this collection speaks to the emergence of much that is new, vital, wondrous, and amazing in the world of assisted reproduction. Yet, many issues are still troubling, ambiguous, ethically questionable, unfair, and unresolved in the second decade of the new millennium. Those who read this volume will have a much better understanding of the multiple issues at stake. Thus, this book is an invaluable resource for clinicians, scholars, and lay readers who care about infertility, assisted reproduction, and reproductive justice in the 21st century.

*Marcia C. Inhorn, PhD, MPH*
*William K. Lanman, Jr. Professor*
*Anthropology and International Affairs*
*Yale University*
*New Haven, Connecticut*

# PREFACE

Fertility and the process of bearing children are a significant experience in most individuals' lives. A substantial number of individuals and couples struggle with challenges with their fertility and ultimately in building the families they desire. Infertility, the inability to conceive after 1 year of unprotected intercourse (Zegers-Hochschild et al., 2009), affects between 49 and 70 million couples around the world (Boivin, Bunting, Collins, & Nygren, 2007; Mascarenhas, Flaxman, Boerma, Vanderpoel, & Stevens, 2012). In the United States, survey studies have found that there are approximately 2 million infertile couples, which is about 9% of the married couples with females aged 15 to 44 years. According to the National Survey of Family Growth (National Center for Health Statistics, n.d.), about 6% of married women are infertile (12 months or longer without birth control and without a pregnancy). Additionally, about 12% of women (both married and single) aged 15 to 44 years had an impaired ability to have children (impaired fecundity) in 2013 (National Center for Health Statistics, n.d.). This latter increase is, in part, likely indicative of the delay in childbearing found in the contemporary couple population base in which significant age-related increases in infertility and impaired fecundity have been reported. The Healthy People 2020 (revised, 2013) goal is to reduce impaired fecundity to 11.4% (Healthypeople.gov, 2013). The medical specialty area known as assisted reproductive technology (ART), encompassing the field of reproductive endocrinology and infertility, has a global goal of improving family building outcomes for those with infertility and fertility challenges.

Although the treatment of infertility is the hallmark of care in ART, advances in physiological sciences have led to novel approaches that are not limited to the specific treatment of infertility. These novel treatment options expand the scope of care to include strategies for the preservation of future fertility and advanced options for examining the genetic structure of embryos before implantation. These ever-expanding treatment options allow a growing number of individuals, especially young women, the ability to preserve fertility (Practice Committees of the American Society for Reproductive Medicine and the Society for Assisted Reproductive Technology, 2013). Individuals with diseases such as cancer, lupus, and sickle cell now have fertility preservation options available to them (Lee et al., 2006; Raptopoulou, Sidiropoulos, & Boumpas, 2004; Roux et al., 2010; Sonmezer & Oktay, 2004). People at risk of transmitting genetic disorders can now opt to have embryos tested during in vitro fertilization (IVF) procedures to decrease the likelihood of transmitting the disorder to future offspring (Baruch, Kaufman, & Hudson, 2008; Hershberger, Schoenfeld, & Tur-Kaspa, 2011). These advances, made possible by cutting-edge breakthroughs in reproductive sciences, were unseen in prior generations. However, as the physiological sciences advance and treatment options become available to more individuals, there is less consideration of the impact of this cutting-edge science on those for whom it is intended to help, nor is there adequate discussion of the contemporary issues that these families, health care professionals, and other interested individuals, scholars, and scientists face.

To fill this critical gap, we set out to explore contemporary health care perspectives related to the health care of individuals, couples, and families dealing with infertility and fertility challenges including, but not limited to, those who are treated with advanced technologies such as IVF, intrauterine insemination, and oocyte preservation. We, as nurses, have had the profound opportunity to provide clinical nursing care for the growing number of people who are struggling with infertility and fertility challenges in today's modern world. We care deeply about people with fertility and infertility challenges and view this book as an extension of that care.

We hope that health care practitioners, public health officials, women's health experts, scientists, students, scholars, and other interested individuals from across the globe will find the information valuable. To that aim, we sought collaborators from a wide range of disciplines to help us enhance awareness, spur discussion, and invoke solutions for improving care of people throughout the world. Our collaborators represent eight countries (Australia, Belgium, Israel, New Zealand, Sweden, The Netherlands, the United Kingdom, and the United States) and nine states within the United States. We also purposely included collaborators who were at various stages in their careers—from those who are well established and leaders in ART, to those who are launching careers, including several students. Their collective voices provide a wealth of perspectives and a broad scope of ideas and information.

The book is organized into four parts (*theory, research and reviews, policy,* and *practice*) where various aspects of health care for those seeking fertility evaluation and treatment are presented. The theoretical part forms the foundation for the book, with chapters that articulate new ways of conceptualizing key concepts and processes that affect infertile people and those at risk of fertility loss. For example, the concept of adaptation is described as a basis for a comprehensive theory of infertility, and the concept of family structure is examined from various theoretical perspectives. The second part, research and reviews, includes chapters in which current research findings and comprehensive reviews provide up-to-date information about contemporary issues in ART. Psychological stress and fertility, delayed parenting, patient and provider perspectives on multifetal pregnancies, and how rabbinic law affects ART procedures are a few of the important topics discussed in this part. The third part advances to chapters covering burgeoning areas in policy that discuss important contemporary considerations such as same-sex relationships and issues related to access to care in the United States and globally. The last section, Part IV, discusses emerging practice considerations including information about treatment options, polycystic ovary syndrome, the unique needs of infertile men, and the specialty practice of fertility nurses in the United Kingdom. The book also offers four case study exemplars that will help readers synthesize areas previously addressed by offering relevant and thought-provoking examples from today's care practices.

Written in response to the ever-evolving science that surrounds the field of ART, this book provides insight about issues and perspectives surrounding contemporary family formation that involve advanced fertility and infertility treatments. We hope readers will find the information valuable and that it will aid in our resolve to improve the health care of the increasing number of individuals and families who find themselves interfacing with the evolving landscape of modern reproductive treatments.

*Eleanor L. Stevenson*
*Patricia E. Hershberger*

## REFERENCES

Baruch, S., Kaufman, D., & Hudson, K. L. (2008). Genetic testing of embryos: Practices and perspectives of US in vitro fertilization clinics. *Fertility and Sterility, 89*(5), 1053–1058.

Boivin, J., Bunting, L., Collins, J. A., & Nygren, K. G. (2007). International estimates of infertility prevalence and treatment-seeking: Potential need and demand for infertility medical care. *Human Reproduction, 22*(6), 1506–1512.

Healthypeople.gov. (2013). *Maternal, infant, and child health.* Retrieved from http://www.healthypeople.gov/2020/topics-objectives/topic/maternal-infant-and-child-health/objectives

Hershberger, P. E., Schoenfeld, C., & Tur-Kaspa, I. (2011). Unraveling preimplantation genetic diagnosis for high-risk couples: Implications for nurses at the front line of care. *Nursing for Women's Health, 15*(1), 36–45.

Lee, S. J., Schover, L. R., Partridge, A. H., Patrizio, P., Wallace, W. H., Hagerty, K., . . . Oktay, K.; American Society of Clinical Oncology. (2006). American Society of Clinical Oncology recommendations on fertility preservation in cancer patients. *Journal of Clinical Oncology, 24*(18), 2917–2931.

Mascarenhas, M. N., Flaxman, S. R., Boerma, T., Vanderpoel, S., & Stevens, G. A. (2012). National, regional, and global trends in infertility prevalence since 1990: A systematic analysis of 277 health surveys. *PLoS Medicine, 9*(12), e1001356.

National Center for Health Statistics. (n.d.). *Key statistics from the national survey of family growth.* Retrieved from http://www.cdc.gov/nchs/nsfg/key_statistics.htm

Practice Committees of the American Society for Reproductive Medicine and the Society for Assisted Reproductive Technology. (2013). Mature oocyte cryopreservation: A guideline. *Fertility and Sterility, 99*, 37–43. doi:10.1016/j.fertnstert.2012.09.028

Raptopoulou, A., Sidiropoulos, P., & Boumpas, D. (2004). Ovarian failure and strategies for fertility preservation in patients with systemic lupus erythematosus. *Lupus, 13*(12), 887–890.

Roux, C., Amiot, C., Agnani, G., Aubard, Y., Rohrlich, P. S., & Piver, P. (2010). Live birth after ovarian tissue autograft in a patient with sickle cell disease treated by allogeneic bone marrow transplantation. *Fertility and Sterility, 93*(7), 2413.e15–2413.e19.

Sonmezer, M., & Oktay, K. (2004). Fertility preservation in female patients. *Human Reproduction Update, 10*(3), 251–266.

Zegers-Hochschild, F., Adamson, G. D., de Mouzon, J., Ishihara, O., Mansour, R., Nygren, K., . . . Vanderpoel, S.; International Committee for Monitoring Assisted Reproductive Technology; World Health Organization. (2009). International Committee for Monitoring Assisted Reproductive Technology (ICMART) and the World Health Organization (WHO) revised glossary of ART terminology, 2009. *Fertility and Sterility, 92*(5), 1520–1524.

# ACKNOWLEDGMENTS

There are many reasons why we wanted to provide a book about worldwide contemporary fertility issues. Foremost, as nurses, we view this book as an extension of our nursing care. In today's contemporary fertility settings, there are a growing number of individuals and couples who seek complex fertility treatments that surround assisted reproductive technologies (ARTs). Ushered in with modern ARTs are a host of issues including the concern that fertility treatments are unobtainable for many individuals and couples worldwide. This book is written to ultimately improve the health care of *all* individuals and couples by presenting a sampling of thoughtful views, novel conceptualizations, research reports, comprehensive reviews, public health and policy perspectives, and innovative care practices to the forefront for discussion by a large global audience. Foremost, we are indebted to each of our collaborators who shared our vision and who were able to contribute their time, effort, and expertise toward our cause of helping those with fertility and infertility challenges in the modern world. We would like to thank them, too, for their willingness to revise and "improve" their chapters, and hope they are aware of our deep gratitude.

We are especially grateful for the intellectual and social support provided by our colleagues at the University of Illinois at Chicago (UIC) and Duke University. I, Patricia, would especially like to thank Drs. Karen Kavanaugh, Agatha Gallo, Carol Estwing Ferrans, Lorna Finnegan, Diana Wilkie, Terri Weaver, and numerous colleagues at the UIC College of Nursing for providing ongoing support and encouragement of my academic research and work. Special thanks to Dr. Bert Scoccia and everyone at the UIC Reproductive Medicine Center. I am grateful, too, to colleagues Drs. Susan Klock (Northwestern University Feinberg School of Medicine) and Ilan Tur-Kaspa (Institute for Human Reproduction) for their continued support of my research and shared commitment to improve patient care. I, Eleanor, would like to especially thank Drs. Anne Derouin, Brigit Carter, Helen Gordon, Diane Holditch-Davis, Catherine Gilliss, Marion Broome, and many others for their support of my academic journey at the Duke University School of Nursing, as well as earlier mentors who helped to shape and support my love of inquiry, in particular Dr. Linda Mayberry and Deborah Chyun. We are both grateful to Dr. Marilyn Oermann for offering insight and guidance to us, two eager and determined nurse scholars.

This book would not be possible without the support of the many women and men who participated in our research studies and allowed us to gain a broader understanding about facing fertility challenges in today's world. We are deeply indebted to them. Our many thanks to Mary Richardson for providing text-editing support and for responding to each of our American Psychological Association (APA) formatting concerns. We also thank our editors at Springer Publishing, Elizabeth Nieginski for her early support and vision of this book, and Jenna Vaccaro for her patience and efforts during its preparation.

Without any doubt, we extend much gratitude to our husbands, children, and families for their patience and ongoing support. We thank them for their understanding and tolerance of our self-imposed work schedules and are grateful for their willingness to carry out our family and social obligations when our schedules took us away. Finally, this book would not have been possible without each other. We are very grateful for the serendipitous events that allowed us to "discover" each other. We hope our mutual vision, motivation, and shared goal of helping individuals and couples from around the world, whose lives have been or could be changed forever through modern ART treatments, will benefit from our meeting and this book.

# PART I

# THEORY: ENGAGING THEORIES AND CONCEPTUAL CONCEPTS IN ART

According to Fawcett (2000), one purpose of a theory is "to provide a relatively concrete and specific structure for the interpretation of initially puzzling behaviors, situations, and events" (p. 19). One of the benefits of articulating theory in research and clinical practice, such as in fertility care, is that the work discovered and carried out can be directly applied in clinical practice, thus improving evidence-based care and providing a structure for evaluation. Because of the importance that theory has to practice, we felt it fitting to lead off this book with a presentation of work that uses theory as its foundation. We take a broad view in our definition of theory and align with eminent scholars such as Sandelowski (1993) by viewing theory not only as a set of statements that specifies relationships between concepts but also as the concepts, conceptual models, and frameworks that describe, organize, and assist with the interpretation of phenomena.

In this part, the chapters approach fertility care issues using a theoretical framework or concepts. In the first chapter, Fawcett, an expert on models and theories within nursing science, applies the Roy Adaptation Model to a comprehensive theory of infertility. Wagner examines the structure of the family from a global perspective through a theoretical lens about the concept of family. Stevenson and Cobb examine the stress of women pregnant through in vitro fertilization (IVF) from a multidimensional theoretical framework, and Hershberger and Yeom consider the dominant unit of analysis—the individual—in research involving fertility populations and challenge scientists to think more broadly in order to understand the phenomenon more comprehensively.

## REFERENCES

Fawcett, J. (2000). *Analysis and evaluation of contemporary nursing knowledge: Nursing models and theories*. Philadelphia, PA: F.A. Davis Company.

Sandelowski, M. (1993). Theory unmasked: The uses and guises of theory in qualitative research. *Research in Nursing and Health, 16*(3), 213–218. doi:10.1002/nur.4770160308

# A TEMPLATE FOR A COMPREHENSIVE THEORY OF INFERTILITY: A ROY ADAPTATION MODEL PERSPECTIVE

*Jacqueline Fawcett*

The purpose of this chapter is to offer a template for developing a comprehensive psychosocial theory of infertility within the context of the Roy Adaptation Model (RAM) of nursing (Roy, 2009). The chapter begins with an overview of the purpose of all research with regard to theory development and the way in which conceptual models guide theory development. The chapter continues with an overview of the RAM and a description of electronic searches for theoretical and empirical literature about psychosocial experiences of infertility. The concepts identified in the retrieved literature are then linked with the concepts of the RAM to create a template for a comprehensive theory. The physiological, psychological, and social factors that may be responsible for infertility; technological advances in treating these conditions; and correlates of options for overcoming infertility, such as adoption, surrogacy, or in vitro fertilization, are beyond the scope of this chapter.

## THEORY DEVELOPMENT, RESEARCH, AND CONCEPTUAL MODELS

Theories, which are made up of relatively concrete and specific concepts and propositions, are typically developed by means of empirical research (Fawcett & Garity, 2009). The starting point for the research that leads to theory development is a conceptual model, which is made up of relatively abstract and general concepts and propositions. The function of the conceptual model is to guide research, and therefore, theory development, by providing a distinctive frame of reference, "a horizon of expectations" (Popper, 1965, p. 47), and to help the researcher to "ask the right questions" (Glanz, 2002, p. 556) throughout all phases of a research project.

### The Roy Adaptation Model

Inasmuch as the RAM (Roy, 2009) has been the guide for my program of research for almost 40 years (Clarke & Fawcett, 2014), I selected this conceptual model to guide the development of a template for a comprehensive theory of infertility. The RAM focuses on changes experienced by human beings as they respond to internal and external environmental stimuli to maintain their physiological, psychic, spiritual, and social integrity. The concepts of the RAM are listed and defined in Box 1.1 and are depicted in Figure 1.1.

## BOX 1.1 SUMMARY OF THE ROY ADAPTATION MODEL

*Environmental Stimuli*—*The pooled effect of the stimuli is the **adaptation level**, that is, the final outcome of adapting to the stimuli.*

- The **focal stimulus** most immediately confronts the human being.
- **Contextual stimuli** are all other environmental factors that influence a situation.
- **Residual stimuli** are factors that have an unknown influence on the situation and, as such, are typically not included in research.

*Coping Processes*—Stimuli pass through two types of coping processes.

- The **regulator coping subsystem** processes stimuli through "neural, chemical, and endocrine coping channels" (Roy, 2009, p. 41) of the autonomic nervous system.
- The **cognator coping subsystem** processes stimuli through "four cognitive-emotive channels: perceptual and information processing, learning, judgment, and emotion" (Roy, 2009, p. 41).

*Modes of Adaptation*—Stimuli are indirectly related to four interrelated modes of adaptation through the coping processes and also are directly related to the four modes.

- The **physiological mode** addresses physical integrity and is concerned with responses to stimuli through "all the cells, tissues, organs, and systems comprising the human body" (Roy, 2009, p. 90).
- The **self-concept mode** addresses psychic and spiritual integrity and pertains "to the personal aspect of human systems" (Roy, 2009, p. 95), including the physical self (body sensations and body image) and personal self (self-consistency, self-ideal, and the moral–ethical–spiritual self).
- The **role function mode** addresses social integrity and pertains to activities that are associated with ascribed and acquired roles (Roy, 2009).
- The **interdependence mode** addresses social integrity and focuses on "interactions related to the giving and receiving of love, respect, and value" (Roy, 2009, p. 45).

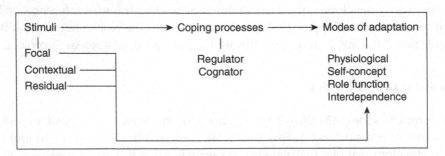

**FIGURE 1.1** The Roy Adaptation Model: concepts and propositions.

## Searches of the Literature

An electronic search of the literature from multiple disciplines yielded an impressively large number of studies of psychosocial aspects of infertility. The report of an initial search of PubMed/MEDLINE is shown in Table 1.1; filters yielded 408 publications. The report of a second search of PubMed/MEDLINE is shown in Table 1.2; this search yielded 225 publications. The report of a search of the Cumulative Index to Nursing and Allied Health Literature (CINAHL Complete), using the search terms [name of conceptual model of nursing] AND infertility, is shown in Table 1.3; this search yielded seven publications. The sources of theory concepts that were

**TABLE 1.1 Results of First Search of PubMed/MEDLINE for Literature About Infertility and Psychological Stress**

| SET # | SEARCH TERMS AND FILTERS | RESULTS |
|---|---|---|
| 1 | "Infertility"[MeSH Major Topic] OR "Reproductive Techniques, Assisted"[MeSH Major Topic] OR infertility[tiab] OR infertile[tiab] | 86,858 |
| 2 | "Stress, Psychological"[MeSH] OR "psychological stress"[tiab] OR "psychologic stress"[tiab] OR "psychological stresses"[tiab] OR "life stress"[tiab] OR "life stresses"[tiab] OR "mental suffering"[tiab] OR "emotional stress"[tiab] OR "emotional stresses"[tiab] OR "distress"[tiab] OR "anxiety"[tiab] | 257,659 |
| 3 | #1 AND #2 | 1,256 |
| 4 | "Randomized controlled trial"[pt] OR randomized[tiab] OR "placebo"[tiab] OR "evaluation studies"[pt] OR "evaluation studies as topic"[MeSH] OR "evaluation study"[tiab] OR "evaluation studies"[tiab] OR "intervention studies"[MeSH] OR "intervention studies"[tiab] OR "intervention study"[tiab] OR "case-control studies"[tiab] OR "case control"[tiab] OR "cohort studies"[MeSH] OR "cohort"[tiab] OR "longitudinal studies"[MeSH] OR "longitudinal"[tiab] OR "longitudinally"[tiab] OR "prospective"[tiab] OR "prospectively"[tiab] OR "retrospective studies"[MeSH] OR "retrospective"[tiab] OR "follow up"[tiab] OR "comparative study"[pt] OR "comparative study"[tiab] OR "systematic"[Subset] OR "meta-analysis"[pt] OR "meta-analysis as topic"[MeSH] OR "meta analysis"[tiab] OR "meta analyses"[tiab] OR "review"[pt] OR interview*[tiab] OR "Interviews as Topic"[MeSH:NoExp] OR experience*[tw] OR "qualitative"[tiab] OR "mixed method"[tiab] OR "mixed methods"[tiab] | 6,672,325 |
| 5 | #3 AND #4 | 830 |
| 6 | #5 NOT (("Animals"[MeSH]) NOT ("Animals"[MeSH] AND "Humans"[MeSH])) | 822 |
| 7 | #6 NOT ("Editorial"[pt] OR "Letter"[pt] OR "Case Reports"[pt] OR "Comment"[pt]) | 802 |
| 8 | #7, Filters: English, 2004- | 408 |

Note: Search conducted by Adrianne Leonardelli, August 12, 2014.

TABLE 1.2 Results of Second Search of PubMed/MEDLINE for Literature About Infertility

| SEARCH TERMS AND FILTERS | RESULTS |
|---|---|
| ("Reproductive Techniques, Assisted/psychology"[MeSH] OR "Infertility/psychology"[MeSH]) AND ("Models, Psychological"[MeSH] OR "Nursing Theory"[MeSH] OR "Psychological Theory"[MeSH] OR model[tiab] OR theory[tiab]) AND (Humans[MeSH] AND English[lang]) | 225 |
| Selected Categories of Results | |
| Core Clinical Journals | 3 |
| Nursing Journals | 39 |
| Systematic Reviews | 7 |
| Prognosis | 38 |
| Etiology/Harm | 18 |
| Therapy (RCT) | 4 |
| Cohort Studies | 32 |

Note: Search conducted by Adrianne Leonardelli, September 11, 2014.

TABLE 1.3 Results of Search of CINAHL Complete for Literature About Nursing Conceptual Models and Infertility

| SEARCH TERMS | RESULTS |
|---|---|
| [Name of Conceptual Model of Nursing] AND infertility | 7 |
| Interaction Model of Client Health Behavior | 1 |
| Johnson's Behavioral System Model | 0 |
| King's Conceptual System | 1 |
| Levine's Conservation Model | 0 |
| Neuman's Systems Model | 1 |
| Orem's Self-Care Framework | 0 |
| Rogers's Science of Unitary Human Beings | 0 |
| Roy's Adaptation Model | 4 |

Note: Search conducted by Jacqueline Fawcett, February 20, 2015.

selected from the plethora of literature were theoretical articles (Cunningham & Cunningham, 2013; Ridenour, Yorgason, & Peterson, 2009); a systematic review of multidisciplinary literature (Greil, 1997); a multidisciplinary meta-analysis (Jordan & Revenson, 1999); reviews of literature included in and/or the findings of studies conducted by nurses or members of other disciplines (Arslan-Özkan, Okumuş, & Buldukoğlu, 2014; Galhardo, Cunha, & Pinto-Gouveia, 2013; Gonzalez, 2000; Hirsch & Hirsch, 1989; Johnson, 1996; Naab, 2011; Özkan, Okumuş, Buldukoğlu, & Watson,

2013; Sandelowski, 1995; van den Akker, 2005); as well as nursing research that was explicitly guided by nursing conceptual models (Ciambelli, 1996; Dağ, Kavlak, & Şirin, 2014; Davis, 1987; DeMasters, 1995; Kelly-Weeder & Cox, 2006; Ko & Chen, 2005; Zbegner, 2003).

## The Template for a Comprehensive Theory

A template for development of a comprehensive theory of the psychosocial experience of infertility is shown in Table 1.4. Given the emphasis in this chapter on the psychosocial experience of infertility, the RAM concepts of the regulator coping subsystem and the physiological mode of adaptation are not considered. In addition, residual stimuli were not considered inasmuch as these, like residual variance in statistics, are not identifiable. As seen in Table 1.4, the RAM concepts provided a way to categorize the theory concepts that were extracted from the literature. The categorization of theory concepts according to the RAM concepts is admittedly arbitrary and not always in keeping with what was done by authors of RAM-guided studies. For example, both Ciambelli (1996) and Zbegner (2003) included theory concepts that they linked with the RAM physiological mode of adaptation (Ciambelli—physical demands and Zbegner—physical energy). For the purposes of this chapter and based on their definitions of those concepts, physical demands were interpreted as functional status and were linked with the role function mode; physical energy was also linked with the role function mode.

Some distinctive theory concepts found in the reviewed literature represent the RAM concept of adaptation level (Box 1.1). These concepts are adjustment, relinquishing infertility, resilience, restitution, and quality of life or subjective well-being. Arslan-Özkan et al. (2014) included *adjustment* as a theory concept in their study of 103 Turkish women. They defined adjustment in women with a diagnosis of infertility as "the ability of individuals to maintain their attitude towards the probability of not having children in behavioural, cognitive and emotional terms" (pp. 1802–1803). In her synthesis of the findings of three qualitative descriptive studies, Sandelowski (1995) discovered that *relinquishing infertility* was experienced as couples who were diagnosed as infertile made "efforts to divest themselves of the identity, thoughts, feelings, and behavior patterns they had developed in response to their encounter with infertility" (p. 123).

Ridenour et al. (2009) included *resilience*, which they defined as "developing strengths in the face of adversity" (p. 35), as the central concept in their theory of infertility. They regarded resilience as both a process and an outcome for couples experiencing infertility, explaining:

> Couple resilience to infertility may be defined as a process, such
> as relationship cohesion or positive communication during the
> ambiguous times following diagnosis. For example, resilience may be
> displayed by remaining close as a couple despite failure to conceive
> a child, or becoming accustomed to the idea that one will never
> have children.... Resilience to infertility also may be considered as
> an outcome of the interconnections between the external factors,

individual influences, and collective interactions and perceptions [of their theory].... Consequently, resilience depends on the individual's and couple's ability to effectively modify previous views, resulting in acceptance of infertility regardless of existent external influences or infertility treatment outcomes. (p. 37)

*Restitution* emerged from Gonzalez's (2000) study of the meaning of infertility for 25 women who had a medical diagnosis of infertility. She explained:

Participants described a process of restitution, in which they accepted the reality of their physical inability to bear a child and attempted to put the pain of the infertility behind them. The participants did not describe themselves as having reached a stage of resolution, a term used historically in the infertility literature to refer to the subsiding of the pain of the loss engendered by infertility.... The participants described this restitutional process as a relinquishing or disengaging from the fantasy of pregnancy and bearing a biological child. (p. 626)

For the purposes of her study of 176 women who had received treatment for infertility, van den Akker (2005) defined *quality of life* as a "multidimensional construct of happiness or satisfaction, from the perspective of 'an individual's sense of well being which stems from satisfaction/dissatisfaction with areas in life that are important to her'" (Ferrans, as cited in van den Akker, 2005, p. 184). Ciambelli (1996) included *subjective well-being* in her RAM-guided test of a middle-range theory of adaptation of marital partners who were experiencing fertility problems. She defined subjective well-being as a health-related outcome focusing on "how people evaluate various domains of their lives, including a summary or overall evaluation of life-as-a-whole ... [and] as their personal assessment of their quality of life-as-a-whole, health and appearance, and personal life" (p. 32).

## Formulating the Theory

The theory concepts shown in Table 1.4 may be used collectively as a comprehensive theory of the psychosocial experience of infertility. Empirical testing of this theory would be guided by the RAM propositions, which are listed here:

- Focal and contextual stimuli are related to coping processes.
- Coping processes are related to the modes of adaptation.
- Focal and contextual stimuli are related to the modes of adaptation.
- The modes of adaptation are interrelated.

Theory propositions, which would be deduced from the RAM propositions, would include all of the theory concepts representing each of the RAM concepts (Table 1.4). Testing a theory with so many concepts would, of course, require a large sample and a large number of questionnaires; therefore, it is most likely not feasible.

TABLE 1.4 Linkage of Roy Adaptation Model Concepts With Potential Concepts for a Comprehensive Theory of Infertility: A Template for Theory Testing

| ROY ADAPTATION MODEL CONCEPTS | FOCAL STIMULUS | CONTEXTUAL STIMULI | COGNATOR COPING PROCESSES | SELF-CONCEPT MODE | ROLE FUNCTION MODE | INTERDEPENDENCE MODE | ADAPTATION LEVEL |
|---|---|---|---|---|---|---|---|
| Theory concepts | Desire for a biological child | Duration of infertility | Ways of coping/coping strategies/coping effectiveness | Lethargy/chronic fatigue | Parenthood motivation | Marital relationships | Adjustment |
| | Involuntary childlessness | Duration of treatment | Cognitive dissonance | Pain | Life roles | Marital satisfaction | Relinquishing infertility |
| | | Gender | Personal expectations | Body image | Career roles | Marital status | Resilience |
| | | Age | Surprise | Personal identity | Self-efficacy | Social interaction | Restitution |
| | | Career stage/employment status | Disbelief | Self-concept | Functional status | Social support | Quality of life/subjective well-being |
| | | Personal finances/socioeconomic status | Frustration | Self-esteem | Physical energy | Social conflict | |
| | | Beliefs about infertility | Disappointment | Self-preservation | Interactions with other parents' children | Social stigmatization | |

(continued)

**TABLE 1.4 Linkage of Roy Adaptation Model Concepts With Potential Concepts for a Comprehensive Theory of Infertility: A Template for Theory Testing** (*continued*)

| ROY ADAPTATION MODEL CONCEPTS | FOCAL STIMULUS | CONTEXTUAL STIMULI | COGNATOR COPING PROCESSES | SELF-CONCEPT MODE | ROLE FUNCTION MODE | INTERDEPENDENCE MODE | ADAPTATION LEVEL |
|---|---|---|---|---|---|---|---|
| | | Culture/social norms | Decision making | Hope | Awareness of loss of desired parental role | Loss of social status | |
| | | | Perceptions of infertility | Psychological distress | Powerlessness | Isolation | |
| | | | | Stress | Feeling less like a woman | Loneliness | |
| | | | | Anxiety | Feeling less like a man | Alienation | |
| | | | | Fear | Feeling less desirable | | |
| | | | | Mourning/grief | Feeling incomplete | | |
| | | | | Denial | Feeling empty | | |
| | | | | Anger | Feeling unworthy | | |
| | | | | Hostility | Feeling defective | | |
| | | | | Desperation | Feelings of failure | | |
| | | | | Guilt | Sexual identity problems | | |
| | | | | Depression | Sexual dysfunction | | |
| | | | | Religiosity/spirituality | | | |

A more feasible approach is to select a few of the concepts that are of particular interest to a researcher for testing. For example, the relations among the theory concepts representing the focal stimulus and one or more of the theory concepts representing the self-concept mode of adaptation could be studied. Or, the relations among some of the theory concepts representing the modes of adaptation could be studied.

Examples of feasible theory testing are the RAM-guided theory development and testing work by Ciambelli (1996) and by Zbegner (2003). They tested the relations among various concepts of their middle-range theories of adaptation to infertility. The theory propositions are listed as hypotheses in Box 1.2.

## BOX 1.2 TWO ROY ADAPTATION MODEL–GUIDED MIDDLE-RANGE THEORIES OF ADAPTATION TO INFERTILITY

*Ciambelli (1996) tested nine hypotheses.*

1. Types of coping strategies and levels of coping effectiveness reported by partners with fertility problems will be related to levels of physical demands; self-esteem; home and work functioning; and social support.
2. Partners' physical demands will be inversely related to subjective well-being and marital satisfaction.
3. Partners' self-esteem levels will be positively related to their subjective well-being and marital satisfaction.
4. Partners' home and work functioning will be positively related to their subjective well-being and marital satisfaction.
5. Partners' social support will be positively related to their subjective well-being and marital satisfaction; and partners' social conflict is inversely related to subjective well-being and marital satisfaction.
6. Partners' subjective well-being will be positively related to their marital satisfaction.
7. Wives' subjective well-being will be positively related to husbands' subjective well-being and wives' marital satisfaction is positively related to husbands' marital satisfaction.
8. Partners' coping use and effectiveness, physical demands, self-esteem, home and work functioning, social support and social conflict, and spousal subjective well-being will explain a significant amount of variance in their subjective well-being.
9. Partners' coping use and effectiveness, physical demands, self-esteem, home and work functioning, social support and social conflict, and spousal marital satisfaction will explain a significant amount of variance in their marital satisfaction.

*Zbegner (2003) tested two hypotheses.*

1. The linear combination of the adaptive mode variables of physical energy level (physical mode), self-esteem (self-concept mode), marital satisfaction (interdependence mode), and parenthood motivation (role function mode) predict coping behaviors better than any one variable alone.
2. The contextual stimuli of age, education, income, and total length of time in treatment are related to the adaptive mode variables of physical energy level, self-esteem, marital satisfaction, and parenthood motivation.

## CONCLUSION

The approach used in this chapter for development of a psychosocial theory of infertility can be replicated using other conceptual models of nursing as overarching frameworks for categorizing theory concepts extracted from the literature and as guides for development of theory propositions that can be empirically tested.

The international, multidisciplinary literature used for development of the RAM-guided theory of the psychosocial experience of infertility spanned several years, from 1987 to 2014. It is noteworthy that few new theory concepts emerged over the years. Apparently, the psychosocial experience of infertility as it relates to adaptation has not changed over time. What has, of course, changed are the technological options now available for women and men who desire a biological child. A review of the psychosocial effects of those options is recommended.

## ACKNOWLEDGMENT

I am indebted to Adrianne Leonardelli, MLIS, for her creative search of much of the literature retrieved for this chapter.

## REFERENCES

Arslan-Özkan, I., Okumuş, H., & Buldukoğlu, K. (2014). A randomized controlled trial of the effects of nursing care based on Watson's theory of human caring on distress, self-efficacy, and adjustment in infertile women. *Journal of Advanced Nursing, 70,* 1801–1812. doi:10.1111/jan.12338

Ciambelli, M. M. (1996). *Adaptation in marital partners with fertility problems: Testing a midrange theory derived from Roy's adaptation model* (Doctoral dissertation). Retrieved from ProQuest Dissertations and Theses. (Dissertation Number 9715826; ProQuest Document ID 304280563.)

Clarke, P. N., & Fawcett, J. (2014). Life as a nurse researcher. *Nursing Science Quarterly, 27,* 37–41. doi:10.1177/0894318413509708

Cunningham, N., & Cunningham, T. (2013). Women's experiences of infertility—Towards a relational model of care. *Journal of Clinical Nursing, 22,* 3428–3437. doi:10.1111/jocn.12338

Dağ, H., Kavlak, O., & Şirin, A. (2014). Neuman systems model and infertility stressors: Review [Abstract]. *Turkiye Klinikleri Hemsirelik Bilimleri, 6*(2), 121–128.

Davis, D. C. (1987). A conceptual framework for infertility. *Journal of Obstetric, Gynecological, & Neonatal Nursing, 16,* 30–35. doi:10.1111/j.1552–6909.1987.tb01435.x

DeMasters, J. (1995). The experience of infertility among women who have sought treatment. *The Missouri Nurse, 64*(2), 12.

Fawcett, J., & Garity, J. (2009). *Evaluating research for evidence-based nursing practice.* Philadelphia, PA: F. A. Davis.

Galhardo, A., Cunha, M., & Pinto-Gouveia, J. (2013). Measuring self-efficacy to deal with infertility: Psychometric properties and confirmatory factor analysis of the Portuguese version of the infertility self-efficacy scale. *Research in Nursing & Health, 36,* 65–74. doi:10.1002/nur.21516

Glanz, K. (2002). Perspectives on using theory. In K. Glanz, B. K. Rimer, & F. M. Lewis (Eds.), *Health behavior and health education: Theory, research, and practice* (3rd ed., pp. 545–558). San Francisco, CA: Jossey-Bass.

Gonzalez, L. O. (2000). Infertility as a transformational process: A framework for psycho-therapeutic support of infertile women. *Issues in Mental Health Nursing, 21,* 619–633. doi:10.1080/01612840050110317

Greil, A. L. (1997). Infertility and psychological distress: A critical review of the literature. *Social Science & Medicine, 45,* 1679–1704. doi:10.1016/S0277-9536(97)00102-0

Hirsch, A. M., & Hirsch, S. M. (1989). The effect of infertility on marriage and self-concept. *Journal of Obstetric, Gynecological, & Neonatal Nursing, 18,* 13–20. doi:10.1111/j.1552-6909.1989.tb01611.x

Johnson, C. L. (1996). Regaining self-esteem: Strategies and interventions for the infertile woman. *Journal of Obstetric, Gynecological, & Neonatal Nursing, 25,* 291–295. doi:10.1111/j.1552-6909.1996.tb02574.x

Jordan, C., & Revenson, T. A. (1999). Gender differences in coping with infertility: A meta-analysis. *Journal of Behavioral Medicine, 22,* 341–358. doi:10.1023/A:1018774019232

Kelly-Weeder, S., & Cox, C. L. (2006). The impact of lifestyle risk factors on female infertility. *Women & Health, 44*(4), 1–23. doi:10.1300/J013v44n04_01

Ko, H. C., & Chen, S. F. (2005). An experience nursing a patient with ovarian hyperstimulation syndrome who has undergone artificial fertilization treatment. *Journal of Nursing, 52*(3), 90–96 [Chinese; English abstract].

Naab, F. (2011). *Women's representations of infertility in Ghana* (Doctoral dissertation). Retrieved from ProQuest Dissertations and Theses (Dissertation Number 3489069; ProQuest Document ID 91200013).

Özkan, İ. A., Okumuş, H., Buldukoğlu, K., & Watson, J. (2013). A case study based on Watson's theory of human caring: Being an infertile woman in Turkey. *Nursing Science Quarterly, 26,* 352–359. doi:10.1177/0894318413500346

Popper, K. R. (1965). *Conjectures and refutations: The growth of scientific knowledge.* New York, NY: Harper & Row.

Ridenour, A. F., Yorgason, J. B., & Peterson, B. (2009). The infertility resilience model: Assessing individual, couple, and external predictive factors. *Contemporary Family Therapy, 31,* 34–51. doi:10.1007/s10591-008-9077-z

Roy, C. (2009). *The Roy Adaptation Model* (3rd ed.). Upper Saddle River, NJ: Pearson.

Sandelowski, M. (1995). A theory of the transition to parenthood of infertile couples. *Research in Nursing & Health, 18,* 123–132. doi:10.1002/nur.4770180206

van den Akker, O. B. A. (2005). Coping, quality of life and psychological symptoms in three groups of sub-fertile women. *Patient Education and Counseling, 57,* 183–189. doi:10.1016/j.pec.2004.05.012

Zbegner, D. K. (2003). *An exploratory retrospective study using the Roy Adaptation Model: The adaptive mode variables of physical energy level, self-esteem, marital satisfaction, and parenthood motivation as predictors of coping behaviors in infertile women.* (Doctoral dissertation). Retrieved from ProQuest Dissertations and Theses (Dissertation Number 3102828; ProQuest Document ID 305228070).

# CHAPTER 2

# SHIFTING FAMILY STRUCTURE: THEORETICAL PERSPECTIVES OF WORLDWIDE POPULATION AND FAMILY COMPOSITION

*Jennie M. Wagner*

The concept of "family," a term that is widely used, can also be a positive or negative emotionally charged term. During the past decade, the concept of family has been changing on national and global levels. In this chapter, we explain and define family from different theoretical perspectives, examine current and future trends, and explore the implications for health care providers in the future.

## THE CONCEPT OF FAMILIES

There has been much debate regarding the definition of a family. The term *family* denotes a certain kinship between individuals and reflects a certain relationship and tasks (Cowen, Field, Hansen, Skolnick, & Swanson, 2014). In addition, the concept of a family depends on the lens used by the discipline; therefore, we examine the definition of a family from an anthropological and sociological perspective.

### Anthropological View of Family

The universality of the concept of family was confirmed by the work of Murdock in his cross-cultural research on kinship (Murdock, 1949; Spiro, 1954). In addition, the term *nuclear family* was also found to be universal and had four functions: sexual, reproductive, economic, and educational (Spiro, 1954). The nuclear family played a valuable role in the preservation of society; therefore, the universality of the term(s) was assumed. Bourdieu (1996) defines a family as a set of individuals related by marriage or adoption who cohabitate. Associated with the concept of family is the presence of two properties: The family has a common vision or attribute that transcends all the members and the view of family as a separate social universe where there is a sanctum from the outside world (Bourdieu, 1996). This inner circle of privacy within a family can also be described as boundaries that are defined by the residence or household to offer protection for this intimate group. Bourdieu (1977, 1996) also researched the societal function of a family in the reproduction of culture within a society through the transfer of social capital. This conceptualization of family as a necessary construct for the preservation of society and to promote the reproduction of culture was the basis for the continued work in the field of sociology.

## Sociological View of Family

At the turn of the century in the midst of the Industrial Revolution, the family was viewed as an endangered species by the prescribed social theories that set out to define and examine the changes in the family concept. Later, in the postwar era in America, families were viewed as an essential structural component of society (Doherty, Boss, LaRossa, Schumm, & Steinmetz, 1993). Therefore, the concept of family is defined by the functional and structural components. A family is any sexually expressive, parent–child, or other kin relationship in which people usually related by ancestry, marriage, or adoption form an economic unit and care for children or other dependents, consider their identity to be significantly attached to the group, and are committed to maintaining their group over time (Lamanna & Riedmann, 2011). The family is important for the socialization of the children, similar to Bourdieu's (1996) concept of the reproduction of culture. A central tenet of Bourdieu's (1977) classic study is the concept of habitus, a method of reproducing the objective framework of a society, such as language, tradition, and culture. The family is a social network whereby social formations tend to reproduce themselves. The societal framework in which the family unit exists has been evolving over the past century, due to unprecedented economic and demographic changes. As the landscape of the United States changed with feminism and diversification, there was an emphasis to take a broader view of the definition of a family. In lieu of using the term *households*, Segalen (1986) elected to use *domestic groups* as a broader and more inclusive term to define a set of people sharing the same living space. The domestic group is a neutral term that can include different nuclear families (mother, father, and children) but also other individuals not related to each other.

The concept of the family from both a functional and structural level has evolved and changed during the last decade (Lamanna & Riedmann, 2011). The legal definition of families has also evolved and an executive order was made granting benefits to same-sex domestic partners of federal employees (Obama, 2010). It has been speculated that there is no *typical* family form today; however, families still provide a place for the members to belong (Lamanna & Riedmann, 2011). The changes in the family structure over the past decade reflect the diversification of the global society. Next we examine the current trends in the family structure from a global and national perspective.

## CURRENT TRENDS

Researchers have documented a significant change in the family structure on international and national levels. Much of this research has focused on the 1950s to the present time with the advances in technology and the diversification of the United

States. Throughout the world, economic, environmental, and policy trends have contributed to the change in family structure. A comparison of these trends in the family structure on global and national levels will be explored.

## Global Trends With Family Structure

On a global basis, there has been an increase in life expectancy. In many countries, this increase in life expectancy is coupled with a corresponding decrease in the overall population. By 2050, the populations of 43 countries are projected to decrease, and 40 of these countries will continue to experience population declines until 2100 (United Nations, Department of Economic and Social Affairs, Population Division, 2013). In addition to the decline in population in Russia and Japan, these countries will experience a significant shift in demographics; both countries are projected to have 30% of their populations composed of individuals aged 65 years or older by 2050 (Ezeh, Bongaarts, & Mberu, 2012). Many factors have been discussed as contributing factors to this shift in population composition.

### Fertility Rates

There has been a corresponding shift in fertility rates on a global level, with the highest fertility rates in sub-Saharan Africa (e.g., 6.1 births per woman in Uganda); moderate rates in the Americas and Oceania (2.1 births per woman); and fertility rates less than population replacement noted in East Asia and Europe (Child Trends, 2014). Although the total fertility rate (TFR), the average number of children born to each woman in Europe, has slowly increased from the early 2000s, the highest rate is observed in Ireland with a replacement level of 2.1; however, the other countries in this region have a TFR ranging from 1.4 to 2.0. In Asia, the TFR continues to drop; in East Asia, the fertility rate is 1.6 or lower and the range is from 3.1 in the Philippines to 1.1 in Taiwan (Child Trends, 2014). The estimated and projected global total fertility calculated by the United Nations as part of the World Populations Project is presented on the world map in Figure 2.1. There is a concern in economically advanced countries that the birthrate below the replacement level will result in a declining economic base as the population ages. With an aging population, the pressure on public pension and the health care system could substantially slow economic growth (Ezeh et al., 2012). An analysis of infertility prevalence among women 20 to 44 years of age in 190 countries reported a rate of 1.9% unable to have a live birth after exposure to the risk of pregnancy (primary infertility), and 10.5% unable to have another child (secondary infertility; Mascarenhas, Flaxman, Boerma, Vanderpoel, & Stevens, 2013). The countries with the highest infertility prevalence were South Asia, sub-Saharan Africa, North Africa/Middle East, Central/Eastern Europe, and Central Asia. The absolute number of couples affected by infertility increased from 42 million in 1990 to 48.5 million in 2010 (Mascarenhas et al., 2013). Research in the area of infertility is sparse; however, it has been reported that the increase in overall infertility rates is due to a decline in male fertility. Since the 1950s, researchers have demonstrated a decrease in semen quality; a linear analysis of these global studies has documented that there is a significant decrease in semen quality (Sengupta, 2014). In addition, the incidence of testicular cancer in

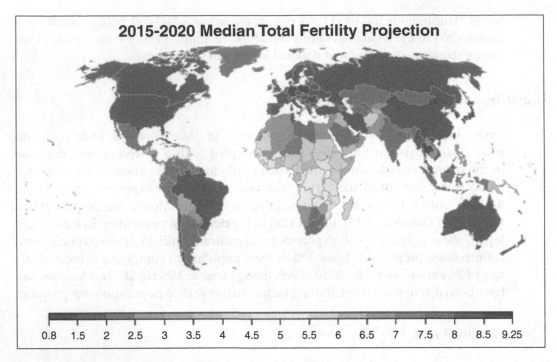

**FIGURE 2.1** Total fertility (average number of children per woman).
From World Populations Project, the United Nations (2012). Used with permission.

men is increasing and there is an associated increase in congenital malformation of the genital tract (Sengupta, 2014). As lifestyles change on a global scale so quickly, it is difficult for researchers to capture the trends in the data that are collected; many questions that reflect this new era are not contained in the old survey formats. Despite a global effort to improve maternal and reproductive health, there remain many unanswered questions in the area of infertility (Mascarenhas et al., 2013).

## Life Expectancy

For the past several decades, there has been a global trend in the increase of life expectancy and in recent years a rise among low-income countries. According to the WHO, the global life expectancy of a child born in 2012 versus 1990 has increased by 6 years. In 2012, a female infant could expect to live until age 72.7 years and a boy until age 68.1 years (WHO, 2014). However, life expectancy is dependent on the country of birth; there is a gap of approximately 15 years in life expectancy between high- and low-income countries (WHO, 2014). The top-five ranked countries in life expectancy are listed in Table 2.1 by sex. Note that the United States is not in this list and is ranked 27th out of 36 among the participating Organization for Economic Cooperation and Development countries (2015).

The shift in the aging structure has contributed to a significant change in family structure. As the life expectancy increases worldwide, the possibility of multiple generations living together also increases. Many middle-aged adults are finding themselves taking care of their parents and even grandparents. The majority

TABLE 2.1  2012 Life Expectancy From Birth for the Top Five Countries, by Gender

| MALE | | | FEMALE | | |
| --- | --- | --- | --- | --- | --- |
| RANK | COUNTRY | AGE (IN YEARS) | RANK | COUNTRY | AGE (IN YEARS) |
| 1 | Iceland | 81.2 | 1 | Japan | 87.0 |
| 2 | Switzerland | 80.7 | 2 | Spain | 85.1 |
| 3 | Australia | 80.5 | 3 | Switzerland | 85.1 |
| 4 | Israel | 80.2 | 4 | Singapore | 85.1 |
| 5 | Singapore | 80.2 | 5 | Italy | 85.0 |

Adapted from World Health Organization (2014). Copyright 2014 by the World Health Organization Reproduction Services.

of middle-aged and older adults having living parents is a phenomenon that has been unprecedented in history (National Institute on Aging, 2007). In the Middle East, Central/South America, and sub-Saharan Africa, it is reported that more than 40% of children live in a household with adults in addition to their parents (Child Trends, 2014). Although many countries have increased extended families that stay together for life, this is not the norm everywhere. For Western countries with a higher divorce rate, remarriage and blended families, delayed childbearing, and more adults in the workforce, an impact is seen on the family structure, including an increase in one-parent households (National Institute on Aging, 2007).

## Family Structure and Cohabitation

The global changes in fertility rates and life expectancy have transcended down to the family unit. Throughout the world, the family composition has changed significantly during the past several decades. There are regional differences in family structure, with more children living in a two-parent household or extended multigenerational households in Asia and the Middle East. In an extended or nuclear family structure, 80% of European children live in a two-parent family, and this ranges from 76% in the United Kingdom to 89% in Italy and Poland. This is in contrast to the two-parent family statistics in the Americas, where 62% of children living in Columbia live in a two-parent household compared with 78% in Canada (Child Trends, 2014).

Marriage has traditionally been an important institution for the promotion of parenthood across the globe. However, the definition of marriage has been shifting and is seen as an option in the Western world; cohabitation has become an acceptable alternative. In Asia and the Middle East, adults aged 18 to 49 years are more likely to be married: 80% in Egypt, 77% in India, and 47% in Singapore. However, there is a downward trend in marriage for the North America and Oceana regions: 45% in the United States, 43% in Canada, and 63% in Mexico (Child Trends, 2014). In a recent study of cohabitation in 15 European countries, the Northern European countries had the highest rates of individuals aged 18 to 45 years reporting a history of cohabitation ranging from 56% to 61% (Kasearu & Kutsar, 2011).

In contrast, Central, Eastern, and Southern European countries are experiencing a significant upward trend in the percent of cohabitating couples. From 2004 to 2008, the change in proportion of cohabitation couples aged 26 to 45 years was 107% in Poland, 75% in Spain, 60% in Slovakia, 48% in Portugal, and 41% in France (Kasearu & Kutsar, 2011). However, there is a notable decrease in the number of children born to cohabitating couples in these 15 European countries, even in the countries with widespread cohabitation practices. The trend to cohabitate has also occurred in the United States; from 1987 to 2010, the percentage of women reporting a history of cohabiting was up 82% (Manning, 2013). There is a trend to cohabitate as a pathway to marriage with more than two thirds of the women in the past decade reporting cohabitation before their first marriage (Manning, 2013). The pattern of increasing cohabitation crosses all ethnic, age, and social economic categories in the United States. Likewise, as with European couples who cohabitate, the cohabitating couples in the United States have lower fertility rates, and this is reported to be related to the less permanent nature of cohabitation relationships versus marriage (Metzger, 2011).

During the past several decades, the pattern of cohabitation has spread across the globe into developing and underdeveloped countries. The extent and rate of cohabitation patterns across countries are dependent on many factors, including religion and cultural traditions and socioeconomic constraints (Kasearu & Kutsar, 2011).

## Family Structure and In Vitro Fertilization/Intracytoplasmic Sperm Injection Treatment

A certain amount of stress is intrinsic to the process of committing to a reproductive plan and taking the steps to become a parent. There are decisions about when to start the process of trying to conceive, how long to wait between offspring, and how many children to have, which are all personal decisions. However, the level of stress intrinsic to the process of conception is even higher for couples who have failed to conceive without intervention and will be employing either in vitro fertilization (IVF) or intracytoplasmic sperm injection (ICSI) treatment.

The latest Centers for Disease Control and Prevention (CDC) survey of family growth in the United States reports infertility as a significant health problem in the United States (Chandra, Copen, & Stephen, 2013). However, a national survey of first-time parents older than 40 years documented that they did not perceive age as a factor that could have a significant negative impact on their ability to conceive (Mac Dougall, Beyene, & Nachtigall, 2013). The women in this study stated that persistent contraception education early in their adolescents gave them the view that fertility would remain at the same level until closer to menopause. The participants who successfully delivered after IVF treatment reported that they felt a sense of alarm and dismay regarding the difficulty they experienced in trying to conceive for the first time beyond the age of 40 years (Mac Dougall et al., 2013). A longitudinal study in Denmark explored the potential for the resulting stress from seeking an infertility examination to affect the relationship with an individual's partner. The researcher followed the Danish women for 12 years and reported that more than 27% of the women were no longer living with the person whom they lived with at the time of the infertility examination. In addition, the pressure of not conceiving a child after a post-infertility evaluation had a larger statistically significant impact on a couple; the odds ratio is 3.89 greater for a divorcee or one who no longer cohabitates with the original partner (Kjaer et al., 2014). Both partners are impacted by the additional stress of seeking an infertility evaluation and subsequent treatment. A study of 214 couples seeking infertility treatment in Portugal explored the impact on the stress levels of the partners. Higher stress levels were noted for both men and women with lower perceived levels of partner support and, in addition, lower levels of family support for women (Martin, Peterson, Almeida, Mesquita-Guimarães, & Costa, 2014). These studies highlight the importance of providing care not only for the individual seeking fertility treatment but also the importance of inclusivity of the partner and other familial supporters. The social and psychological ramifications of infertility treatment are diffused through the patient and the partner.

Finally, there have been positive research results in the long-term outcomes of IVF/ICSI childbirth in the family. According to Blake, Richards, and Golombok (2014), there is no empirical support for a bio-normative viewpoint as preferable in relation to the family, whether a couple chooses infertility treatment or adoption. In post-IVF/ICSI studies of families, there was no long-term psychological stress or negative impact on the child's behavior noted (Beukers et al., 2012). In addition, a study of IVF/ICSI couples by Jongbloed-Pereboom et al. (2012) reported no long-term parental well-being and anxiety 1 year after childbirth. Although there is a potential for additional tension and strain on the individual and his or her partner seeking infertility evaluation and treatment, this impact is noted on a short-term versus a long-term basis. Therefore, it is important to support the individual and his or her partner during the infertility process to minimize any negative impact on the couple. The need for support for an individual and his or her partner during infertility treatment is a global phenomenon.

Thus far, we have explored and assessed families from a global perspective. The trends in the family structure have changed significantly on an international level and in the United States. In the next section, the changes in family structure and composition are explored on the national level.

## National Trends With Family Structure

The United States has experienced a significant change in demographics and this trend is projected to continue in the future (Table 2.2). The United States has become more ethnically and racially diverse; according to the 2010 U.S. Census, the percent of individuals identifying themselves as Hispanic was 17%; Black, 13%; Asian, 5%; and White, 62% (U.S. Census Bureau, 2014). It is worth noting that, in the latest census, the multiracial category grew by the largest percent of any single racial/ethnic group; there was a 32% increase from 2000 to 2010 (Jones & Bullock, 2012). The top three states in the United States that report more than 200,000 individuals of a dual race are California, Texas, and New York (Jones & Bullock, 2012). A second demographic milestone that has been reached in the United States is that the ethnic and racial minority births present almost 50% of the annual births (U.S. Census Bureau, 2012). The United States of the future is projected to be very different with

TABLE 2.2 U.S. Population Facts, 2013

| U.S. POPULATION ESTIMATE, 2013 | TOTAL POPULATION ESTIMATES: 316,497,531 (%) |
|---|---|
| Persons younger than 5 years | 6.3 |
| Persons younger than 18 years | 23.3 |
| Persons 65 years or older | 14.1 |
| Females | 50.8 |
| Percent of population reporting racial/ethnic affiliation | |
| White, alone, not Hispanic or Latino | 62.6 |
| Hispanic or Latino, alone | 17.1 |
| Black or African American, alone | 13.2 |
| Asian, alone; American Indian/Alaska, alone | 5.3 |
| Native Hawaiian or other Pacific Islander, alone | 0.2 |
| Two or more races | 2.4 |

Adapted from U.S. Census Bureau (2014).

demographic shifts where the White category will be in the minority and there will be no clear single ethnic category as the majority in the nation (Kotkin, 2010). These changes in demographics have transcended into the family structure in the United States.

## U.S. Families, Past and Future

There have been significant changes in the structure of families in the United States during the last century. The households of today are 50% smaller than those in the 1850s (Salcedo, Schoellman, & Tertilt, 2012). The typical American family has changed significantly since the 1950s, when the majority of children were being raised in male-breadwinner families with married parents (Cohen, 2014). In addition, only approximately 18% of the children resided in households with dual working parents (Cohen, 2014). Today, there is no majority category that defines a typical family in the United States (Cohen, 2014; Vespa, Lewis, & Kreider, 2013). The proportion of family households declined from 81% in 1970 to 66% in 2012; for the same time period, the share of households that had married couples with children declined from 40% to 20% and one-person households increased from 17% to 27% (Vespa et al., 2013). In addition, the average number of people per household in the United States has declined from 3.1 in 1970 to 2.6 in 2012 (Vespa et al., 2013). The changes in family structure have been attributed to economic changes and technological advancements. Currently, U.S. women are better educated and are more likely to work outside of the household than at any point in history.

## Fertility

Despite the national decrease in household size, the U.S. fertility rate is higher than the rates for other countries. By 2050, the population in the United States is expected to increase by 100 million people and will be slightly older, with 20% of the population older than 65 years compared with the current 13% (Vincent & Velkoff, 2010). However, immigration will account for a substantial portion of this projected population increase.

There has been controversy regarding the fertility rates calculated for the United States. Regarding infertility estimates, the National Center for Health Statistics presented data from the 1982 to 2010 National Survey of Family Growth survey and defined *infertility* as a lack of pregnancy 12 months before the survey, despite having unprotected sexual intercourse with the same husband or partner for those months; fecundity was defined as a physical challenge in getting pregnant or maintaining the pregnancy to a live birth (Chandra et al., 2013). Using these definitions, the percentage of married women aged 18 to 44 years who reported being infertile decreased from 8.5% in 1982 to 6% in 2006 to 2010. And impaired fecundity for married women aged 18 to 44 years was reported as 11% in 1982, 15% in 2002, and 12% in 2006 to 2010 (Chandra et al., 2013).

However, other researchers have rebuked these estimates as being inaccurate due to the definitions used to classify infertility. The traditional definition does not include cohabiting couples; therefore, another statistical approach for gathering the infertility data is recommended. The current duration approach includes a construct for measuring derived from questions regarding sexual activity, contraceptive use, relationship status, and pregnancy, as well as a measurement based on the individual's estimated time to pregnancy based on the current duration of attempt to become pregnant (Thoma et al., 2013). Using the current duration approach to obtain infertility estimates in the United States, the levels are almost twofold higher: 15.5% infertility rate versus 7% fertility rate using just the traditional measurement (Thoma et al., 2013). According to the researchers, these new estimates are aligned with an increase in non-married women giving birth, an increase in cohabiting couples, and a decline in first marriages (Thoma et al., 2013). An accurate rate of reporting and tracking infertility is needed due to socioeconomic implications, increase in health risks, and adverse impact on population growth in the future.

## Family Structure and Cohabitation

Regarding families, marriage, and cohabitation, there have been significant trends during the second half of the 21st century in the United States. There is a notable increase in cohabitation, delay in marriage, and age at first birth. The median age at first marriage has increased from 20 years for women and 23 years for men in the 1950s to 26 years for women and 28 years for men by 2010 (Lundberg & Pollak, 2013). During the same time period, there has been a corresponding increase in cohabitation in addition to an increase in the number of births that take place outside of marriage; only 59% of births in the United States occurred to married women in 2009 (Hayford, Guzzo, & Smock, 2014). There is also a notable trend to delay childbirth after marriage (or to be childless), which is related to the higher educational levels of women. Interestingly, in 2009, the median age of first birth was lower than the median age of first marriage (Hayford et al., 2014). Cohabitation is viewed as a precursor to marriage in highly educated couples, but cohabitation with multiple partners is related to less economically and educational advanced individuals (Hayford et al., 2014). Overall, in the United States, the traditional two-parent family is no longer the norm and many other alternative arrangements have occurred. There are blended families with different parents and offspring, as well as childless and same-sex couples. Marriage has been viewed from an economic perspective as an investment in children, but this view has changed as more children are raised in nontraditional households.

The changes in the family structure during the past several decades have an impact on the nation in many dimensions. There are social, economic, and health implications that are important and need to be considered regarding how they will impact the future generation. In addition, the trends in marriage, family, and births need to be considered by health care providers to determine how best to meet the needs of the new American families.

## IMPLICATIONS FOR HEALTH CARE PROVIDERS

Health care providers in this era of influx and constant change must be adaptable to the need and concerns of their clientele. With the changes in demographics in the United States, health care providers must take steps to provide culturally sensitive patient care.

### Cultural Competency

Cultural competency has been defined as the knowledge, attitude, and skills needed to provide therapeutic intervention with a vast array of clients from different racial and ethnic backgrounds (American Association of Colleges of Nursing [AACN], 2008). The concept of cultural competency is not new; it was integrated into the AACN Baccalaureate Essentials of Nursing Competencies in 2008 and was the focus of the Institute of Medicine in 2002 highlighting the unequal treatment in health care for racial and ethnic groups (AACN, 2008). A culturally competent practitioner is aware of how his or her own attitudes, knowledge, and beliefs can impact the care he or she provides to the client. By increasing awareness of the health beliefs, practices, cultures, and linguistic needs of an ethnically and racially diverse patient population, the health care provider can establish a framework to meet the needs of all individuals. Research has demonstrated that increasing cultural competency among practitioners results in a decrease in health care disparities and improves patient outcomes (National Institutes of Health, n.d.). During the past decade, there has been a focus on education and practice to increase the cultural competency of practitioners at all levels.

The need for cultural competency to reduce health care disparity also applies to the area of infertility. For both African American and Hispanic clients, there has been a delay in seeking and obtaining treatment for infertility. According to the literature,

African American and Hispanic women waited 1.5 years longer to obtain treatment for infertility (Missmer, Seifer, & Jain, 2011). Reasons for this delay in seeking infertility treatment included difficulty in getting an appointment, taking time off of work, and paying for treatment. There were also cultural differences; African American women were more likely to be concerned about disappointing their spouses, whereas for Asian American women, the stigma associated with infertility was a major concern (Missmer et al., 2011). A culturally competent practitioner recognizes and appreciates the uniqueness of each individual he or she encounters. Willingness to ask questions, increasing knowledge of different cultures, and being open to opportunities to seek and learn more regarding the different ethnic and racial characteristics of the individuals and families encountered increase cultural competence. Increasing your own personal awareness of how you define a typical family will assist you in responding openly to the variety of family structures you encounter in practice. In this new era, where change is the only constant, health care providers must remain open to the fluid definition of family and embrace flexibility within their own practice. There have been significant demographic changes within the United States and the ability to reduce barriers to seeking equitable health care begins with each practitioner.

## CONCLUSION

An increase in cultural competency will assist in reducing the health care disparities among racial and ethnic groups. The United States has become more ethnically and racially diverse and this trend will continue in the future. The future U.S. population will be slightly older and more ethnically and racially diverse than at any other point in recent history. In addition, the conceptualization of what constitutes a family is fluid and assumptions by health care providers cannot be made. The U.S. census has documented the substantial changes in the American family in the past 50 years (see Box 2.1 for a summary of changes in families and living arrangements). There is no quintessential American family structure; therefore, the health care provider must approach each client without any predisposing assumptions. This exchange can be mutually beneficial to the client who receives culturally competent care and the health care provider who is open to new learning

### BOX 2.1 CHANGES IN AMERICAN FAMILIES

- Households are smaller, with a decrease in the average number of persons from 3.1 in 1970 to 2.6 in 2012.
- Married households are older and are declining as a percent of all households; non-married households constituted one third of the American households in 2012.
- There has been an increase in one-person households (32 million in 2011) versus married couples (37 million in 2011).
- The age for first marriage for men and women has been rising.

Adapted from Vespa, Lewis, and Kreider (2013). Copyright 2013 by the U.S. Census Bureau.

opportunities. Adjusting to the transitions occurring within American families is a challenge for health care and health care providers. However, remaining flexible in practice and incorporating the cultural needs of clients will assist health care providers in providing excellent patient care to the individual and families they encounter in practice.

## REFERENCES

American Association of Colleges of Nursing. (2008). *Cultural competency in baccalaureate nursing education*. Retrieved from http://www.aacn.nche.edu/leading-initiatives/education-resources/competency.pdf

Beukers, F., Houtzager, B. A., Paap, M. C. S., Middelburg, K. J., Hadders-Algra, M., Bos, A. F., & Kok, J. H. (2012). Parental psychological distress and anxiety after a successful IVF/ICSI procedure with and without preimplantation genetic screening: Follow-up of a randomised controlled trial. *Early Human Development, 88*, 725–730. doi:10.1016/j.earlhumdev.2012.03.001

Blake, L., Richards, M., & Golombok, S. (2014). The families of assisted reproduction and adoption. In F. Baylis & C. McLeod (Eds.), *Family making: Contemporary ethical challenges* (pp. 64–88). Oxford, UK: Oxford University Press.

Bourdieu, P. (1977). *Outline of a theory of practice* (R. Nice, Trans.). Cambridge, UK: Cambridge University Press.

Bourdieu, P. (1996). On the family as a realized category. *Theory, Culture & Society, 13*(3), 19–26. doi:10.1177/026327696013003002

Chandra, A., Copen, C. E., & Stephen, E. H. (2013). *Infertility and impaired fecundity in the United States, 1982–2010: Data from the National Survey of Family Growth* (Report No. 67). Retrieved from http://www.cdc.gov/nchs/products/nhsr.htm

Child Trends. (2014). World family map 2014: Mapping family change and child well-being outcomes. Retrieved from http://worldfamilymap.org/2014

Cohen, P. (2014). *Family diversity is the new normal for America's children*. Retrieved from https://contemporaryfamilies.org/the-new-normal

Cowan, P. A., Field, D., Hansen, D. A., Skolnick, A., & Swanson, G. E. (2014). *Family, self, and society: Toward a new agenda for family research*. New York, NY: Routledge.

Doherty, W., Boss, P. G., LaRossa, R., Schumm, W., & Steinmetz, S. (1993). Families theories and methods: A contextual approach. In P. Boss, W. J. Doherty, R. LaRossa, W. R. Schumm, & S. K. Steinmetz (Eds.), *Sourcebook of family theories and methods: A contextual approach* (pp. 3–30). New York, NY: Springer.

Ezeh, A. C., Bongaarts, J., & Mberu, B. (2012). Global population trends and policy options. *The Lancet, 380*, 142–148. doi:10.1016/S0140-6736(12)60696-5

Hayford, S. R., Guzzo, K. B., & Smock, P. J. (2014). The decoupling of marriage and parenthood? Trends in the timing of marital first births, 1945–2002. *Journal of Marriage and Family, 76*, 520–538. doi:10.1111/jomf.12114

Jones, N. A., & Bullock, J. (2012). *The two or more races population: 2012* (Issue Brief No. C2010BR-13). Retrieved from http://www.census.gov/prod/cen2010/briefs/c2010br-13.pdf

Jongbloed-Pereboom, M., Middelburg, K. J., Heineman, M. J., Bos, A. F., Haadsma, M. L., & Hadders-Algra, M. (2012). The impact of IVF/ICSI on parental well-being and anxiety 1 year after childbirth. *Human Reproduction, 27*, 2389–2395. doi:10.1093/humrep/des163

Kasearu, K., & Kutsar, D. (2011). Patterns behind unmarried cohabitation trends in Europe. *European Societies, 13*(2), 307–325. doi:10.1080/14616696.2010.493586

Kjaer, T., Albieri, V., Jensen, A., Kjaer, S. K., Johansen, C., & Dalton, S. O. (2014). Divorce or end of cohabitation among Danish women evaluated for fertility problems. *Acta Obstetricia et Gynecologica Scandinavica, 93*, 269–276. doi:10.1111/aogs.12317

Kotkin, J. (2010, August). The changing demographics of America. *Smithsonian Magazine*. Retrieved from http://www.smithsonianmag.com/40th-anniversary/the-changing-demographics-of-america-538284

Lamanna, M. A., & Riedmann, A. (2011). *Marriages, families, and relationships: Making choices in a diverse society* (11th ed.). Belmont, CA: Wadsworth, Cengage Learning.

Lundberg, S., & Pollak, R. A. (2013). *Cohabitation and the uneven retreat from marriage in the U.S., 1950–2010* (Working Paper No.19413). Retrieved from http://www.nber.org/papers/w19413

Mac Dougall, K., Beyene, Y., & Nachtigall, R. D. (2013). Age shock: Misperceptions of the impact of age on fertility before and after IVF in women who conceived after age 40. *Human Reproduction, 28*, 350–356. doi:10.1093/humrep/des409

Manning, W. D. (2013). *Trends in cohabitation: Over twenty years of change, 1987–2010* (FP-13-12). Retrieved from http://www.bgsu.edu/content/dam/BGSU/college-of-arts-and-sciences/NCFMR/documents/FP/FP-13-12.pdf

Martin, M. V., Peterson, B. D., Almeida, V., Mesquita-Guimarães, J., & Costa, M. E. (2014). Dyadic dynamics of perceived social support in couples facing infertility. *Human Reproduction, 29*, 83–89. doi:10.1093/humrep/det403

Mascarenhas, M. N., Flaxman, S. R., Boerma, T., Vanderpoel, S., & Stevens, G. A. (2013). National, regional, and global trends in infertility prevalence since 1990: A systematic analysis of 277 health surveys. *PLoS Medicine, 9*(12), e1001356. doi:10.1371/journal.pmed.1001356

Metzger, E. L., III. (2011). Falling fertility rates: The offspring of the contraceptive mentality. *Notre Dame Journal of Law, Ethics & Public Policy, 24*, 425–453. Retrieved from http://scholarship.law.nd.edu/ndjlepp/vol24/iss2/7/

Missmer, S. A., Seifer, D. B., & Jain, T. (2011). Cultural factors contributing to health care disparities among patients with infertility in midwestern United States. *Fertility and Sterility, 95*, 1943–1949. doi:10.1016/j.fertnstert.2011.02.039

Murdock, G. P. (1949). *Social structure*. New York, NY: Macmillan.

National Institute on Aging. (2007). Why population aging matters: A global perspective. Retrieved from http://www.nia.nih.gov/sites/default/files/WPAM.pdf

National Institutes of Health. (n.d.). Cultural competency. Retrieved from http://www.nih.gov/clearcommunication/culturalcompetency.htm

Obama, B. (2010). *Presidential memorandum-extension of benefits to same-sex domestic partners of federal employees*. Retrieved from https://www.whitehouse.gov/the-press-office/presidential-memorandum-extension-benefits-same-sex-domestic-partners-federal-emplo

Organization for Economic Cooperation and Development. (2015). Better life index: Health. Retrieved from http://www.oecdbetterlifeindex.org/topics/health

Salcedo, A., Schoellman, T., & Tertilt, M. (2012). Families as roommates: Changes in U.S. household size from 1850 to 2000. *Quantitative Economics, 3*, 133–175. doi:10.3982/QE76

Segalen, M. (1986). *Historical anthropology of the family* (J. C. Whitehouse & S. Matthews, Trans.). New York, NY: Cambridge University Press.

Sengupta, P. (2014). Current trends of male reproductive health disorders and the changing semen quality. *International Journal of Preventive Medicine, 5*, 1–5. Retrieved from http://ijpm.mui.ac.ir/index.php/ijpm/article/view/1266/1325

Spiro, M. E. (1954). Is the family universal? *American Anthropologist, 56*, 839–846. doi:10.1525/aa.1954.56.5.02a00080

Thoma, M. E., McLain, A. C., Louis, J. F., King, R. B., Trumble, A. C., Sundaram, R., & Louis, G. M. B. (2013). Prevalence of infertility in the United States as estimated by the current duration approach and a traditional constructed approach. *Fertility and Sterility, 99*, 1324–1331.

United Nations, Department of Economic and Social Affairs, Population Division. (2013). *World population prospects: The 2012 revision, highlights and advance tables.* Working Paper No. ESA/P/WP.228. Retrieved from http://esa.un.org/wpp/Documentation/pdf/WPP2012_HIGHLIGHTS.pdf

U.S. Census Bureau. (2012). Most children younger than age 1 are minorities, census bureau reports [Press Release (Release No. CB12–90)]. Retrieved from https://www.census.gov/newsroom/releases/archives/population/cb12–90.html

U.S. Census Bureau. (2014). *State and country quickfacts.* Retrieved from http://quickfacts.census.gov/qfd/states/00000.html

Vespa, J., Lewis, J. M., & Kreider, R. M. (2013). *America's families and living arrangements: 2012 Population characteristics* (Report No. P20–570). Retrieved from http://www.census.gov/library/publications/2013/demo/p20–570.html

Vincent, G. K., & Velkoff, V. A. (2010). *The next four decades: The older population in the United States: 2010 to 2050* (Report No. P25–1138). Retrieved from https://www.census.gov/prod/2010pubs/p25-1138.pdf

World Health Organization. (2014). *World health statistics 2014: A wealth of information on global public health.* Retrieved from http://apps.who.int/iris/bitstream/10665/112739/1/WHO_HIS_HSI_14.1_eng.pdf?ua=1

# CHAPTER 3

# A THEORETICAL APPROACH TO MULTIDIMENSIONAL STRESS EXPERIENCED DURING PREGNANCY BY WOMEN WHO CONCEIVE VIA IN VITRO FERTILIZATION

*Eleanor L. Stevenson and Kristina Cobb*

In vitro fertilization (IVF) has been available in most developed nations for just more than three decades, with larger numbers of women using IVF in roughly the past 15 years due to refinement of the science and greater insurance coverage (Reddy, Wapner, Rebar, & Tasca, 2007). Even as the number of IVF procedures and success of these procedures increase, many women who become pregnant through IVF are simply told to "go home and have a healthy baby" (Klock & Greenfeld, 2000, p. 1159). Given the increasing number of IVF pregnancies, researchers need to develop a greater understanding of these pregnancies, particularly the stress that may be associated with them. DiPietro, Ghera, Costigan, and Hawkins (2004) state that one significant, but largely unrecognized, methodological issue in the measurement of stress during pregnancy is the fact that pregnancy has unique psychological and social challenges. Failure to measure pregnancy-specific sources of stress can lead to underestimating maternal distress. Although limited, some researchers have begun to assess pregnancy-related anxiety, specifically the potential impact on adverse pregnancy outcomes (Wadhwa, Sandman, Porto, Dunkel-Schetter, & Garite, 1993; Yali & Lobel, 2002). This review is concerned with both general and pregnancy-specific stress.

The general pregnancy literature has examined stress extensively (Giurgescu, Penckofer, Maurer, & Bryant, 2006; Jomeen & Martin, 2005; Lobel & Dunkel-Schetter, 1990; Stark & Brinkley, 2007; Yali & Lobel, 2002), but little is known, conceptually or methodologically, about stress in women who become pregnant via IVF. The data that are available on stress in the IVF population are conflicting, with some disagreement over whether this population experiences more stress than those who conceive without assistance. Sufficient data do indicate that getting pregnant via IVF is a stressful experience (Coughlan, Walters, Ledger, & Li, 2014; Lawson et al., 2014; Turner et al., 2013). This stress might disappear once pregnancy is achieved, leaving women with an experience similar to that of a woman who conceives without assistance. However, there are no data to either support or reject this hypothesis.

Both qualitative and quantitative research indicates that women with IVF pregnancies perceive and experience their pregnancies differently from women who conceive unassisted. For instance, researchers of one qualitative study found that infertile couples put forth significant effort to normalize their pregnancies and to make themselves feel special; these couples described their pregnancies as equal to, more complicated than, or even superior to pregnancies achieved by those able to conceive naturally (Sandelowski, Harris, & Black, 1992). Other qualitative researchers found that the majority of the sample (75%) of women who became pregnant through fertility treatments perceived their pregnancies differently from those without fertility issues (Hjelmstedt, Widström, Wramsby, & Collins, 2003a). In particular, the women believed that those without fertility issues could achieve another pregnancy again but that the current pregnancy was probably the only pregnancy they themselves would be able to achieve. One participant stated, "for us it is so complicated to start again" (p. 159). Similar to the qualitative research, quantitative data also indicate that the women pregnant via IVF experience their pregnancies differently from other women; however, the differences are challenging to quantify. When examining stress from a quantitative perspective, even defining stress in a standardized way is difficult. As leading stress researchers have noted, inconsistencies in both the conceptual and operational definitions of stress lead to difficulties in drawing meaningful conclusions about it (Lobel, 1994; Lobel, Dunkel-Schetter, & Scrimshaw, 1992).

One approach to defining stress in a robust way is to use a multidimensional construct. Lobel et al. (Lobel, 1994; Lobel et al., 1992) conceptualize stress as being composed of three components: stimulus/environmental, perceptual, and emotional response, all of which fit into Lazarus's transactional model (Lazarus, 1966). These components, measured collectively, create a comprehensive evaluation of stress. Currently, no single measure exists that accounts for the multiple dimensions of stress; therefore, this chapter examines the existing literature about stress during pregnancies conceived by IVF in order to ascertain the extent to which this literature supports Lobel et al.'s conceptualization of stress.

## THEORETICAL MODEL

Research indicates that IVF is stressful. However, it is unknown whether the stress of the IVF procedure carries into the pregnancies that result, and it is also unknown whether the stress levels are higher than those of women who conceive without assistance. A multidimensional conceptualization of stress proposed by Lobel et al. (1992), as described earlier, can be used to understand the stress women may experience during pregnancies after undergoing IVF. The multidimensional definition of pregnancy stress proposed by Lobel et al. (Lobel, 1994; Lobel & Dunkel-Schetter, 1990; Lobel et al., 1992) forms the conceptual framework for this review. Lobel et al.'s work was based on that of Lazarus and Folkman, whose transactional model of stress and coping (Lazarus, 1966; Lazarus & Folkman, 1984; Lazarus & Launier, 1978) defines stress as the product of a dynamic interaction or relationship between the individual and the environment that takes into account both the characteristics of the person and the nature of the environmental event (Lazarus, 1966; Lazarus & Folkman, 1984; Lazarus & Launier, 1978). In Lobel's conceptualization (1992), the three components of stress, when taken together, represent an individual's overall level of stress. The relationships found by Lobel and Dunkel-Schetter (1990) between the three components may be the result of various relationships, both unidirectional and bidirectional, between each of these variables.

The first component of the multidimensional stress model, the stimulus/ environmental element, is typically measured in terms of life events that require the individual to make major changes or adjustments. The second component, the perceptual, involves an individual's perception of an event or events as stressful (Lobel, 1994; Lobel & Dunkel-Schetter, 1990; Lobel et al., 1992). As Cohen, Kamarck, and Mermelstein (1983) state, "perceived stress can be viewed as an outcome variable, measuring the experienced level of stress as a function of objective stressful events, coping processes, personality factors, etc." (p. 386). The third component of the stress model is the emotional response, which occurs when an individual is confronted with an event that she perceives as stressful. The most frequently measured negative emotional response is anxiety (Lobel, 1994), with the contextually related form of anxiety being pregnancy-related anxiety.

## RESULTS

After an exhaustive search of the literature, 13 studies were designed to measure at least one of the three components of stress in women who were pregnant via IVF. These 13 studies were evaluated in terms of whether and how they measured stress in women with IVF pregnancies. Of the studies, none considered the environmental component of stress; one study evaluated the perceptual component, and 13 considered the emotional response component. The only one of the three stress dimensions that has been evaluated by multiple researchers in women with IVF pregnancies is the emotional response component, which encompasses both general and pregnancy-related anxiety. Of those that examined emotional response, 10 studied *general anxiety* and eight studied *pregnancy-specific anxiety* (see Tables 3.1 and 3.2 for more detail about these studies). In the review of these studies, the factors of interest were as follows: whether the women in the samples had previous pregnancies, which country was the setting of the study, and when in the pregnancy the variables were measured.

### Perceptual Component

Only one study examined perceived stress in a sample of women who had become pregnant via IVF (Darwiche et al., 2014). In the study, researchers were interested in stress levels in an IVF population before prenatal testing as compared with a control sample of women who became pregnant without assistance. The IVF group had more perceived stress than controls as measured at 11 weeks gestation (Darwiche et al., 2014).

### Emotional Response Component

The emotional response component is the only one of the three stress dimensions that was evaluated by multiple researchers in samples of women with IVF pregnancies.

**TABLE 3.1 Summary of Studies Included in Review**

| STUDY | DESIGN | PURPOSE | SAMPLE | METHODS | MEASURES | RESULTS |
|---|---|---|---|---|---|---|
| Darwiche et al. (2014) | Prospective Study | To compare levels of general and pregnancy-specific anxiety related to well-being of child and psychological stress before noninvasive screening. | Fifty-one nulliparous women pregnant via IVF/ICSI compared with 54 women who conceived spontaneously during first trimester | Participants completed questionnaires about their general and pregnancy-specific anxiety, and psychological stress at one time point. Demographic, obstetrical, and medical histories were obtained at recruitment. | Spielberger State and Trait Anxiety Inventory (STAI) for state anxiety; Pregnancy-Related Anxiety Questionnaire (PRAQ-R) for anxiety about well-being of child; Psychological Stress Measure (PSM) for psychological stress; Prenatal Psychosocial Profile (PPP) for stress related to psychosocial issues | Anxiety scores were higher in IVF/ICSI group; higher pregnancy-related anxiety about well-being of child in control group, but regression showed no difference in groups; higher psychological stress in IVF/ICSI group. |
| McMahon et al. (2013) | Longitudinal Cohort Study | To compare the prevalence of nausea and vomiting of pregnancy (NVP) in singleton and twin gestations conceived via IVF, and to analyze the impact of associated psychological factors. | Forty-five singleton gestations and 12 twin gestations, studied after confirmation of pregnancy (baseline), 10 to 12 weeks gestation, and 20 to 22 weeks gestation | Participants completed three questionnaires evaluating NVP, anxiety, and depression during each encounter. Demographic, obstetrical, and medical histories were obtained at recruitment. | Pregnancy-Unique Quantification of Emesis and Nausea, Center for Epidemiologic Studies Depression Scale, and the STAI | Anxiety scores, but not depression, are higher in women with twin gestations who underwent IVF as compared with singleton gestations. |

*(continued)*

| STUDY | DESIGN | PURPOSE | SAMPLE | METHODS | MEASURES | RESULTS |
|---|---|---|---|---|---|---|
| McMahon et al. (2011) | Prospective Study | To examine the impact of mode of conception and maternal age on adjustment during the transition to parenthood. | Women in their third trimester of pregnancy who conceived through ART (n = 297) or spontaneously (n = 295), stratified into three different age groups: "younger" (≤ 20–30 years); "middle" (31–36 years); and "older" (≥ 37 years) | Participants completed an interview, as well as questionnaires assessing socioeconomic status, personality, state and trait anxiety, pregnancy-focused anxiety, quality of partner relationship, and maternal–fetal attachment. | Socioeconomic and reproductive history variables (collected through phone interview), STAI, Edinburgh Postnatal Depression Scale, Baby Schema Questionnaire, and Maternal–Fetal Attachment Scale | No significant age group differences in the proportions of women with anxiety levels (state and pregnancy focused) in the clinical range (p > .10). |
| Jahangiri et al. (2011) | Longitudinal Pilot Study | To compare the prevalence of NVP in singleton and twin gestations conceived via IVF, and to analyze the impact of associated psychological factors. | Forty-five singleton gestations and 12 twin gestations, studied after confirmation of pregnancy (baseline), 10 to 12 weeks gestation, and 20 to 22 weeks gestation | Participants completed three questionnaires evaluating NVP, anxiety, and depression during each encounter. Demographic, obstetrical, and medical histories were obtained at recruitment. | Pregnancy-Unique Quantification of Emesis and Nausea, Center for Epidemiologic Studies Depression Scale, and the STAI | Anxiety scores, but not depression, are higher in women with twin gestations who underwent IVF as compared with singleton gestations. |

*(continued)*

TABLE 3.1 Summary of Studies Included in Review  (continued)

| STUDY | DESIGN | PURPOSE | SAMPLE | METHODS | MEASURES | RESULTS |
|-------|--------|---------|--------|---------|----------|---------|
| Gameiro, Moura-Ramos, Canavarro, and Soares (2010) | Longitudinal Prospective Study | To examine the psychosocial adjustment of couples who conceived via artificial reproductive technologies. | Thirty-five couples who conceived via ART and 31 couples who conceived spontaneously studied at week 24 of pregnancy and 4 months postpartum | Participants completed questionnaires separately regarding perceptions of pregnancy and parenthood, psychological distress, quality of life, marital relationship, and parenting stress. Demographic and obstetrical history obtained through medical charts. | Perceptions questionnaire, Brief Symptom Inventory, World Health Organization Quality of Life brief instrument, ENRICH marital inventory, and Parenting Stress Index | No multivariate effects found regarding parents' psychological distress or parenting stress. Couples who conceived through ART perceived their pregnancies to be more demanding and riskier, but also more rewarding than those who conceived spontaneously. |
| Cox, Glazebrook, Sheard, Ndukwe, and Oates (2006) | Limited Prospective Study | To examine self-esteem, anxiety, and parenting self-efficacy in IVF pregnancies. | Seventy women who conceived via ART and 111 women who conceived spontaneously, assessed at 18 and 28 weeks gestation and 6 weeks postpartum. | Participants completed postal questionnaires regarding self-esteem and anxiety at 18 and 28 weeks gestation and were interviewed at 6 weeks postpartum | Self-Concept Questionnaire, Hospital Anxiety, and Depression Scale, Parenting Self-Efficacy Scale | No significant differences between groups in levels of anxiety during pregnancy and postpartum period. Self-esteem scores significantly increased between 18 and 28 weeks for both groups [$F(1,142) = 15.0$, $p < .001$]. |

*(continued)*

| STUDY | DESIGN | PURPOSE | SAMPLE | METHODS | MEASURES | RESULTS |
|---|---|---|---|---|---|---|
| Poikkeus et al. (2006) | Prospective Study | To compare the prevalence of severe fear of childbirth and pregnancy-related anxiety in second trimester in groups of ART and spontaneously conceiving women with singleton pregnancies. | Three hundred and sixty-seven women (260 nulliparous) who conceived via ART and 379 women (135 nulliparous) who conceived spontaneously, studied during second trimester of pregnancy | Participants completed a set of questionnaires at a mean of 20 weeks gestation. Medical and obstetric histories were obtained, including previous infertility treatments. | Fear of Childbirth Questionnaire, Pregnancy Anxiety Scale, demographic data, obstetric history, and somatic symptoms | Frequency of severe fear of childbirth and anxiety did not differ between groups. Nulliparity associated with increases in severe anxiety only in controls. In nulliparous, partnership of more than 5 years decreased risk of severe fear of childbirth. In nulliparous ART group (OR: 0.3, 95% CI [0.2–0.7]), 7 or more years if increased risk of severe fear of childbirth (OR: 4.4, 95% CI [1.2–16.9]). |
| Hjelmstedt, Widström, and Collins (2006) | Subset of a Larger Longitudinal Project. | To compare prenatal attachment and its relationship with psychosocial variables. | Fifty-six IVF women from IVF clinics and 41 control women from antenatal clinics assessed in gestational weeks 26 and 36 | Participants completed self-rating scales that measured prenatal attachment, personality, marital relationship, anxiety, and depression. | Prenatal Attachment Inventory, STAI, Karolinska Scales of Personality, Edinburgh Postnatal Depression Scale, Barnett Scale, Emotional Responses to Pregnancy Scale | State anxiety was not correlated with prenatal attachment at either week 26 or 36; anxiety about losing the pregnancy ($R = -0.22$, $p = .024$) was only correlated at 36 weeks and not 26 weeks. No associations between prenatal attachment and trait anxiety or depression were found. |

(continued)

**TABLE 3.1 Summary of Studies Included in Review** *(continued)*

| STUDY | DESIGN | PURPOSE | SAMPLE | METHODS | MEASURES | RESULTS |
|---|---|---|---|---|---|---|
| Hjelmstedt et al. (2003a) | Longitudinal Study | To compare emotional response to pregnancy and expectations of and attitudes toward pregnancy, parenthood, and children. | Fifty-seven IVF women and 43 controls at gestational week 13; 56 IVF women and 41 controls at gestational week 26; and 52 IVF women and 38 controls at gestational week 36 | Participants completed a psychological assessment at pregnancy weeks 13, 26, and 36. The IVF group was recruited from IVF units between two hospitals in Stockholm. The control group was recruited nonrandomly from four separate antenatal clinics in the suburbs and inner city of Stockholm. | Emotional Responses to Pregnancy Scale, Wikman Attitude Scale, single question regarding anxiety about whether the baby would be injured during birth, nonstandardized scale regarding the experience of the pregnancy, and the Infertility Reaction Scale | Study group had higher anxiety about losing pregnancy ($F = 15.60$, df = 1, $p < .001$). Both groups had decrease in anxiety as pregnancy progressed, with significance between weeks 13 and 26 ($p < .0001$) and 13 and 36 ($p < .0001$). |
| Hjelmstedt Widström, Wramsby, Matthiesen, and Collins (2003b) | Prospective Study | To compare personality factors and emotional responses to pregnancy among women who conceived after IVF and those that conceived spontaneously. | Fifty-seven women pregnant after IVF and 43 women who conceived spontaneously, studied between 11 and 17 weeks of gestation | Participants completed scales of personality traits, anxiety, emotional responses to pregnancy, marital adjustment, and reactions to recalled infertility. These participants were recruited from IVF and antenatal clinics in Stockholm. | Infertility Reaction Scale, Barnett Scale, Karolinska Scales of Personality, STAI, Emotional Responses to Pregnancy Scale | No differences between groups in mean state or trait anxiety (IVF women: $33.2 \pm 6.7$, control women: $31.1 \pm 6.3$); the study group was more anxious about losing the pregnancy ($F = 31.58$, df = 1, $p < .0001$) and was less anxious over the baby not being healthy ($F = 4.01$, df = 1, $p < .05$) than the control group. |

*(continued)*

| STUDY | DESIGN | PURPOSE | SAMPLE | METHODS | MEASURES | RESULTS |
|-------|--------|---------|--------|---------|----------|---------|
| Klock and Greenfeld (2000) | Prospective Longitudinal Study | To determine whether women who conceived via IVF differ psychologically from women who conceived spontaneously. | Seventy-four women pregnant via IVF and 40 women who conceived without any medical intervention, assessed at 12 and 28 weeks gestation | Participants completed self-report questionnaires that were mailed to be received during weeks 12 and 28 of pregnancy. Participants were recruited from outpatient infertility and obstetric practices. | Demographic questionnaire, health history, marital adjustment, Beck Depression Inventory, STAI, Rosenberg Self-Esteem Scale, and Rewards and Concerns of Pregnancy | No significant differences between groups on anxiety. Within-group changes over time indicated that women pregnant via IVF had an increase in self-esteem and decrease in anxiety during pregnancy. |
| McMahon, Ungerer, Beaurepaire, Tennant, and Saunders (1997) | Prospective Longitudinal Study | To compare the prevalence of anxiety and quality of prenatal attachment during IVF and spontaneously conceived pregnancies. | Seventy women who conceived via IVF and 63 matched controls, studied around 30 weeks gestation and again at 4 and 12 months postpartum | Participants were mailed questionnaires regarding anxiety and prenatal attachment that were to be filled out independently at home and brought in for structured interview between 28 and 33 weeks gestation. Participants were later assessed again at 4 and 12 months postpartum. Participants were recruited from IVF units and through an obstetrician at the same hospital. | STAI, Baby Schema, Antenatal Bonding Questionnaire, Courtauld Emotional Control Scale, and obstetric history | State anxiety higher in IVF group ($F = 3.36$, df = 1,123, $p = .07$); specific anxiety about pregnancy higher in IVF group ("anxieties concerning health and defects in child" [$F = 7.23$, df = 1,120, $p = .008$]; trusted the survival of the pregnancy later [$F = 14.2$, df = 1,120, $p = .000$]; delayed telling others about the pregnancy later [$F = 4.59$, df = 1,120, $p = .034$]; threats to child during birth process [$F = 12.93$; df = 1,120, $p = .000$]; more negative feelings toward birth [$F = 8.99$, df = 1,120, $p = .003$]) |

(continued)

TABLE 3.1 Summary of Studies Included in Review  *(continued)*

| STUDY | DESIGN | PURPOSE | SAMPLE | METHODS | MEASURES | RESULTS |
|-------|--------|---------|--------|---------|----------|---------|
| Stanton and Golombok (1993) | Prospective Study | To examine the degree of anxiety experienced by women pregnant via IVF as well as their attitudes toward pregnancy and the strength of their prenatal attachment. | Fifteen women who conceived via IVF and 20 women who conceived spontaneously, participating at 20 weeks of gestation | Participants were randomly selected or recruited from various clinics after 20 weeks gestation. Participants were asked to complete questionnaires regarding anxiety and prenatal attachment. | STAI, Maternal–Fetal Attachment Scale, and Childbearing Attitudes Questionnaire | No statistically significant differences between the groups were found for state or trait anxiety. Furthermore, there were no statistically significant associations between state or trait anxiety and either maternal–fetal attachment or adjustment to motherhood. |

ART, assisted reproductive technology; ENRICH, Evaluating and Nurturing Relationship Issues, Communication, Happiness; ICSI, intra-cytoplasmic sperm injection; IVF, in vitro fertilization.

TABLE 3.2  Summary of Findings Regarding Stress Outcomes During IVF-Initiated Pregnancies Versus Non-IVF-Initiated Pregnancies

| OUTCOME MEASURED | SUMMARY OF FINDINGS |
|---|---|
| Perceived stress | Higher psychological stress in IVF/ICSI group (Darwiche et al., 2014) |
| General anxiety | IVF/ICSI group had higher levels of state anxiety than group that conceived without assistance (Darwiche et al., 2014) |
| Pregnancy-related anxiety | No differences between groups in state or trait anxiety over time (Hjelmstedt et al., 2003b; Klock & Greenfeld, 2000; Stanton & Golombok, 1993) |
| | No significant differences between the IVF and control group in terms of anxiety during pregnancy and in the postpartum period (Cox et al., 2006) |
| | Significant decrease in state anxiety during pregnancy within the IVF group over time (T1 = 35.2, T2 = 32.0, $t$ = 2.62, $p$ < .03) (Klock & Greenfeld, 2000) |
| | Women who conceived via ART had significantly lower STAI scores in their third trimester of pregnancy (state, $p$ < .01, trait, $p$ < .05). (Coughlan et al., 2014) |
| | State anxiety higher in IVF group ($F$ = 3.36, df = 1,123, $p$ = .07) (McMahon et al., 1997) |
| | A trend toward higher anxiety scores among twin pregnancies starting at 10 to 12 weeks ($p$ = .05), which became significant at 20 to 22 weeks ($p$ = .035). These scores did not differ throughout the study period. Scores for singleton pregnancies decreased significantly from baseline to 20 to 22 weeks ($p$ = .027) (Jahangiri et al., 2011) |
| | No associations between prenatal attachment and trait anxiety, state anxiety, or depression were found (Hjelmstedt et al., 2006) |
| | Lesser tendency for IVF mothers to report feelings of anxiety and depression (McMahon et al., 1997) |
| | No significant differences between groups (Darwiche et al., 2014; Poikkeus et al., 2006) |
| | Anxiety about losing the pregnancy ($R$ = 0.24, $p$ = .016) was only correlated at 36 weeks and not 26 weeks (Hjelmstedt et al., 2006) |
| | IVF group was more anxious about losing the pregnancy ($F$ = 31.58, df = 1, $p$ < .0001; $F$ = 15.60, df = 1, $p$ < .001, respectively) (Hjelmstedt et al., 2003a, 2003b) |
| | IVF group was less anxious over the baby not being healthy ($F$ = 4.01, df = 1, $p$ < .05) than the control group (Hjelmstedt et al., 2003b) |
| | Specific anxiety about pregnancy was higher in the IVF group ("anxieties concerning health and defects in child" [$F$ = 7.23, df = 1,120, $p$ = .008]; the IVF group trusted the survival of the pregnancy later [$F$ = 14.2, df = 1,120, $p$ = .000], delayed telling others about the pregnancy later [$F$ = 4.59, df = 1,120, $p$ = .034], had concerns about threats to child during birth process [$F$ = 12.93; df = 1,120, $p$ = .000], and had more negative feelings toward birth [$F$ = 8.99, df = 1,120, $p$ = .003) than the control group (McMahon et al., 1997) |

(continued)

TABLE 3.2 Summary of Findings Regarding Stress Outcomes During IVF-Initiated Pregnancies Versus Non-IVF-Initiated Pregnancies  (continued)

| OUTCOME MEASURED | SUMMARY OF FINDINGS |
| --- | --- |
| | Numerous previous IVF attempts (≥4) decreased the risk of severe fear of childbirth (OR: 0.06, 95% CI [0.005–0.07]) (Poikkeus et al., 2006) |
| | No differences in psychosocial adjustment between couples that conceived via ART versus couples that conceived spontaneously, with no multivariate effects regarding psychological distress or parenting stress (Gameiro et al., 2010) |
| | No significant age group differences in women with pregnancy-related anxiety during pregnancies conceived via ART (McMahon et al., 2011) |

ART, assisted reproductive technology; ICSI, intra-cytoplasmic sperm injection; IVF, in vitro fertilization; STAI, Spielberger State and Trait Anxiety Inventory.

The research investigated both general and pregnancy-related anxiety in terms of three factors that impact general and pregnancy-related anxiety levels in women with IVF pregnancies: previous pregnancies; country of origin, ethnicity, and cultural identity; and gestational age. The following section discusses these three factors in turn, first in terms of general anxiety and then pregnancy-specific anxiety.

## Impact of Previous Pregnancies on Anxiety

Researchers have investigated whether previous pregnancies impact a woman's levels of general anxiety in 10 studies, and findings are mixed. Two found IVF samples to experience increased general anxiety compared with controls (Darwiche et al., 2014, McMahon et al., 1997), whereas others in this review found no difference in general anxiety (Cox et al., 2006; Gameiro et al., 2010; Hjelmstedt et al., 2003b; Klock & Greenfeld, 2000) even when assessed at multiple time points throughout pregnancy. However, the higher age of the women in the IVF group was statistically significant, as was the fact that they had more previous miscarriages or ectopic pregnancies and fewer previous abortions than controls (Hjelmstedt et al., 2003b).

Interestingly, some research suggested that women pregnant through IVF actually experience less general anxiety than the controls do (Coughlan et al., 2014). In one study, women in the IVF group had more previous miscarriages than the controls, and reported more complications in the current pregnancy, such as bleeding, hypertension, and gestational diabetes; the general state anxiety was lower during the third trimester in this group (McMahon et al., 2011, 2013).

The two other studies that evaluated general anxiety during pregnancy recruited samples of women who were either nulliparous or multiparous (Jahangiri et al., 2011; Stanton & Golombok, 1993). Because researchers of one of these studies found IVF samples to have more anxiety (Jahangiri et al., 2011) and the other found no difference (Stanton & Golombok, 1993), the mixed parity of the recruited sample may have influenced results; women who had previous births may have had a different experience of pregnancy than women who were pregnant with their first child.

Although 10 studies dealt with general anxiety, only eight studies examined whether women pregnant via IVF had different levels of pregnancy-specific anxiety than comparison groups of women who conceived without assistance. Overall, many researchers found increases in pregnancy-specific anxiety in women in the IVF groups over controls. Researchers compared pregnancy-specific anxiety between women pregnant via IVF to comparison women and found that the IVF group had more anxiety, with no differences across age groups (McMahon et al., 2011, 2013). In another study, researchers found that their IVF group members had more anxiety about losing their pregnancies. Furthermore, they found a weak correlation in the IVF group between recalled infertility distress and higher anxiety about losing the pregnancy (Hjelmstedt et al., 2003b).

The pregnancy-specific anxiety measured indicated that when women are pregnant via IVF, they are more likely to negatively perceive various aspects of the pregnancy or upcoming birth, such as health and health defects of the baby, fears about damaging the baby during birth, negative feelings toward birth (McMahon et al., 1997), and about losing the pregnancy (Hjelmstedt et al., 2003a, 2006). Women with long durations of infertility (greater than or equal to 7 years) had more severe fears of childbirth, although numerous IVF attempts (four or more) decreased this risk (Poikkeus et al., 2006). In only one of the studies did the control have higher levels of anxiety about the child's well-being, although the regression analysis showed no difference between the groups (Darwiche et al., 2014). Pregnancy-specific anxiety seems to be higher in samples of women pregnant via IVF.

## Impact of Country of Origin, Ethnicity, and Cultural Identity on Anxiety

Ten studies examined general stress among pregnant women in various countries and cultures around the world. When conducting this literature review, it was important to identify the country in which each study of anxiety was conducted because the cultural differences among study populations may impact the ability to compare study results.

Of the two studies that recruited women from a U.S. population, researchers of one found some indication of differences in general anxiety levels between the two groups, particularly halfway through the pregnancy (Jahangiri et al., 2011) whereas the other found no difference (Klock & Greenfeld, 2000). These two studies were the only ones reviewed to provide data about the racial breakdown of the study sample, which is likely reflective of the increased diversity in the United States compared with many more homogeneous countries (Jahangiri et al., 2011; Klock & Greenfeld, 2000). In the two studies conducted in the United Kingdom (Cox et al., 2006; Stanton & Golombok, 1993), data showed no differences in general anxiety scores. Additionally, data from three studies conducted in Australia showed no increase in anxiety in those pregnant via IVF versus without assistance (McMahon et al., 1997, 2011, 2013). Three other studies dealing with general anxiety were conducted in Sweden, Switzerland, and Portugal, and showed mixed results: with no difference in the Swedish study (Hjelmstedt et al., 2003b) and more anxiety in the IVF group in the Swiss and Portuguese studies (Darwiche et al., 2014; Gameiro et al., 2010). Ultimately, in comparing the studies on general anxiety during pregnancy, no clear trend within or between countries was found. Even among studies conducted within the same country, there was no definitive trend in anxiety levels between women who became pregnant with or without IVF.

In addition to general anxiety, eight studies (none in the United States or United Kingdom) looked at pregnancy-specific anxiety. Data from several studies using Swedish and Australian samples showed that women who were pregnant through IVF had more pregnancy-specific anxieties than their counterparts who did not require assistance to conceive (Hjelmstedt et al., 2003a, 2003b; McMahon et al., 1997, 2011, 2013).

## Impact of Gestational Age on Anxiety

Ten of the 13 studies examined the general anxiety of women pregnant via IVF at varying points in pregnancy, with fetuses at different gestational ages. In the first half of pregnancy, women pregnant with twins through IVF experienced more anxiety than singletons (Jahangiri et al., 2011), those with singletons conceived via IVF had similar levels of anxiety to those pregnant without assistance (Cox et al., 2006; Hjelmstedt et al., 2003b; Klock & Greenfeld, 2000; Stanton & Golombok, 1993), and sometimes anxiety was even less in women pregnant through IVF (McMahon et al., 2011, 2013). The eight studies that examined pregnancy-specific anxiety at various points in the pregnancy suggest that women pregnant via IVF have more pregnancy-specific anxiety than those who conceive without assistance, and this holds in all three trimesters (Darwiche et al., 2014; Hjelmstedt et al., 2003a, 2003b, 2006; McMahon et al., 1997, 2011, 2013).

## DISCUSSION

The purpose of this review was to examine the existing literature about stress during pregnancies conceived by IVF and to ascertain the extent to which this literature supports Lobel et al.'s three-pronged conceptualization of stress as having environmental/stimulus, perceptual, and emotional response components (Lobel, 1994; Lobel et al., 1992). Of the 13 studies that were designed to measure stress in populations of women pregnant by IVF, none was designed using Lobel's (1994) multidimensional approach. In terms of individual treatment of the three dimensions of stress, no studies evaluated the environmental component, one study evaluated the perceptual component, and 13 studies evaluated the emotional component. Of the emotion studies, some considered general anxiety, others considered pregnancy-specific anxiety, and some considered both, with a general trend of no difference in general anxiety between groups and those in IVF groups experiencing increases in pregnancy-specific anxiety. The lack of research involving the first two components of stress during pregnancy (environmental/stimulus and perceptual) indicates a discernable deficiency in researchers' understanding of stress during the IVF experience, particularly during the pregnancy that results from a successful IVF procedure.

Of the 13 studies included in this analysis, it is difficult to draw conclusions about the perceptual component of stress because only one study examined this component, and that study had a relatively small sample size (IVF = 51, control = 54). However, several studies did examine the emotional response component: 10 evaluated general anxiety and eight evaluated pregnancy-specific anxiety. The majority of researchers found no differences in general anxiety between IVF and control groups, although there were differences in samples including parity, country of origin, and time during pregnancy when they were evaluated. Furthermore, the majority of researchers found higher pregnancy-specific anxiety in pregnant IVF groups than those who conceived without assistance. Again, there were variations within the studies in terms of parity, country of origin, and time during pregnancy at which the measurement was conducted. The stress component that has been most widely measured in the pregnant IVF population, albeit not extensively, is the emotional component. Studies have investigated both general and pregnancy-related anxiety. However, it is challenging to draw significant conclusions about these women's experience of anxiety due to the limited number of studies; the discrepancies among studies; the equivocal results of some studies; and the differences among samples in terms of previous pregnancy, country of origin, instrument used to assess anxiety, and time during pregnancy that anxiety was measured.

The review found that recent research on general anxiety in pregnancy does not adequately capture the full intensity and depth of the experience (Buss, Davis, Hobel, & Sandman, 2011; Huizink, Mulder, Robles de Medina, Visser, & Buitelaar, 2004); for this reason, a more appropriate variable for researchers to study in pregnant women may be pregnancy-specific anxiety. Indeed, the literature on preterm birth shows a positive relationship between pregnancy-related anxiety and preterm birth (Dominguez, Dunkel-Schetter, Glynn, Hobel, & Sandman, 2008; Dunkel-Schetter, 2011; Glynn, Schetter, Hobel, & Sandman, 2008), although this relationship has not been studied in the pregnant IVF population. It is possible that the pregnant IVF population may be at greater risk of pregnancy-specific anxiety based on the length of time required and the procedures undergone to achieve the pregnancy. Researchers performing qualitative work have indicated that women who become pregnant by IVF may view their pregnancies differently from women who conceive without assistance (McMahon, Tennant, Ungerer, & Saunders, 1999; Sandelowski et al., 1992). Other researchers indicated that these pregnancies were perceived as hard-won, special, and devastating to lose (Olshansky, 1990). The process of conception was described as distressing, and those feelings often extended well into the second trimester of pregnancy (Sandelowski, Harris, & Holditch-Davis, 1990). Moreover, women who conceived by IVF were more anxious about the pregnancy and baby than their nonassisted counterparts (Hjelmstedt et al., 2003b).

The stress of non-infertile pregnant women has been studied extensively and very often from a multidimensional perspective, with particular attention to poor obstetrical and neonatal outcomes. The researchers have found relationships between psychological stress and adverse outcomes such as difficulty transitioning to motherhood and attaching to the infant (Bernstein, Lewis, & Seibel, 1994; Niemelä, 1992; Stanton & Golombok, 1993); poor outcomes in the baby, such as delayed motor development, cognitive disorders, and behavioral disorders (Huizink, Robles de Medina, Mulder, Visser, & Buitelaar, 2003; Kinsella & Monk, 2009); neonatal stress reactivity after birth (Leung et al., 2010); and emotional problems (O'Connor, Heron, Golding, Beveridge, & Glover, 2002). Researchers have found associations between stress (measured by pregnancy-related anxiety) and both lower motor maturity in neonates (Standley, Soule, & Copans, 1979) and greater infant irritability (Van den Bergh, 1990). Increased stress has been found to increase the risk of premature delivery (Dailey, 2009; Hedegaard, Henriksen, Sabroe, & Secher, 1993; Kramer et al., 2009; Mackey, Williams, & Tiller, 2000; Nkansah-Amankra, Luchok, Hussey, Watkins, & Jiu, 2010; Tegethoff, Greene, Olsen, Meyer, & Meinlschmidt, 2010), and increased anxiety has been associated with low birth weight (Nkansah-Amankra et al., 2010; Pagel, Smilkstein, Regen, & Montano, 1990; Tegethoff et al., 2010; Wadhwa et al., 1993). Researchers approaching stress multidimensionally have frequently found a relationship between increases in stress and increased risk of premature delivery (Copper et al., 1996; Hedegaard et al., 1993; Lobel et al., 1992). Such research into stress during pregnancy is necessary because nurses and other health care practitioners need to be able to identify patients at risk of such stress.

Although considerable attention has been given to adverse obstetrical and neonatal outcomes in the general pregnancy population, little work has been done to measure, from a multidimensional approach, the stress of women pregnant through IVF. Such research would provide a more robust understanding of stress during IVF pregnancies. Although data indicate that pregnancies conceived after the assistance of IVF are at increased risk of delivering prematurely (Helmerhorst, Perquin, Donker, & Keirse, 2004; Jackson, Gibson, Wu, & Croughan, 2004; McDonald, Murphy, Beyene, & Ohlsson, 2005; McGovern, Llorens, Skurnick, Weiss, & Goldsmith, 2004), no reason has been found to account for this trend. This problem may become more widespread as IVF becomes increasingly more popular.

Although this review was comprehensive, it should be reviewed with caution. An important limitation to point out is the age of the majority of research cited in this review. Much of the research that has examined the experience of pregnancy that follows successful IVF treatment was conducted in the 1990s and 2000s. This time period parallels the point during the IVF technology at which success rates dramatically began to improve and usage of this treatment increased (Society for Assisted Reproductive Technology, 2013); therefore, it was logical and appropriate for scientists to try to understand the psychosocial aspects of this emerging technology. The challenge, however, is making those conclusions relevant today in the ever-changing landscape that includes complex variables such as expanded technologies, reimbursement changes, and even shifting focus on family dynamics and structure.

## CONCLUSION

As science advances, so do the success rates of IVF, resulting in more pregnancies conceived via IVF each year (Society for Assisted Reproductive Technology, 2013). At present, no current standards exist in nursing or in medicine for identifying increases in stress during the IVF process and resulting pregnancies. Very often, patients are not seen by clinical psychologists as part of their treatments unless the patients are considering the use of donor eggs, sperm, or gestational carriers. Meanwhile, research is unclear as to whether a woman who becomes pregnant by IVF is the same as the one who conceives without assistance, and thus, whether common wisdom about pregnancy applies to these women.

The gap in research and practice hinders the work of health care providers caring for this population, who must adequately be able to assess patients' psychological adaptation to pregnancy after IVF. The care team interacts with women extensively during prenatal visits while patients are under the care of reproductive endocrinologists, obstetricians, and midwives. If women are experiencing significant amounts of stress during the infertility process and resulting pregnancy, providers can intervene directly with the patient and provide appropriate referrals as they transition to their primary obstetrician or midwife, who can then follow the patient through the course of the pregnancy. Women who experience stress during pregnancy are at risk of a difficult transition to motherhood and attachment to their infant may be impaired (Bernstein et al., 1994; Niemelä, 1992; Stanton & Golombok, 1993), but early identification can help women to deal with this stress early on in the pregnancy, thus preventing potential negative outcomes. In this context, well-designed studies can contribute to research and practice in improving identification of and treatment for increases in stress. It is essential that research determine whether standardization of care is necessary for managing the psychological needs of women who become pregnant through IVF, so that stress does not exact long-term harm on women and their babies.

# REFERENCES

Bernstein, J., Lewis, J., & Seibel, M. (1994). Effect of previous infertility on maternal-fetal attachment, coping styles, and self-concept during pregnancy. *Journal of Women's Health, 3*, 125–133. doi:10.1089/jwh.1994.3.125

Buss, C., Davis, E. P., Hobel, C. J., & Sandman, C. A. (2011). Maternal pregnancy-specific anxiety is associated with child executive function at 6–9 years age. *Stress, 14*(6), 665–676.

Cohen, S., Kamarck, T., & Mermelstein, R. (1983). A global measure of perceived stress. *Journal of Health and Social Behavior, 24*(4), 385–396.

Copper, R. L., Goldenberg, R. L., Das, A., Elder, N., Swain, M., Norman, G., . . . Meier, A. M. (1996). The preterm prediction study: Maternal stress is associated with spontaneous preterm birth at less than thirty-five weeks' gestation. National Institute of Child Health and Human Development Maternal-Fetal Medicine Units Network. *American Journal of Obstetrics and Gynecology, 175*(5), 1286–1292.

Coughlan, C., Walters, S., Ledger, W., & Li, T. C. (2014). A comparison of psychological stress among women with and without reproductive failure. *International Journal of Gynaecology and Obstetrics, 124*(2), 143–147.

Cox, S. J., Glazebrook, C., Sheard, C., Ndukwe, G., & Oates, M. (2006). Maternal self-esteem after successful treatment for infertility. *Fertility and Sterility, 85*(1), 84–89

Dailey, D. E. (2009). Social stressors and strengths as predictors of infant birth weight in low-income African American women. *Nursing Research, 58*(5), 340–347.

Darwiche, J., Lawrence, C., Vial, Y., Wunder, D., Stiefel, F., Germond, M., . . . de Roten, Y. (2014). Anxiety and psychological stress before prenatal screening in first-time mothers who conceived through IVF/ICSI or spontaneously. *Women & Health, 54*(5), 474–485.

DiPietro, J. A., Ghera, M. M., Costigan, K., & Hawkins, M. (2004). Measuring the ups and downs of pregnancy stress. *Journal of Psychosomatic Obstetrics and Gynaecology, 25*(3–4), 189–201.

Dominguez, T. P., Dunkel-Schetter, C., Glynn, L. M., Hobel, C., & Sandman, C. A. (2008). Racial differences in birth outcomes: The role of general, pregnancy, and racism stress. *Health Psychology, 27*(2), 194–203.

Dunkel-Schetter, C. (2011). Psychological science on pregnancy: Stress processes, biopsychosocial models, and emerging research issues. *Annual Review of Psychology, 62,* 531–558. doi:10.1146/annurev.psych.031809.130727

Gameiro, S., Moura-Ramos, M., Canavarro, M. C., & Soares, I. (2010). Psychosocial adjustment during the transition to parenthood of Portuguese couples who conceived spontaneously or through assisted reproductive technologies. *Research in Nursing & Health, 33*(3), 207–220.

Giurgescu, C., Penckofer, S., Maurer, M. C., & Bryant, F. B. (2006). Impact of uncertainty, social support, and prenatal coping on the psychological well-being of high-risk pregnant women. *Nursing Research, 55*(5), 356–365.

Glynn, L. M., Schetter, C. D., Hobel, C. J., & Sandman, C. A. (2008). Pattern of perceived stress and anxiety in pregnancy predicts preterm birth. *Health Psychology, 27*(1), 43–51.

Hedegaard, M., Henriksen, T. B., Sabroe, S., & Secher, N. J. (1993). Psychological distress in pregnancy and preterm delivery. *BMJ, 307*(6898), 234–239.

Helmerhorst, F. M., Perquin, D. A., Donker, D., & Keirse, M. J. (2004). Perinatal outcome of singletons and twins after assisted conception: A systematic review of controlled studies. *BMJ, 328*(7434), 261.

Hjelmstedt, A., Widström, A.-M., & Collins, A. (2006). Psychological correlates of prenatal attachment in women who conceived after in vitro fertilization and women who conceived naturally. *Birth, 33*(4), 303–310.

Hjelmstedt, A., Widström, A.-M., Wramsby, H., & Collins, A. (2003a). Patterns of emotional responses to pregnancy, experience of pregnancy and attitudes to parenthood among IVF couples: A longitudinal study. *Journal of Psychosomatic Obstetrics & Gynecology, 81,* 153–162. doi:10.3109/01674820309039669

Hjelmstedt, A., Widström, A.-M., Wramsby, H., Matthiesen, A. S., & Collins, A. (2003b). Personality factors and emotional responses to pregnancy among IVF couples in early pregnancy: A comparative study. *Acta Obstetricia et Gynecologica Scandinavica, 82*(2), 152–161.

Huizink, A. C., Mulder, E. J., Robles de Medina, P. G., Visser, G. H., & Buitelaar, J. K. (2004). Is pregnancy anxiety a distinctive syndrome? *Early Human Development, 79*(2), 81–91.

Huizink, A. C., Robles de Medina, P. G., Mulder, E. J., Visser, G. H., & Buitelaar, J. K. (2003). Stress during pregnancy is associated with developmental outcome in infancy. *Journal of Child Psychology and Psychiatry, and Allied Disciplines, 44*(6), 810–818.

Jackson, R. A., Gibson, K. A., Wu, Y. W., & Croughan, M. S. (2004). Perinatal outcomes in singletons following in vitro fertilization: A meta-analysis. *Obstetrics and Gynecology, 103*(3), 551–563.

Jahangiri, F., Hirshfeld-Cytron, J., Goldman, K., Pavone, M. E., Gerber, S., & Klock, S. C. (2011). Correlation between depression, anxiety, and nausea and vomiting during pregnancy in an in vitro fertilization population: A pilot study. *Journal of Psychosomatic Obstetrics and Gynaecology, 32*(3), 113–118.

Jomeen, J., & Martin, C. R. (2005). Self-esteem and mental health during early pregnancy. *Clinical Effectiveness in Nursing, 9,* 92–95. doi:10.1016/j.cein.2004.09.001

Kinsella, M. T., & Monk, C. (2009). Impact of maternal stress, depression and anxiety on fetal neurobehavioral development. *Clinical Obstetrics and Gynecology, 52*(3), 425–440.

Klock, S. C., & Greenfeld, D. A. (2000). Psychological status of in vitro fertilization patients during pregnancy: A longitudinal study. *Fertility and Sterility, 73*(6), 1159–1164.

Kramer, M. S., Lydon, J., Séguin, L., Goulet, L., Kahn, S. R., McNamara, H., . . . Platt, R. W. (2009). Stress pathways to spontaneous preterm birth: The role of stressors, psychological distress, and stress hormones. *American Journal of Epidemiology, 169*(11), 1319–1326.

Lawson, A. K., Klock, S. C., Pavone, M. E., Hirshfeld-Cytron, J., Smith, K. N., & Kazer, R. R. (2014). Prospective study of depression and anxiety in female fertility preservation and infertility patients. *Fertility and Sterility, 102*(5), 1377–1384.

Lazarus, R. S. (1966). *Psychological stress and the coping process.* New York, NY: McGraw Hill.

Lazarus, R. S., & Folkman, S. (1984). *Stress, appraisal, and coping.* New York, NY: Springer.

Lazarus, R. S., & Launier, R. (1978). Stress-related transactions between person and environment. In L. A. Pervin & M. Lewis (Eds.), *Perspectives in interactional psychology* (pp. 287–327). New York, NY: Plenum.

Leung, E., Tasker, S. L., Atkinson, L., Vaillancourt, T., Schulkin, J., & Schmidt, L. A. (2010). Perceived maternal stress during pregnancy and its relation to infant stress reactivity at 2 days and 10 months of postnatal life. *Clinical Pediatrics, 49*(2), 158–165.

Lobel, M. (1994). Conceptualizations, measurement, and effects of prenatal maternal stress on birth outcomes. *Journal of Behavioral Medicine, 17*(3), 225–272.

Lobel, M., & Dunkel-Schetter, C. (1990). Conceptualizing stress to study effects on health: Environmental, perceptual, and emotional components. *Anxiety Research, 3,* 213–230. doi:10.1080/08917779008248754

Lobel, M., Dunkel-Schetter, C., & Scrimshaw, S. C. (1992). Prenatal maternal stress and prematurity: A prospective study of socioeconomically disadvantaged women. *Health Psychology, 11*(1), 32–40.

MacKey, M. C., Williams, C. A., & Tiller, C. M. (2000). Stress, pre-term labour and birth outcomes. *Journal of Advanced Nursing, 32*(3), 666–674.

McDonald, S. D., Murphy, K., Beyene, J., & Ohlsson, A. (2005). Perinatal outcomes of singleton pregnancies achieved by in vitro fertilization: A systematic review and meta-analysis. *Journal of Obstetrics and Gynaecology Canada, 27*(5), 449–459.

McGovern, P. G., Llorens, A. J., Skurnick, J. H., Weiss, G., & Goldsmith, L. T. (2004). Increased risk of preterm birth in singleton pregnancies resulting from in vitro fertilization-embryo transfer or gamete intrafallopian transfer: A meta-analysis. *Fertility and Sterility, 82*(6), 1514–1520.

McMahon, C. A., Boivin, J., Gibson, F. L., Hammarberg, K., Wynter, K., Saunders, D., & Fisher, J. (2011). Age at first birth, mode of conception and psychological wellbeing in pregnancy: Findings from the parental age and transition to parenthood Australia (PATPA) study. *Human Reproduction, 26*(6), 1389–1398.

McMahon, C. A., Boivin, J., Gibson, F. L., Hammarberg, K., Wynter, K., Saunders, D., & Fisher, J. (2013). Pregnancy-specific anxiety, ART conception and infant temperament at 4 months post-partum. *Human Reproduction, 28*(4), 997–1005.

McMahon, C. A., Tennant, C., Ungerer, J. A., & Saunders, D. (1999). "Don't count your chickens": A comparative study of the experience of pregnancy after IVF conception. *Journal of Reproductive and Infant Psychology, 17,* 345–356. doi:10.1080/02646839908404600

McMahon, C. A., Ungerer, J. A., Beaurepaire, J., Tennant, C., & Saunders, D. (1997). Anxiety during pregnancy and fetal attachment after in-vitro fertilization conception. *Human Reproduction, 12*(1), 176–182.

Niemelä, P. (1992). Working through ambivalence about parenthood. In K. Wijma & B. von Schoultz (Eds.), *Reproductive life* (pp. 128–133). Park Ridge, NJ: The Parthenon Publishing Group.

Nkansah-Amankra, S., Luchok, K. J., Hussey, J. R., Watkins, K., & Jiu, X. (2010). Effects of maternal stress on low birth weight and preterm birth outcomes across neighborhoods of South Carolina, 2000–2003. *Maternal and Child Health Journal, 14,* 215–226. doi:10.1007/s10995-009-0447-4

O'Connor, T. G., Heron, J., Golding, J., Beveridge, M., & Glover, V. (2002). Maternal antenatal anxiety and children's behavioural/emotional problems at 4 years. Report from the Avon Longitudinal Study of Parents and Children. *The British Journal of Psychiatry, 180,* 502–508.

Olshansky, E. F. (1990). Psychosocial implications of pregnancy after infertility. *NAACOG's Clinical Issues in Perinatal and Women's Health Nursing, 1*(3), 342–347.

Pagel, M. D., Smilkstein, G., Regen, H., & Montano, D. (1990). Psychosocial influences on new born outcomes: A controlled prospective study. *Social Science & Medicine, 30*(5), 597–604.

Poikkeus, P., Saisto, T., Unkila-Kallio, L., Punamaki, R. L., Repokari, L., Vilska, S., ... Tulppala, M. (2006). Fear of childbirth and pregnancy-related anxiety in women conceiving with assisted reproduction. *Obstetrics and Gynecology, 108*(1), 70–76.

Reddy, U. M., Wapner, R. J., Rebar, R. W., & Tasca, R. J. (2007). Infertility, assisted reproductive technology, and adverse pregnancy outcomes: Executive summary of a National Institute of Child Health and Human Development workshop. *Obstetrics and Gynecology, 109*(4), 967–977.

Sandelowski, M., Harris, B. G., & Black, B. P. (1992). Relinquishing infertility: The work of pregnancy for infertile couples. *Qualitative Health Research, 2,* 282–301. doi:10.1177/104973239200200303

Sandelowski, M., Harris, B. G., & Holditch-Davis, D. (1990). Pregnant moments: The process of conception in infertile couples. *Research in Nursing & Health, 13*(5), 273–282.

Society for Assisted Reproductive Technology. (2013). *Clinic summary reports.* Retrieved from https://www.sartcorsonline.com/rptCSR_PublicMultYear.aspx?ClinicPKID=0

Standley, K., Soule, B., & Copans, S. A. (1979). Dimensions of prenatal anxiety and their influence on pregnancy outcome. *American Journal of Obstetrics and Gynecology, 135*(1), 22–26.

Stanton, F., & Golombok, S. (1993). Maternal-fetal attachment during pregnancy following in vitro fertilization. *Journal of Psychosomatic Obstetrics and Gynaecology, 14*(2), 153–158.

Stark, M. A., & Brinkley, R. L. (2007). The relationship between perceived stress and health-promoting behaviors in high-risk pregnancy. *The Journal of Perinatal & Neonatal Nursing, 21*(4), 307–314.

Tegethoff, M., Greene, N., Olsen, J., Meyer, A. H., & Meinlschmidt, G. (2010). Maternal psychosocial adversity during pregnancy is associated with length of gestation and offspring size at birth: Evidence from a population-based cohort study. *Psychosomatic Medicine, 72*(4), 419–426.

Turner, K., Reynolds-May, M. F., Zitek, E. M., Tisdale, R. L., Carlisle, A. B., & Westphal, L. M. (2013). Stress and anxiety scores in first and repeat IVF cycles: A pilot study. *PLoS One, 8,* 1–6. doi:10.1371/journal.pone.0063743

Van den Bergh, B. (1990). The influence of maternal emotions during pregnancy on fetal and neonatal behavior. *Prenatal & Perinatal Psychology, 5,* 119–130.

Wadhwa, P. D., Sandman, C. A., Porto, M., Dunkel-Schetter, C., & Garite, T. J. (1993). The association between prenatal stress and infant birth weight and gestational age at birth: A prospective investigation. *American Journal of Obstetrics and Gynecology, 169*(4), 858–865.

Yali, A. M., & Lobel, M. (2002). Stress-resistance resources and coping in pregnancy. *Anxiety Stress Coping, 15,* 289–309. doi:10.1080/10615800021000020743

# CHAPTER 4

# EXAMINING THE UNIT OF ANALYSIS IN ASSISTED REPRODUCTION: CONCEPTUAL INSIGHTS INTO INDIVIDUAL, COUPLE, AND FAMILY RESEARCH IN EDUCATION AND COUNSELING

*Patricia E. Hershberger and Sooyoung Yeom*

Over the past few decades, our knowledge of reproductive technologies has substantially broadened through active and vibrant clinical research and practice around the world. There is no doubt that state-of-the-art reproductive technologies have led to remarkable advancements in the field of fertility treatments. Perhaps the best evidence of these advancements lies in the most recent data from 55 participating countries where more than 200,000 babies were born as a direct result of assisted reproductive technology (ART) in a 1-year period alone (Ishihara et al., 2015). Suffice to say, since 1978, when Louise Brown, the first in vitro fertilization (IVF) baby, ushered in a new era of fertility care, a myriad of individuals, couples, and families have benefited from the remarkable advancements in the field.

As the use of ARTs grew, an increasing awareness of the need for education and counseling among those who were infertile or at risk of fertility loss was recognized (Greenfeld, 1997). Likewise, because of the social nature of people and the effects that reproduction has on individuals, couples, and often the family at large, we wanted to obtain knowledge about how investigators have conceptualized the focus of the research. Therefore, in this chapter we take a close, but succinct, look at how investigators have approached research designs by examining the unit of analysis (i.e., individual, couple, and family) used by investigators to advance the science and practice of education and counseling in the field of ART. Because there is very little in the scholarly literature about the unit of analysis in research designs, our aim is to provide a beginning foundation for researchers, clinicians, and others in the ART field as they approach future research and address counseling and education in the clinical setting.

To focus our discussion and provide a concise sample of the types of individual, couple, and family research completed in the field of ART, we searched the online database PubMed using the phrase, "in vitro fertilization" in June 2015. The search identified more than 16,800 articles. In order to obtain a feasible sample, we

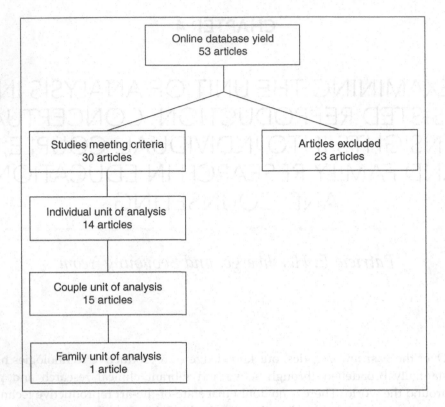

**FIGURE 4.1** Retrieval and identification of articles.

limited the search by using the search phrase, "in vitro fertilization AND education AND counseling." Using this phrase, a sample of 53 published articles was obtained. We read each of the 53 articles to determine which were: (a) research based and (b) directly involved infertile participants. Of the 53 articles, we identified 14 reports where the individual was the unit of analysis, 15 reports where the couple was the unit of analysis, and one report where the family was the unit of analysis (Figure 4.1). Many of the remaining 23 articles were informative or review articles, committee reports, or research reports in which the sample was composed of health care providers or clinic managers. Because we were interested in understanding the unit of analysis used by investigators in educational and counseling research in the population of patients that use ART, our analysis, to a great extent, is centered on research reports where current, future, or former participants were patients. In the following, we provide an overview of our analysis and discussion of the findings.

## INDIVIDUAL UNIT OF ANALYSIS FINDINGS

We identified 14 reports in which the individual was the unit of analysis. Noteworthy, in the majority of articles ($n = 12$, 86%) where the unit of analysis was at the individual level, women were the focus of the research reports as compared with men. No reports where children were the focus of the research were identified.

Women have historically been the target of reproductive research and our findings support this notion. Within the 12 identified articles where women were the focus of the individual unit of analysis, various types of research were completed including physiological, qualitative, and quantitative. In the one physiological report identified in our sample, investigators evaluated 116 infertile women's physiological (i.e., serum anti-Müllerian) levels and age on pregnancy outcomes (Lee, Wu, Lin, Lin, & Hwu, 2011). Another report identified was a case study delineating an esophageal atresia in an IVF pregnant woman (Whitman-Elia, Plouffe, Craft, & Khan, 1997). Two of the studies focused on understanding women's lived experiences. In the first, Su and Chen (2006) examined the concept of "hope" among 24 infertile women who had unsuccessfully undergone IVF and subsequently terminated IVF treatment. In the second, 22 childless women from India were interviewed to understand the experience of women who were planning to undergo IVF treatment (Widge, 2005). Many of the remaining research articles that had an individual unit of analysis focused on understanding women's psychosocial concerns. Because "counseling" was used in the search phrase, it was expected that psychological concerns would be a primary focus. However, "education" was also included in the search phrase and it was often a secondary outcome of the research rather than the aim of the investigation. For example, in a study by Lok et al. (2002), 372 women who underwent IVF or ovulation induction and who were unsuccessful in achieving pregnancy were evaluated for psychiatric morbidity. Lee, Liu, Kuo, and Lee (2011) examined postpartum depression in 60 women who received IVF treatment. Likewise, Gürhan, Oflaz, Atici, Akyüz, and Vural (2007) examined the effects of nurse counseling on coping and depression in 67 women who were undergoing IVF treatment. And Kariminia, Saunders, and Chamberlain (2002) sought to understand "regret" in 97 women who had previously undergone a tubal ligation for voluntary sterilization and who sought out IVF treatment to conceive a biological child. Wang et al. (2007) wanted to understand psychological characteristics and marital quality of 100 infertile women who were scheduled for IVF with intracytoplasmic sperm injection (ICSI). Noteworthy is that women who were planning or had undergone IVF were not the only female population included in the sample of our identified studies. Women who had applied to become egg donors ($n = 40$) were also the focus in one study (Zenke & Chetkowski, 2002).

Of the 14 studies identified that targeted the individual as the unit of analysis, only two targeted men exclusively (Li, Zhang, Zeng, Li, & Cui, 2013; Ting-Ting, Xian-Ping, Xia, Jing, & Li-Yuan, 2013). Regarding these two studies, Li et al. (2013) examined depression in 844 men who were undergoing assisted reproduction in China; and in a physiological study, also completed in China, investigators examined microdeletions in the Y chromosomes of 203 infertile men (Ting-Ting et al., 2013). Grey, Thompson, Jenkins, and Payne (2012) queried clinicians from the United Kingdom about their management of men who had sought care to reverse a previous vasectomy in order to improve clinical practice. However, only the studies completed by Li and colleagues (2013) and Ting-Ting et al. (2013) included men with fertility concerns in their samples; therefore, the Grey et al. (2012) study was not included in the number of reports identified in this review. It is mentioned here because of the low number of reports identified where men were the target of the individual unit of analysis. Noteworthy, too, is that in this dataset the first report addressing the fertility needs of men exclusively was in 2012 (Grey et al., 2012) and the remaining two that targeted infertile men exclusively (Li et al., 2013; Ting-Ting et al., 2013) were reported in 2013.

## Discussion About the Individual Unit of Analysis

We found the overwhelming number of studies completed at the individual, or person, level of analysis involved women. Men were the focus of only two research studies in our sample and these studies were reported in 2013. Although completing research at the individual level of analysis can be beneficial as the previously described studies have shown, gaps remain, especially for men and children conceived through IVF.

Regarding the use of an individual level unit of analysis, it is understandable that many investigators target individuals. In the United States, the individual has a long social and cultural history and is valued in society (Hofstede, 1980). Often the medical treatment goal is to target the problem (e.g., disease, condition, disorder) at the individual level. Additionally, the field of psychology, a major discipline in education and counseling, emphasizes the individual before other potentially higher levels of analysis like those where relationships and interactions between an individual and group members are examined (Bond & Kenny, 2002). These factors have contributed to the frequency of research where the individual is the unit of analysis. From a pragmatic view, collecting data from one individual source is less costly and creates fewer recruitment and statistical analysis challenges than collecting data from multiple sources (Uphold & Strickland, 1989).

A subtle, yet necessary need to complete research at the individual level that emerged from the sample presented here was that in some instances the security, safety, or stigma that women in particular faced from partners or even other family members as a result of their inability to bear children should be considered when designing research. These considerations may be especially important for highly sensitive reproductive research centered on education and counseling that involves ART. In the Wang et al. (2007) study, although the sample consisted of married women who used ICSI, which is typically performed to treat male-related fertility problems, the investigators discussed the importance of family in Chinese society including the major role that women's in-laws play in marriages. Although the emphasis on family can be beneficial to women, some women may be at risk of abuse, being deserted, or even sued for divorce if they are unable to provide children for their husbands (Wang et al., 2007). Widge (2005) also noted the stigma that infertile women in India face and how the inability to produce a biological child can affect a woman's status and security in society. In these instances, research completed at the individual level may not only be more feasible in terms of the resources and analytic processes needed to conduct the study but may also uncover more veracity about the phenomena while keeping women safe. If women understand that the information they share with investigators is confidential and their partners or other family members are not involved in the study, the women may be more apt to participate and report their true perceptions about their experiences.

## COUPLE AND FAMILY UNIT OF ANALYSIS FINDINGS

We identified 15 research reports that focused on couples as the unit of analysis; however, one study was reported in Sweden and because neither of the authors are fluent in Swedish, we have not discussed this article in our analysis. We did identify one study that used the family as the unit of analysis. There was little variation in how investigators constructed the unit of analysis among the couple studies and in the family study (i.e., most investigators used a standard dyadic design) where participating individuals were measured on the same variables (Kenny, Kashy, & Cook, 2006) or participated in interviews where the same interview questions were asked of each individual in the dyad.

Some variation was noted in the composition of the sample of couples by sex. Even though the focus of the research was on couples, in five of the studies, women participants outnumbered men by a fairly large margin. The aim of these studies was primarily to understand the needs and behaviors of couples to ultimately improve the quality of care. For example, in the research by Hawkins et al. (2014), 138 couples (138 women and 70 men) were queried about their perceptions of lifestyle behaviors (e.g., yoga, exercise, rest after embryo transfer) in order to better understand how couples' perceptions of behavior might affect IVF success rates; whereas Tarlatzis et al. (1993) sought to examine the psychosocial effects (e.g., stress, anxiety, and depression) of couples (69 women and 18 men) who were undergoing infertility treatment. In the earliest identified study in our analysis, Brinsmead et al. (1986) obtained their sample of 147 women and 134 men from couples who presented to their clinic for IVF treatment. The aim of this study was to understand demographic and personality characteristics of the couples who were planning to undergo IVF treatment to improve the quality of care (Brinsmead et al., 1986). The remaining two studies targeted understanding the intentions of infertile couples in order to increase knowledge about behavior. In the first of these studies, McMahon and Saunders (2009) examined the attitudes of couples (78 women and 55 men) with stored frozen embryos about their intentions toward donating embryos through a conditional embryo donation process. In this study, each individual member of the couple dyads completed the survey questions via the Internet. In the second study that focused on intentions, Daniluk, Pattinson, Zouvez, and Mitchell (1993) sampled couples (51 females and 41 males) about their intentions to undergo a subsequent IVF treatment cycle after experiencing a successful IVF cycle. The investigators mailed potential participants questionnaires and asked them to complete the questionnaires independently from their partner.

Other couple studies ($n = 7$) reported an equal or almost equal number of women and men participants. However, women in all but one of these studies remained the higher number of participants when the sample differed slightly by gender. The aim of the studies was often on improving patient care in the clinic, understanding psychosocial characteristics of infertile couples including their attitudes about genetic risk, or examining gender difference. Thia, Vo Thanh, and Loh (2007) obtained data from 50 couples to understand the psychosocial experiences of couples before and during IVF treatment. The aim of the study was to delineate strategies to improve couples' experiences during IVF treatment. Another study with almost equal numbers of male and female participants (117 women and 101 men) also queried participants about how best to provide support for couples in IVF clinics (Laffont &

Edelmann, 1994). Two of the six studies used an experimental design to examine interventions aimed at improving patient care (Connolly et al., 1993; Terzioglu, 2001). In the Connolly et al. (1993) study, 152 couples that were undergoing IVF treatment were recruited and randomly assigned to an experimental or control group. The investigators examined whether an experimental counseling intervention resulted in better outcomes on stress, relationship effects, and satisfaction with counseling compared with the control group (Connolly et al., 1993). Moreover, Terzioglu (2001) examined the effectiveness of nurse counseling on IVF outcomes (e.g., pregnancy rates) among 30 infertile couples in an experimental group and 30 infertile couples in a control group. One study sought to understand how 55 IVF couples managed genetic risks (Schover, Thomas, Falcone, Attaran, & Goldberg, 1998). The couple interviews for this study were obtained as part of the "normal clinical services" (p. 863) where coping skills and partner support for genetic treatment decisions were assessed (Schover et al., 1998). Wischmann, Stammer, Scherg, Gerhard, and Verres (2001) sought to understand whether infertile couples differed from other couples on psychosocial characteristics. Data were obtained from about 500 out of 564 couples where psychosocial measures of infertile couples were compared with a representative sample. Last, in one study (Pottinger et al., 2006) where the aim was to examine gender differences in coping behaviors among infertile couples, the sample was slightly skewed toward men ($n = 25$ women, $n = 26$ men). According to the authors, one woman declined to participate even though her husband opted to participate in the study (Pottinger et al., 2006).

There were two studies where the sample composition of "couples" was more unique. In the first, investigators used an individual unit of analysis as a proxy for "couples" (Salakos, Roupa, Sotiropoulou, & Grigoriou, 2004). In this study, 235 infertile women were queried about the types of psychological and emotional support that family planning centers could provide to infertile couples (Salakos et al., 2004). The second study was a case report about the spontaneous, natural conception of a couple following failed IVF + ICSI treatment (Codreanu et al., 2013).

Our analysis identified one research study that conceptualized the "family" as the unit of analysis (Nachtigall, Mac Dougall, Lee, Harrington, & Becker, 2010). In this study, the investigators sampled 106 families (110 women, 74 men) who had an average of six frozen embryos in storage. In another report, Hay et al. (1990) discussed the information that multiple birth families should receive before, during, and after the birth of their multiples. This report is an informational article rather than a report of research findings. The article is framed so that the target of care is the family (Hay et al., 1990).

## Discussion About the Couple and Family Unit of Analysis

Our analysis identified 16 research articles that used a couple or family focus, as compared with the 14 studies that focused on an individual level. This finding from our concise sample dataset is promising, as multi-informant research is complex and challenging (Kenny et al., 2006; McHale, Amato, & Booth, 2014). Some of the challenges arise from the lack of available quantitative and qualitative tools that capture the couple or family dynamics. For example, summing or averaging the scores on quantitative measures such as perceived marital stress by the partners within a couple may be inappropriate. When investigating multigenerational couples or families, obtaining data from various ages and developmental stages represented within the couple or family involves extra effort and expertise (McClement & Woodgate, 1998). Another challenge is the increased effort required to prepare, incorporate, and maintain human subjects' protection and institutional review board approval for complex couple and family studies.

Despite the challenges, there have been multiple calls from several scientific experts regarding the need for knowledge about and involving dyadic and family research, which will inform future research and practice about education and counseling for patients that consider or use IVF treatment. One area that has received attention is the area of study examining differences between the sexes (male/female) because of the growing evidence about differences in brain activity by sex. Leaders in the field have called for an examination of male–female differences in all research (Cahill, 2012; Stevens & Hamann, 2012). Another area is decision science. In this field, experts have reported that most decision research has targeted decision making at the individual level, which leaves a large gap in knowledge about how interrelated partners with potentially disparate views formulate a decision (Elwyn, Stiel, Durand, & Boivin, 2011). In this analysis of couple and family research, we identified one study that had a primary aim to examine sex differences (Pottinger et al., 2006) and one study that had a primary aim to examine decision making (Daniluk et al., 1993). Two additional studies were identified that sought to understand couples' attitudes (McMahon & Saunders, 2009; Schover et al., 1998) and one study examined the family's needs regarding the disposition of embryos (Nachtigall et al., 2010). These latter three studies have application into understanding how couples and families make decisions that can advance the science in both ART and dyadic and family decision research.

The low number of studies that used the family as the unit of analysis identified in our sample was disappointing. We are also aware of a focus on heterosexual couples in our identified studies that used the couple as the unit of analysis. We acknowledge that our analysis is a snapshot of the completed research in ART and is limited. Yet, it provides a starting point for scholars and others interested in advancing educational and counseling research in the field. The critical gaps we identified warrant design considerations by future investigators. The low number of studies that focused on the family or couples other than heterosexuals may be due to the difficulty in conceptualizing the diverse families or couples in ART (Parke, 2013, Chapter 5). Or, it may be that the emphasis of research has been on clinical care when families are forming and the normative population is heterosexual. Yet, a broader conceptualization and inclusion of more diverse families and couples are needed to improve clinical care of these patients despite the challenges of carrying out couple and family research.

## CONCLUSION

Fertility concerns and the desire to bring a child into the world affects the would-be-parent(s) but it also affects egg and sperm donors, surrogates, would-be-grandparents, potential aunts and uncles, cousins, and the life of the yet-to-be-born child.

Our analysis found that most research in this area has focused on the individual or couple as the unit of analysis with a dearth of studies conceptualizing the analysis from the family unit. Although research on individuals and couples is important, and in some studies preferred, the limited number of studies that examine the family unit highlights the need for future research in this area. Education and counseling of individuals, couples, and families that are involved with ARTs could benefit from a wider breadth of research with representation from more diverse individuals, couples, and families, which would advance understanding. When planning future studies, informed and careful selection of the appropriate unit of analysis with full awareness of the gaps in knowledge and the benefits and challenges of each approach would help us to advance the science and, ultimately, the care of the many individuals, couples, and families that are affected by ARTs.

## REFERENCES

Bond, C. F., & Kenny, D. A. (2002). The triangle of interpersonal models. *Journal of Personality and Social Psychology, 83*(2), 355–366.

Brinsmead, M., Guttmann, S., Oliver, M., Stanger, J., Clark, L., & Adler, R. (1986). Demographic and personality characteristics of couples undergoing in vitro fertilisation. *Clinical Reproduction and Fertility, 4*(6), 373–381.

Cahill, L. (2012). A half-truth is a whole lie: On the necessity of investigating sex influences on the brain. *Endocrinology, 153*(6), 2541–2543.

Codreanu, D., Coricovac, A., Mirzan, L., Dracea, L., Marinescu, B., & Boleac, I. (2013). Natural conception following total fertilization failure with intracytoplasmic sperm injection in a couple with unexplained infertility: A case report. *Revista medico-chirurgicală a Societăţii de Medici şi Naturalişti din Iaşi, 117*(2), 431–438.

Connolly, K. J., Edelmann, R. J., Bartlett, H., Cooke, I. D., Lenton, E., & Pike, S. (1993). An evaluation of counselling for couples undergoing treatment for in-vitro fertilization. *Human Reproduction, 8*(8), 1332–1338.

Daniluk, J., Pattinson, T., Zouvez, C., & Mitchell, J. (1993). Factors related to couples' decisions to attempt in vitro fertilization. *Journal of Assisted Reproduction and Genetics, 10*(4), 310–316.

Elwyn, G., Stiel, M., Durand, M. A., & Boivin, J. (2011). The design of patient decision support interventions: Addressing the theory-practice gap. *Journal of Evaluation in Clinical Practice, 17*(4), 565–574.

Greenfeld, D. A. (1997). Does psychological support and counseling reduce the stress experienced by couples involved in assisted reproductive technology? *Journal of Assisted Reproduction and Genetics, 14*(4), 186–188.

Grey, B. R., Thompson, A., Jenkins, B. L., & Payne, S. R. (2012). UK practice regarding reversal of vasectomy 2001–2010: Relevance to best contemporary patient management. *BJU International, 110*(7), 1040–1047.

Gürhan, N., Oflaz, F., Atici, D., Akyüz, A., & Vural, G. (2007). Effectiveness of nursing counseling on coping and depression in women undergoing in vitro fertilization. *Psychological Reports, 100*(2), 365–374.

Hawkins, L. K., Rossi, B. V., Correia, K. F., Lipskind, S. T., Hornstein, M. D., & Missmer, S. A. (2014). Perceptions among infertile couples of lifestyle behaviors and in vitro fertilization (IVF) success. *Journal of Assisted Reproduction and Genetics, 31*(3), 255–260.

Hay, D. A., Gleeson, C., Davies, C., Lorden, B., Mitchell, D., & Paton, L. (1990). What information should the multiple birth family receive before, during and after the birth? *Acta Geneticae Medicae et Gemellologiae, 39*(2), 259–269.

Hofstede, G. (1980). *Culture's consequences: International differences in work-related values.* Thousand Oaks, CA: Sage.

Ishihara, O., Adamson, G. D., Dyer, S., de Mouzon, J., Nygren, K. G., Sullivan, E. A., ... Mansour, R. (2015). International committee for monitoring assisted reproductive technologies: World report on assisted reproductive technologies, 2007. *Fertility and Sterility, 103*(2), 402–13.e11.

Kariminia, A., Saunders, D. M., & Chamberlain, M. (2002). Risk factors for strong regret and subsequent IVF request after having tubal ligation. *The Australian & New Zealand Journal of Obstetrics & Gynaecology, 42*(5), 526–529.

Kenny, D. A., Kashy, D. A., & Cook, W. L. (2006). *Dyadic data analysis.* New York, NY: Guilford Press.

Laffont, I., & Edelmann, R. J. (1994). Perceived support and counselling needs in relation to in vitro fertilization. *Journal of Psychosomatic Obstetrics and Gynaecology, 15*(4), 183–188.

Lee, R. K. K., Wu, F. S. Y., Lin, M.-H., Lin, S.-Y., & Hwu, Y.-M. (2011). The predictability of serum anti-Müllerian level in IVF/ICSI outcomes for patients of advanced reproductive age. *Reproductive Biology and Endocrinology, 9*, 115. doi:10.1186/1477-7827-9-115

Lee, S. H., Liu, L. C., Kuo, P. C., & Lee, M. S. (2011). Postpartum depression and correlated factors in women who received in vitro fertilization treatment. *Journal of Midwifery & Women's Health, 56*(4), 347–352.

Li, L., Zhang, Y., Zeng, D., Li, F., & Cui, D. (2013). Depression in Chinese men undergoing different assisted reproductive technique treatments: Prevalence and risk factors. *Journal of Assisted Reproduction and Genetics, 30*, 1161–1167. doi:10.1007/s10815-013-0057-3

Lok, I. H., Lee, D. T., Cheung, L. P., Chung, W. S., Lo, W. K., & Haines, C. J. (2002). Psychiatric morbidity amongst infertile Chinese women undergoing treatment with assisted reproductive technology and the impact of treatment failure. *Gynecologic and Obstetric Investigation, 53*(4), 195–199.

McClement, S. E., & Woodgate, R. L. (1998). Research with families in palliative care: Conceptual and methodological challenges. *European Journal of Cancer Care, 7*(4), 247–254.

McHale, S. M., Amato, P., & Booth, A. (Eds.). (2014). *Emerging methods in family research.* New York, NY: Springer.

McMahon, C. A., & Saunders, D. M. (2009). Attitudes of couples with stored frozen embryos toward conditional embryo donation. *Fertility and Sterility, 91*(1), 140–147.

Nachtigall, R. D., Mac Dougall, K., Lee, M., Harrington, J., & Becker, G. (2010). What do patients want? Expectations and perceptions of IVF clinic information and support regarding frozen embryo disposition. *Fertility and Sterility, 94*(6), 2069–2072.

Parke, R. D. (2013). *Future families: Diverse forms, rich possibilities.* Chichester, UK: Wiley-Blackwell.

Pottinger, A. M., McKenzie, C., Fredericks, J., DaCosta, V., Wynter, S., Everett, D., & Walters, Y. (2006). Gender differences in coping with infertility among couples undergoing counselling for in vitro fertilization treatment. *The West Indian Medical Journal, 55*(4), 237–242.

Salakos, N., Roupa, Z., Sotiropoulou, P., & Grigoriou, O. (2004). Family planning and psychosocial support for infertile couples. *European Journal of Contraception & Reproductive Health Care, 9*(1), 47–51.

Schover, L. R., Thomas, A. J., Falcone, T., Attaran, M., & Goldberg, J. (1998). Attitudes about genetic risk of couples undergoing in-vitro fertilization. *Human Reproduction, 13*(4), 862–866.

Stevens, J. S., & Hamann, S. (2012). Sex differences in brain activation to emotional stimuli: A meta-analysis of neuroimaging studies. *Neuropsychologia, 50*(7), 1578–1593.

Su, T. J., & Chen, Y. C. (2006). Transforming hope: The lived experience of infertile women who terminated treatment after in vitro fertilization failure. *The Journal of Nursing Research, 14*(1), 46–54.

Tarlatzis, I., Tarlatzis, B. C., Diakogiannis, I., Bontis, J., Lagos, S., Gavriilidou, D., & Mantalenakis, S. (1993). Psychosocial impacts of infertility on Greek couples. *Human Reproduction, 8*(3), 396–401.

Terzioglu, F. (2001). Investigation into effectiveness of counseling on assisted reproductive techniques in Turkey. *Journal of Psychosomatic Obstetrics and Gynaecology, 22*(3), 133–141.

Thia, E. W., Vo Thanh, L. A., & Loh, S. K. (2007). Study on psychosocial aspects and support of in vitro fertilisation programme in an Asian population. *Singapore Medical Journal, 48*(1), 61–68.

Ting-Ting, H., Xian-Ping, D., Xia, W., Jing, R., & Li-Yuan, Z. (2013). Analysis of Y chromosome microdeletion in non-obstructive male infertile patients with azoospermia and severe oligozoospermia. *Journal of Sichuan University. Medical Science Edition, 44*(2), 188–192.

Uphold, C. R., & Strickland, O. L. (1989). Issues related to the unit of analysis in family nursing research. *Western Journal of Nursing Research, 11*(4), 405–417.

Wang, K., Li, J., Zhang, J. X., Zhang, L., Yu, J., & Jiang, P. (2007). Psychological characteristics and marital quality of infertile women registered for in vitro fertilization-intracytoplasmic sperm injection in China. *Fertility and Sterility, 87*(4), 792–798.

Whitman-Elia, G. F., Plouffe, L., Craft, K., & Khan, I. (1997). Esophageal atresia in an in vitro fertilization pregnancy. *Southern Medical Journal, 90*(1), 86–88.

Widge, A. (2005). Seeking conception: Experiences of urban Indian women with in vitro fertilisation. *Patient Education and Counseling, 59*(3), 226–233.

Wischmann, T., Stammer, H., Scherg, H., Gerhard, I., & Verres, R. (2001). Psychosocial characteristics of infertile couples: A study by the "Heidelberg Fertility Consultation Service." *Human Reproduction, 16*(8), 1753–1761.

Zenke, U., & Chetkowski, R. J. (2002). Inclusion of heterozygotes for cystic fibrosis in the egg donor pool. *Fertility and Sterility, 78*(3), 557–561.

# CHAPTER 5

## *Exemplar:* USING AN EGG DONOR: INSIGHTS INTO AN INFERTILE WOMAN'S EXPERIENCE

*Patricia E. Hershberger*

In 1984, the first successful treatment of an infertile woman with ovarian failure by using a donated egg from another woman was reported by scientists in Australia (Lutjen et al., 1984). Since then, women from around the world have used donor eggs to achieve pregnancy and establish or complete their families. In fact, the use of donor eggs to establish pregnancy in infertile women has grown exponentially since 1984 and is now available in more than 40 countries, with recent data reporting 36,272 donor-egg procedures or transfers carried out in one calendar year alone (Mansour et al., 2014). In addition, novel applications for donor-egg use are on the horizon (e.g., donor eggs for mitochondrial gene replacement; Amato, Tachibana, Sparman, & Mitalipov, 2014; Bredenoord & Braude, 2010; Paull et al., 2013). Women who receive donor eggs do not typically share a genetic lineage with their donor-conceived children, although in some instances women have had their biological sisters or other close family members serve as egg donors.

Informing the donor-conceived children about the origins of conception has been debated (Pacey, 2010); however, there is steady support for disclosing the true nature of the conception to children (Ethics Committee of American Society for Reproductive Medicine, 2013; Pruett, 1992) including legislation to allow donor-conceived offspring access to donors' identities (Human Fertilisation and Embryology Authority, 2004). Yet, in some countries, such as the United States, where no governmental mandate exists and in countries where data were collected before current mandates, not all egg recipients opt to disclose (Hershberger, Klock, & Barnes, 2007; Murray & Golombok, 2003). Building on the content of the prior theoretical chapters, the following case study provides an exemplar of one hypothetical egg-donor-recipient woman and her dilemma with egg donation and disclosure.

## CASE STUDY

C.M. is a 38-year-old woman living just outside of Pittsburgh, Pennsylvania, who desperately wants to have a child. She is longing to become pregnant, experience everything about pregnancy and childbirth, and have a little baby to love, raise, and parent. Unfortunately, C.M. and her husband have been trying to have children since she was about 32 years old, at which time she stopped using her oral birth control pills. At the age of about 34 years, C.M. sought medical treatment as she was not yet pregnant. Soon after, C.M. was diagnosed with infertility as a result of polycystic ovary syndrome. Despite multiple infertility treatments over several years, including taking time off from treatment to rest and regain a sense of normalcy, and, according to C.M., doing "everything humanly possible" to achieve a biological pregnancy, C.M. has been unable to become pregnant. Then, several months ago when C.M. was celebrating her 38th birthday, her physician recommended that she consider using donor eggs to establish pregnancy. C.M.'s husband has been by his wife's side during the infertility treatments, although he has started to feel stressed and is having trouble sleeping at night.

Over the past 4 months as C.M. and her husband have considered using donor-egg treatment, C.M. finds that she has not mentioned her physician's recommendation about using an egg donor to anyone other than her husband—except her sister. C.M. recalls that many of her close friends and family members are aware of her strong and heartfelt desire to become a mother and experience pregnancy. Most of these individuals know that she is undergoing infertility treatment. C.M. herself was one of four children and grew up in a Roman Catholic family, attending catholic elementary and high schools. However, she decided to withhold information about using an egg donor to all but her sister whom she had always shared details of her life with and her sister in turn shares details of her life with C.M. In addition to her sister, C.M. simply feels that she does not want to provide any further details about her health history or her infertility treatment to her family and friends at this time.

Recently, while talking about her infertility treatment and the need to use an egg donor with her sister, C.M.'s sister offers to provide eggs to her via egg donation. At first, C.M. is shocked by this generous offer but grateful at the same time. She likes the idea of knowing the health history, personality traits, and just about everything regarding her sister, a potential would-be egg donor. Plus, she loves her sister very much and the thought of having children like her sister, a direct genetic link to her own biology, is also appealing. In the conversation C.M. and her sister have about her sister providing eggs to C.M., her sister states only one request: If she is to be the egg donor, she would not want any resulting children to know. C.M.'s sister states that "she would like to be the aunt and *only* the aunt" to any future children of C.M. even if she is the egg donor. At present, C.M. is in the midst of deciding whether to have her sister as an egg donor. Although there are aspects of having her sister as an egg donor that C.M. views as beneficial, she is worried and stressed about the thought of not telling any future children about the nature of the conception. C.M.'s husband is not sure what is best to do.

## Sample Discussion Questions

1. Can Fawcett's *Comprehensive Theory of Infertility* be applied to the aforementioned case study? If so, how?
2. Do the circumstances for C.M., her husband, and her sister fit within Wagner's shifting family structure? Why or why not?

3. How does the application of stress as described by Stevenson and Cobb play into the situation that C.M. and her husband are experiencing?

## REFERENCES

Amato, P., Tachibana, M., Sparman, M., & Mitalipov, S. (2014). Three-parent in vitro fertilization: Gene replacement for the prevention of inherited mitochondrial diseases. *Fertility and Sterility, 101*, 31–35. doi:10.1016/j.fertnstert.2013.11.030

Bredenoord, A. L., & Braude, P. (2010). Ethics of mitochondrial gene replacement: From bench to bedside. *BMJ, 341*, c6021. doi:10.1136/bmj.c6021

Ethics Committee of American Society for Reproductive Medicine. (2013). Informing offspring of their conception by gamete or embryo donation: A committee opinion. *Fertility and Sterility, 100*, 45–49. doi:10.1016/j.fertnstert.2013.02.028

Hershberger, P., Klock, S. C., & Barnes, R. B. (2007). Disclosure decisions among pregnant women who received donor oocytes: A phenomenological study. *Fertility and Sterility, 87*, 288–296. doi:10.1016/j.fertnstert.2006.06.036

Human Fertilisation and Embryology Authority (Disclosure of Donor Information) Regulations 2004. (2004). SI 2004/1511. Retrieved from http://www.legislation.gov.uk/uksi/2004/1511/contents/made

Lutjen, P., Trounson, A., Leeton, J., Findlay, J., Wood, C., & Renou, P. (1984). The establishment and maintenance of pregnancy using in vitro fertilization and embryo donation in a patient with primary ovarian failure. *Nature, 307*, 174–175. doi:10.1038/307174a0

Mansour, R., Ishihara, O., Adamson, G. D., Dyer, S., de Mouzon, J., Nygren, K. G., ... Zegers-Hochschild, F. (2014). International Committee for Monitoring Assisted Reproductive Technologies world report: Assisted reproductive technology 2006. *Human Reproduction, 29*, 1536–1551. doi:10.1093/humrep/deu084

Murray, C., & Golombok, S. (2003). To tell or not to tell: The decision-making process of egg-donation parents. *Human Fertility, 6*, 89–95. doi:10.1080/1464770312331369123

Pacey, A. (2010). Sperm donor recruitment in the UK. *The Obstetrician & Gynaecologist, 12*, 43–48. doi:10.1576/toag.12.1.043.27557

Paull, D., Emmanuele, V., Weiss, K. A., Treff, N., Stewart, L., Hua, H., ... Egli, D. (2013). Nuclear genome transfer in human oocytes eliminates mitochondrial DNA variants. *Nature, 493*, 632–637. doi:10.1038/nature11800

Pruett, K. D. (1992). Strange bedfellows? Reproductive technology and child development. *Infant Mental Health Journal, 13*, 312–318. doi:10.1002/1097–0355(199224)13:4<312::AID-IMHJ2280130406>3.0.CO;2-Q

# PART II

# RESEARCH AND REVIEWS: DELINEATING THE STATE OF THE SCIENCE IN ART

Carper (1978) developed the fundamental ways of knowing, which is a framework containing different sources from which knowledge and beliefs in professional practice can be derived. She stated, "It is the general conception of any field of inquiry that ultimately determines the kind of knowledge that field aims to develop as well as the manner in which that knowledge is to be organized, tested and applied" (p. 13). One of the essential components of this framework is empirical knowledge, essential in any clinical science in order to provide evidence-based care. In this part, thought leaders have provided an opportunity to explore some of the many important areas of the science that supports care for individuals and couples with fertility challenges.

These authors present current information about how individuals and couples experience the role of a patient: Lawson provides a comprehensive review of the literature, including more than 100 references, about stress that is experienced during the process of infertility, and Indekeu and Daniels present data from research examining pregnancy, birth, and breastfeeding following oocyte donation. As the age of those having their first pregnancies continues to rise, we are in need of understanding the parenthood phenomena for those seeking fertility treatment who ultimately become parents. There is an opportunity to critically consider this experience: Woodward and MacDuffie provide an overview of what is known about the parenting experience for those older than 40 years, and Romain and Nachtigall delve a little deeper by reporting their findings about how older parenthood can impact certain aspects of life such as work and play. As with all clinical areas, patient populations are unique and diverse, and therefore they have specific care needs. Hershberger considers the needs of special populations in the fertility setting and presents a review of the reasons young women with cancer choose whether or not to undergo fertility preservation treatment. Ivry presents fertility care considerations for Jewish populations adhering to rabbinic law. Finally, Cooper, Flynn, and Duthie present data about the divergent goals of multifetal pregnancies between patient and provider.

## REFERENCE

Carper, B. A. (1978). Fundamental patterns of knowing in nursing. *Advances in Nursing Science, 1,* 13–24. doi:10.1097/00012272–197810000-00004

# CHAPTER 6

# PSYCHOLOGICAL STRESS AND FERTILITY

## Angela K. Lawson

*"Just relax. It will happen."* It is a phrase commonly heard by women struggling to get pregnant. Although the statement is likely intended to let women know that others are optimistic about their chances of having a baby, at its core it blames women for being too stressed to conceive. For generations, many women and men have believed that the experience of psychological stress caused by physiological changes interfered with a woman's chances of conceiving. Although anecdotal stories of women relaxing and getting pregnant have been widely shared, research examining the role of stress in the etiology of infertility is limited. This chapter includes a discussion of the role of stress as a cause and/or as a consequence of infertility and infertility treatment.

## OVERVIEW OF THE PHYSIOLOGY OF STRESS

Stress can be defined as an internal state, which differs from one's normal state of rest, caused by an external or internal stressor (Selye, 1955). The human body reacts to such changes in state by engaging in automatic physiological responses intended to aid the individual in adequately responding to the noxious stimuli (Cannon, 1994; Galatzer-Levy et al., 2014; Selye, 1955). Responses to stress can either be positive or negative; positive responses lead to eustress that can enhance performance; negative responses lead to distress or disease (Hargrove, Quick, Nelson, & Quick, 2011). The response to stress and the resulting experience of eustress or distress are influenced by biological factors such as genetic predisposition and sociobehavioral factors, such as social support (Hargrove et al., 2011).

Coined by Walter B. Cannon as "the fight or flight response," the physiological response to acute stress is thought to involve the activation of the sympathetic nervous system and the inhibition of the parasympathetic nervous system to defend against harm (Cannon, 1994). This physiological response begins when the hypothalamus, recognizing a state of stress, stimulates the secretion of the neurotransmitters epinephrine (i.e., adrenalin) and norephinephrine (i.e., noradrenalin) into the blood from the adrenal medulla of the autonomic nervous system (ANS), part of the sympathetic–adrenal–medullary (SAM) pathway (Figure 6.1; Lynch, Sundaram, Maisog, Sweeney, & Buck Louis, 2014; McCorry, 2007). These neurotransmitters

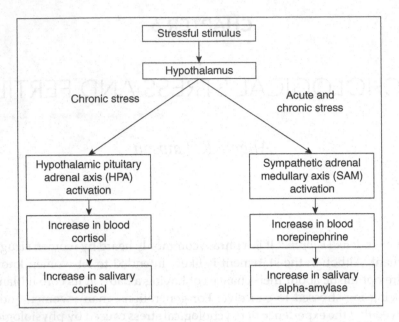

**FIGURE 6.1** Measuring the human stress response. Used with permission from Lynch et al. (2014).

stimulate the sympathetic nervous system to enhance or accelerate (a) blood pressure and heart rate, thereby pushing nutrient-rich blood to muscles; (b) the rate and depth of breathing (to increase oxygen and decrease carbon dioxide in the body); (c) muscle contraction; (d) sweating (for thermoregulation); (e) metabolism (to provide metabolic energy); and (f) sensory (e.g., hearing and vision) awareness. Additionally, vasoconstriction occurs and serves to move blood away from the body's extremities and digestive system and is diverted to large muscle groups in preparation for defense.

Increases in norepinephrine are also associated with increases in salivary alpha amylase (sAA; Lynch et al., 2014). Investigators have demonstrated that, as with norepinephrine, sAA levels increase in the context of psychological stressors (e.g., sAA was found to be higher in individuals preparing to skydive as compared with controls) and there is a moderate correlation between sAA and measures of state anxiety. Thus, sAA levels may be an indirect indicator of the stress response; as such, sAA has been frequently used as a biomarker of stress (Nater & Rohleder, 2009; Stegmann, 2011).

The secretion of epinephrine and norepinephrine also triggers the inhibition of the parasympathetic nervous system, sometimes referred to as the "rest and digest" or "breed and feed" system, which reduces activity in digestion, reproduction, growth, tissue repair, and the immune system (Cannon, 1994; Hargrove et al., 2011; McCorry, 2007). Although the autonomic system is activated and the parasympathetic system is reduced in times of stress, and the opposite is true at times of rest, neither system is ever completely shut down and both systems constantly provide input to the body (McCorry, 2007).

In situations of chronic stress, both the SAM and hypothalamic–pituitary–adrenal (HPA) axis pathways are activated. When the HPA is activated, the hypothalamus stimulates the pituitary gland to secrete multiple hormones including adrenocorticotropic hormone (ACTH). ACTH then stimulates the adrenal glands to produce cortisol (Greenberg, Carr, & Summers, 2002; Lynch et al., 2014; Selye, 1955). Cortisol is hypothesized to inhibit the sympathetic nervous system ("fight or flight") response once a threat is no longer imminent, thus aiding the return of homeostasis. Indeed, research on cortisol has found that higher levels of cortisol post-stressor are protective against emotional distress (Galatzer-Levy et al., 2014).

## BIOLOGICAL PLAUSIBILITY OF STRESS AND REDUCED FECUNDITY

It is hypothesized that fecundity will be impaired during times of stress due to inhibition of the parasympathetic nervous system. Stimulation of the HPA axis may in turn inhibit the hypothalamic–pituitary–gonadal (HPG) axis (Figure 6.2; Whirledge & Cidlowski, 2013; Young, Midgley, Carlson, & Brown, 2000). The hypothalamus is responsible for the production and release of gonadotropin-releasing hormone (GnRH) in women and men. GnRH, in turn, triggers the pituitary gland to release luteinizing hormone (LH) and follicle-stimulating hormone (FSH). LH and FSH play a vital role in the maturation of ovarian follicles, oocyte (egg) ovulation,

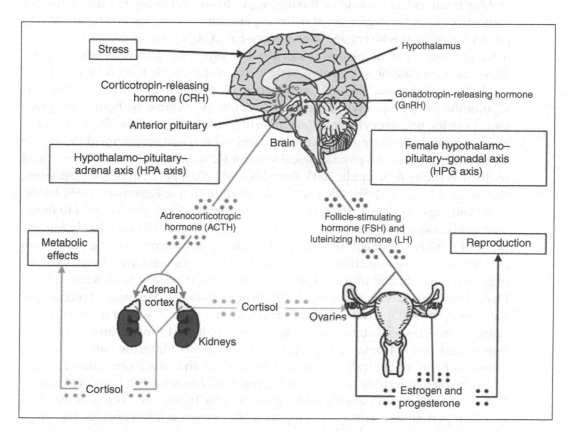

**FIGURE 6.2** The HPA axis and female HPG axis. © Pablo Nepomnaschy and Katrina Salvante (2012). Used with permission.

HPA, hypothalamic–pituitary–adrenal; HPG, hypothalamic–pituitary–gonadal.

and the production of sperm (i.e., spermatogenesis). Therefore, it is postulated that if the HPG axis is inhibited during times of stress, LH and FSH are also inhibited and fertility could be impaired (Maeda et al., 2010; Whirledge & Cidlowski, 2013). Overall, however, limited research has examined stress as a cause of infertility whereas a significant amount of literature supports infertility and infertility treatment as a cause of distress.

## REVIEW OF LITERATURE

### Distress as a Consequence of Infertility

Many studies on the development and consequences of fertility treatment–related psychological distress (Berghuis & Stanton, 2002; Hansell, Thorn, Prentice-Dunn, & Floyd, 1998; Jordan & Revenson, 1999; Lawson et al., 2014; Miles, Keitel, Jackson, Harris, & Licciardi, 2009; Peterson, Newton, Rosen, & Skaggs, 2006; Terry & Hynes, 1998) have framed their analyses within Lazarus and Folkman's (1984) landmark theory of the relationship between stress, appraisal, and coping. With this theoretical framework, infertility patients who negatively appraise their infertility diagnosis and/or treatment as harmful or threatening to them, and engage in inadequate or ineffective coping strategies, are at risk of experiencing depression and/or anxiety. In particular, patients who engage in avoidance-based coping strategies such as denial of the problem are at the greatest risk of negative psychological outcomes during fertility treatment (Berghuis & Stanton, 2002; Lawson et al., 2014; Terry & Hynes, 1998).

It is well known that the experience of primary infertility (defined as 12 months of appropriately timed unprotected intercourse without conception and no prior pregnancy); secondary infertility (defined as difficulty conceiving after previously becoming pregnant); and any subsequent engagement in infertility treatment serves as a psychological stressor for women and men that may lead to distress (Bitler & Schmidt, 2006; Brandes et al., 2009; Farr, Anderson, Jamieson, Warner, & Macaluso, 2009; Gleicher et al., 1996; Jordan & Revenson, 1999; Klock, 2006; Verberg et al., 2008). The term *distress* is often used as a generic term to represent mild-to-severe emotional reactions to stressors. Research finds that before the onset of fertility treatment, most infertile patients report experiencing some form of emotional distress, including increased feelings of sadness and decreased feelings of self-worth, and impaired sexual functioning (Downey & McKinney, 1992; Dyer, Lombard, & Van der Spuy, 2009; Dyer, Abrahams, Mokoena, Lombard, & van der Spuy, 2005). The inability to conceive may also result in divorce, ostracism, decreased social status, isolation, feelings of loss of control, and stigmatization (Cousineau & Domar, 2007; Dyer et al., 2005). Most infertile patients are not found to be more clinically depressed or anxious that their non-infertile peers before beginning fertility treatment (Downey & McKinney, 1992; Dyer et al., 2009). However, research on patients undergoing fertility treatment has found that 40% to 50% report mild to moderate symptoms of depression, 2% report severe symptoms of depression, and 15% to 56% experience significant anxiety symptoms; these symptoms worsen over time and particularly so after failed treatment cycles (Berghuis & Stanton, 2002; Cousineau & Domar, 2007; Demyttenaere et al., 1998;

Lawson et al., 2014; Pasch et al., 2012; Volgsten, Skoog Svanburg, Ekselius, Lundkvist, & Poromaa, 2010). Furthermore, patients undergoing even the earliest and least invasive forms of fertility treatment (e.g., intrauterine insemination [IUI]) have been found to be more emotionally distressed than patients attempting to conceive naturally (Vahratian, Smith, Dorman, & Flynn, 2011). This experience of emotional distress is the primary cause of many patients who prematurely terminate fertility treatment before achieving pregnancy (Brandes et al., 2009; Custers et al., 2013; Domar, 2004; Farr et al., 2009; Gameiro, Boivin, Peronace, & Verhaak, 2012; Gleicher et al., 1996; Olivius, Friden, Borg, & Bergh, 2004; Rajkhowa, McConnell, & Thomas, 2006; Smeenk, Verhaak, Stolwijk, Kremer, & Braat, 2004; Verberg et al., 2008). The experience of emotional distress among female infertility patients may be so severe that it has been found to be comparable to the emotional experiences of patients with other serious medical conditions such as cancer (Domar, Zuttermeister, & Friedman, 1993; Lawson et al., 2014). Furthermore, the lack of a birth following fertility treatment has been associated with a 17% increased risk of psychiatric hospitalization (Baldur-Felskov et al., 2013).

## Stress as a Cause of Infertility

Support for the relationship between stress and reproductive function is evident in research on the causes of delayed pubertal onset and functional hypothalamic amenorrhea. Although much of the research on stress and delayed pubertal onset has been conducted in animal models (Whirledge & Cidlowski, 2013), some literature supports the effect of potentially stressful environments (e.g., food insecurity, excessive exercise) and delayed puberty onset in girls (Belachew et al., 2011; Warren & Stiehl, 1999). However, research on humans is inconclusive as to any amount of unique variance explained in puberty delay as a result of psychological stress rather than by physiological stressors such as poor nutrition. Given that stressors such as food insecurity and excessive exercise can lead to both poor nutrition and psychological distress (Belachew et al., 2011), and the methodological design flaws such as the use of cross-sectional studies of stress and reproductive function (Bleil et al., 2012), it is difficult to determine the amount of variance in pubertal delay assigned to either physiological or psychological causes. It is similarly difficult to assess the primacy of physical or psychological causes of functional hypothalamic amenorrhea following engagement in excessive exercise and/or women with poor nutrition (e.g., among women with eating disorders; Gidwani, 1999; Warren & Stiehl, 1999).

Early studies on the relationship between psychological factors and fertility, rather than reproductive function, generally focused on female personality characteristics and ambivalence for motherhood as the cause of medically unexplained infertility (Greil, 1997). Referred to as "psychogenic infertility," these early studies on the psychological causes of unexplained infertility have since been largely rejected by researchers due to methodological and other study flaws (Greil, 1997; Wischmann, 2003). Furthermore, as the medical evaluation and diagnosis of infertility has advanced, an increasing number of patients have been found to have a medical cause for their infertility. However, a large number of patients currently are assigned an unidentified medical diagnosis for their infertility. Although some argue that a diagnosis of unexplained infertility is inappropriate as such a diagnosis is dependent on the limited quantity and quality of medical tests performed (Gleicher & Barad, 2006; Kamath & Bhattacharya, 2012), others argue that the physiological consequences of psychological stress or distress are the cause of unexplained infertility. Such research focuses on the assessment of perceived stress, biomarkers of stress, or on stress-reducing activities that are hypothesized to affect fertility (Wischmann, 2003).

## Survey-Based Assessment of Stress and Infertility

Many investigators examining the effect of stressors on fertility focus on research participants' survey responses regarding self-reported perceptions of stress and/or the number of stressful events an individual has experienced. Although some researchers have identified a relationship between psychological stress or negative life events and in vitro fertilization (IVF) and donor insemination outcomes (An, Sun, Li, Zhang, & Ji, 2013; Boivin & Schmidt, 2005; Demyttenaere et al., 1998; Ebbesen et al., 2009; Gourounti, Anagnostopoulos, & Vaslamatzis, 2011; Quant et al., 2013; Sejbaek, Hageman, Pinborg, Hougaard, & Schmidt, 2013; Smeenk et al., 2001, 2005; Turner et al., 2013; Williams, Marsh, & Rasgon, 2007), several recent meta-analyses of patients beginning IVF found no relationship between psychological stress and IVF outcomes (Boivin, Griffiths, & Venetis, 2011; Matthiesen, Frederiksen, Ingerslev, & Zachariae, 2011). Additionally, investigators in two recent prospective studies of IVF patients also found no relationship between symptoms of clinical depression and/or anxiety and IVF outcomes despite the majority of participants experiencing such symptomatology (Lawson et al., 2014; Pasch et al., 2012). It appears that investigators who found no relationship between psychological stress and fertility treatment outcomes utilized more rigorous study designs, which examined patients during their first IVF treatment cycle, included validated objective measures of psychological distress, had larger sample sizes, used appropriate statistics for data that are not normally distributed, and/or controlled for other variables likely to influence pregnancy rates (e.g., age; Anderheim, Holter, Bergh, & Möller, 2005; Boivin et al., 2011; Lawson et al., 2014; Lintsen, Verhaak, Eijkemans, Smeenk, & Braat, 2009; Matthiesen et al., 2011; Pasch et al., 2012). However, limited survey-based research has examined whether there is a relationship between self-reported stress and pregnancy outcomes by fertility diagnosis. Such research is warranted.

Much of the existing survey-based research on stress and infertility has focused on women's outcomes; however, research specifically with both fertile and infertile men has also identified inconsistent relationships between measures of psychological stress, coping, decreased testosterone levels, and semen parameters (Clarke, Klock, Geoghegan, & Travassos, 1999; Gollenberg et al., 2010; Hall & Burt, 2012; Hjollund et al., 1998, 2004; Janevic et al., 2014; Li, Lin, Li, & Cao, 2011; Pook, Tuschen-Caffier, Kubek, Schill, & Krause, 2005; Ragni & Caccamo, 1992; Sheiner, Sheiner, Carel, Potashnik, & Shoham-Vardi, 2002; Vellani et al., 2013; Zorn, Auger, Velikonja, Kolbezen, & Meden-Vrtovec, 2008). For example, some studies have identified a relationship between symptoms of depression, low testosterone, and semen parameters (Schweiger et al., 1999; Zorn et al., 2008). However, it remains unknown if depression is the cause or effect of low testosterone and there are limited data regarding the relationship between psychological distress, decreased semen parameters (i.e., concentration, morphology, and motility), and pregnancy rates. The inconsistencies in the research on semen parameters and psychological stress are limited by cross-sectional study design, with small samples, that fail to control for relevant variables (e.g., lifestyle, occupation, toxic exposure, age, etc.) and other methodological flaws. Furthermore, limited studies have examined the relationship, if any, between changes in semen parameters with differences in pregnancy rates. Two such studies, however, did not find a relationship between male psychological stress and pregnancy (Hjollund et al., 1998; Zorn et al., 2008). Finally, an alternative and plausible hypothesis as to one of the primary causes of male factor infertility, exposure to toxins and other sources of excessive oxidative stress, has been shown to be associated with male-factor infertility (Agarwal, Durairajanayagam, Halabi, Peng, & Vazquez-Levin, 2014; Ko, Sabanegh, & Agarwal, 2014). Furthermore, oxidative stress is hypothesized to cause some symptoms of anxiety and/or depression, which may at least partially explain such symptoms seen in infertile individuals (Bouayed, Rammal, & Soulimani, 2009; Grases, Colom, Fernandez, Costa-Bauzá, & Grases, 2014). It should be noted, however, that use of antioxidants has not been supported as an effective treatment for male or female factor infertility (Showell, Brown, Clarke, & Hart, 2013; Showell et al., 2014).

Overall, self-report studies are inherently problematic as they often rely on cross-sectional and correlational studies of subjective perceptions of stress, the number of negative life events, and IVF pregnancy chances. Although providing valuable insight into women's and men's emotional experiences during family building, such studies have limited ability to account for participants' bias in recalling historical events, widely varying subjective perceptions of stress, and the inability to generalize correlational results to causative factors. Although still unable to answer the question of causation, more objective examinations of the experience of stress/distress have used hormonal biomarkers of stress/distress as proxy indicators of stress.

## Hormonal Biomarkers of Stress and Infertility

Alpha amylase and cortisol are two of the most commonly studied hormones found to increase in concentration when individuals are exposed to stressful stimuli. Although both can be measured via blood draw, salivary assessment of these hormones is often easier for participants and salivary stress hormone levels have been found to correlate highly with concentrations of other stress hormones measured via blood assay (Nater & Rohleder, 2009). Studies of sAA and cortisol have been conducted primarily on female study participants with and without a diagnosis of infertility.

### Alpha Amylase
The first documented study of sAA and psychological distress found a positive relationship between increased level of sAA and psychological distress in subjects

who had been exposed to hyperbaric pressure (Nater & Rohleder, 2009). More recent research has explored the relationship between sAA concentrations and fecundity. One such study of women who denied having a history of infertility and had been trying to get pregnant for less than 3 months completed one morning assay of sAA and cortisol on day 6 of each menstrual cycle for six cycles. After controlling for multiple variables including but not limited to age, intercourse frequency, and alcohol consumption, women who were found to have increased levels of sAA had lower daily conception chances in the first month but no effect was found for fecundability. Furthermore, no relationship between cortisol and fecundity was found and there was no relationship among fecundity, stress hormones, and any of the psychological measures included in the study (Louis et al., 2011; Lynch, Sundaram, Buck Louis, Lum, & Pyper, 2012). However, the findings of this study are limited as there was no formal assessment of the participant's fertility and no assessment of the cause of increased levels of sAA or cortisol. It is possible that the lack of a relationship among psychological measures, fecundity, and hormonal biomarkers may be attributable to the administration of measures that were not sensitive enough to assess psychological stress and/or the measures may have been administered at a wrong time of the month (Louis et al., 2011; Lynch et al., 2012). Similar methodological concerns are evident in another study of couples in the early stages of natural family building (less than or equal to 2 months) who denied a history of infertility and were followed for a maximum of 12 months or through pregnancy (Lynch et al., 2014). sAA was collected twice from study participants, once the morning after enrollment and once on the morning of the participant's first menstrual cycle. Additionally, a self-report assessment of stress was administered. Participants were asked to self-monitor ovulation and a longer time to pregnancy (TTP) was found among women with higher levels of sAA but not cortisol. These women also had a lower daily probability of conception in the first cycle; however, almost all women (87%) got pregnant during the study period. Furthermore, individuals in the highest tertile of sAA levels were found to have an increased risk of infertility (Lynch et al., 2014). The lack of medical evaluation of study participants, the self-report nature of measures of stress and ovulation, the inability to identify stress as the cause of increases in sAA and cortisol, and the inability to determine the ultimate cause of differences in TTP limit the study findings.

Additional studies of stress and sAA levels have found sAA levels to be influenced by sAA collection and storage techniques, certain medications, nature of the stressor, individual coping strategies, nicotine and caffeine intake, and food intake. Furthermore, because exercise can also stimulate the sympathetic nervous system, it is not surprising that sAA has been found to increase during exercise and may remain high for long after the exercise stops (Nater & Rohleder, 2009; Rohleder & Nater, 2009; Stegmann, 2011). A one-to-one relationship between stress and hormonal biomarkers has not been found; thus, there are likely additional unknown variables that can influence levels of sAA (Nater & Rohleder, 2009). Therefore, the inconsistent findings, methodological flaws, and limits of current studies of sAA and fertility make interpretation of study findings unclear.

*Cortisol*

Multiple studies of women without a diagnosis of infertility have found no relationship between cortisol and fecundity or psychological measures included in the studies (Louis et al., 2011; Lynch et al., 2012, 2014). Additional studies of cortisol and fecundity have found no relationship between cortisol and stress levels or TTP in non-infertile women trying to conceive (Tiplady, Jones, Campbell, Johnson, & Ledger, 2013). Furthermore, in a longitudinal prospective study of women undergoing their first cycle in IVF, no relationship was found between salivary cortisol (morning and evening samples) and treatment outcomes (e.g., number of oocytes retrieved, hormone levels, and live birth rate) nor between salivary cortisol concentrations and psychological distress as measured by the Fertility Problem Inventory ([FPI]; Nouri et al., 2011). In contrast, one prospective study of new IVF patients found a relationship between lower cortisol levels on the day of oocyte retrieval (but not before IVF treatment) and increased chance of pregnancy success (An et al., 2013). Although data on the role of cortisol in men and fertility are limited, one study of male psychiatric inpatients found a relationship among cortisol levels, depression, and decreased testosterone in men (Schweiger et al., 1999).

As with sAA, factors other than stress may influence cortisol levels. For example, food intake and exercise have been found to correlate with increased levels of cortisol (Garde et al., 2009). Furthermore, hormones important to female and male fertility (e.g., estradiol and testosterone) are decreased in times of depression, and thus, it may be that clinical depression (not measured in any identified studies of stress, cortisol, and fecundity) increases levels of cortisol. However, data on the relationship between depression and cortisol are inconsistent (Vammen et al., 2014) and more research on the relationship of cortisol, sAA, and fertility are needed to provide a clearer understanding of any association.

## Relaxing Conditions/Activities and Fertility

If, as hypothesized, psychological stress or distress can interfere with fertility, then it could be argued that activities that produce a relaxation response could improve pregnancy chances. Indeed, multiple studies have examined the positive effects of relaxation or relaxing activities and the cessation of stress-inducing activities (e.g., fertility treatment) on both fertility and the reduction of emotional distress.

## Acupuncture and Other Nontraditional Medicines

Acupuncture is the most commonly studied form of complementary and alternative medicine (CAM) among infertile patient populations. Traditional Chinese acupuncture treatment focuses in part on 14 main meridians, which are networked channels that allow the circulation of energy throughout the human body. These channels are marked by 400 acupuncture points (acupoints) where "vital energy (Qi and blood) of the viscera infuses" (Zheng, Huang, Zhang, & Wang, 2012, p. 600). Imbalances in Qi are believed to result in disease that can be alleviated via the stimulation of acupoints (Moy et al., 2011). Acupuncture is believed to treat the disease of infertility by "improving blood circulation to the ovaries and uterus; neurohormonal modulation; cytokine modulation and improving implantation; and reducing stress, anxiety, and depression" (Anderson & Rosenthal, 2013, p. 3). It has also been proposed that acupuncture can lessen the physical side effects (e.g., bloating and fluid retention) of exogenous hormones administered during fertility treatment (Anderson & Rosenthal, 2013). During acupuncture, disposable needles are inserted into the desired acupoints and stimulated for 15 to 30 minutes by hand or electrical current (Zheng et al., 2012). One of the common acupuncture protocols for infertility is the Paulus protocol, which includes an acupuncture session 25 minutes before and after embryo transfer (Anderson & Rosenthal, 2013).

Multiple individual trials and meta-analyses have been conducted over the years to better understand the relationship between acupuncture and fertility (see, e.g., Meldrum, Fisher, Butts, Su, & Sammel, 2013 for a review; Zheng et al., 2012). The findings from both meta-analyses and individual trials are inconsistent in nature, with one study finding that acupuncture led to elevated levels of cortisol and prolactin, which was associated with increased pregnancy rates (Magarelli, Cridennda, & Cohen, 2009), a finding that contradicts the theory that increased cortisol limits pregnancy chances. Overall, some studies suggest that acupuncture could increase pregnancy rates, could have no effect on pregnancy rates, or could reduce pregnancy rates.

A recent meta-analysis (Zheng et al., 2012) of acupuncture and pregnancy found a pregnancy benefit for acupuncture. However, the study data were reanalyzed in an effort to address multiple criticisms of the previous work by limiting studies with heterogeneity and by separately comparing studies with and without control groups. This secondary analysis of the data revealed no relationship between acupuncture and pregnancy rates with some concern for a negative relationship between acupuncture and pregnancy when the acupuncture is perceived by patients as aggressive and/or stressful (Meldrum et al., 2013).

Unfortunately, rigorous research with limited design flaws on the effects of acupuncture and fertility appears to be limited. Regardless of the rigor of study trials on the relationship between acupuncture and pregnancy, concern remains about the failure of such protocols to individualize treatment as it is typical in the practice of Chinese medicine but not in research protocols, problems with low dosage (e.g., too few treatment sessions and number of acupoints needled), differences in patient populations, and heterogeneity in study designs (Anderson & Rosenthal, 2013). More research on acupuncture and fertility is warranted. However, given that acupuncture, which is not perceived as stressful by the patient, could improve emotional well-being during fertility treatment and may have a small placebo effect on pregnancy, it has been recommended that physicians appropriately counsel patients regarding the limited support for acupuncture and pregnancy but allow patients to obtain such treatment if so desired (Meldrum et al., 2013).

In addition to acupuncture, mindfulness meditation and other mind–body interventions have been studied as a means to reduce emotional distress during fertility treatment. Mind–body interventions often focus on acceptance without judgment and conscious awareness of internal and external experiences. These interventions also may include a focus on improvement of lifestyle behaviors (e.g., diet). Research on mind–body interventions have generally found an improvement in emotional and spiritual well-being among women who participate in such programs (Galhardo, Cunha, & Pinto-Gouveia, 2013). In addition, some studies have found an increased chance of pregnancy associated with participation in mind–body treatment. Although studies also show that pregnancy rates are similar between mind–body intervention and other support groups, mind–body interventions have been found to result in greater improvement in emotional well-being (Domar et al., 2011). However, given the limited research on mind–body interventions and pregnancy, the inclusion of lifestyle habit intervention in mind–body studies, and the known relationship between lifestyle factors and fertility (Rooney & Domar, 2014), more research on the possible effect of mind–body intervention and pregnancy is needed. Overall, current research provides support for mind–body intervention as a means for improving emotional well-being during fertility treatment. It is unclear if such interventions have any effect on pregnancy.

Another CAM employed during fertility treatment is yoga. Yoga is based on a spiritual philosophy and involves the practice of physical poses and breathing techniques intended to liberate its practitioners from the limits of the physical world and connect them with the "Supreme Being" (Valoriani et al., 2014). Yoga has been hypothesized to improve individual resilience to stress, muscle strength, and flexibility, as well as "stabilize the autonomic nervous system with a tendency toward parasympathetic dominance" (Valoriani et al., 2014, p. 159). Limited research has explored the relationship between yoga practice and fertility. Only one study was identified in which the investigators examined the effect of yoga on women pursuing fertility treatment. The study included women who were waiting to start their first cycle of IVF and who were offered a free 3-month course of yoga classes. Results of the study indicate that women who were more distressed were more likely to participate in yoga and that participation in yoga was associated with a reduction in symptoms of anxiety. The study did not examine any relationship between yoga and pregnancy rates (Valoriani et al., 2014).

## Psychotherapy and Psychological Intervention

Psychological counseling is often recommended to patients pursuing fertility treatment. Multiple studies have examined the relationship between counseling and emotional well-being as well as counseling and pregnancy rates. The quality of such studies as well as therapeutic approaches employed varies and most studies, with the noticeable exception of one meta-analysis (Hämmerli, Znoj, & Barth, 2009), have generally found that counseling was associated with decreased emotional distress, although more improvement was seen in anxious versus depressive symptomatology. Furthermore, greater improvement was seen for interventions that focused on education and skill building rather than expression of emotions (Boivin, 2003; de Liz & Strauss, 2005; Wischmann, 2008). Recent studies suggest that carefully designed online psychoeducational programs may also reduce emotional distress in infertile patients (Cousineau et al., 2008; Haemmerli, Znoj, & Berger, 2010). Both individual trials and meta-analyses would benefit from the exploration of the relationship between psychological intervention and distress reduction, which includes the use of control groups and high-quality therapeutic applications such as cognitive behavioral therapy; separates individual, group, and face-to-face service provision as compared with technology-driven therapeutic approaches; and includes validated measures of distress.

Research on the effects of psychological intervention on pregnancy rates has found an inconsistent relationship between pregnancy and counseling that is confounded by the fact that the studied patient populations were often undergoing fertility treatment that could reasonably account for pregnancy rates and/or included data from nonrandomized controlled trials (Boivin, 2003; Cousineau & Domar, 2007; Domar et al., 2000; Frederiksen, Farver-Vestergaard, Skovgard, Ingerslev, & Zachariae, 2015; Hämmerli et al., 2009). Pre-fertility treatment psychological counseling has been found to be acceptable to most patients; patients often reported gaining greater benefit from counseling than they had expected (Hakim, Newton, MacLean-Brine, & Feyles, 2012). Thus, although results from individual trials and meta-analyses are conflicting, continued recommendation of psychological support appears to be warranted because (a) many infertile patients report experiencing psychological distress that should not go untreated, (b) there does not appear to be a negative effect of psychological intervention in infertile patient populations, and (c) patients are receptive to and generally report benefit from such interventions; whether or not such benefit rises to clinical significant levels remains to be determined.

## Adoption as a Cause of Relaxation

Anecdotal data regarding spontaneous conception following adoption have been documented for decades (Mai, 1971; Sandler, 1965). The presumed belief is that stopping the effort to achieve pregnancy and engaging in adoption eliminates the stress associated with attempts to conceive and therefore increases one's chances of conception. However, parenthood is also anecdotally described as a chronic life stressor (see, e.g., Senior, 2015), and thus, adoption could hypothetically have a bidirectional effect on the experience of stress. Furthermore, it appears that there is a bias toward sharing stories of successful versus unsuccessful conception following adoption.

Early research conducted before the advent of modern fertility treatment, although methodologically flawed, found wildly varying rates of spontaneous conception after adoption ranging from 4% to 65% (Mai, 1971; Sandler, 1965). More recent and rigorous research has found no relationship between adoption and spontaneous conception (Wischmann, 2003). For example, in a 5-year longitudinal study of 817 Danish women referred for fertility treatment between 2000 and 2001, less than 1% of the 48 women who adopted had a spontaneous conception after adoption (Pinborg, Hougaard, Nyboe Andersen, Molbo, & Schmidt, 2009). In another study of 123 French women who discontinued IVF treatment in 1998 without a live birth, only one out of 56 women who adopted achieved spontaneous conception after adoption by 2006 (de La Rochebrochard, Quelen, Peikrishvili, Guibert, & Bouyer, 2009). In another study of 226 German couples who had engaged in fertility treatment between 1987 and 1997, only five out of 22 (23%) couples who applied for adoption after fertility treatment reported a spontaneous conception (Kupka et al., 2003). Thus, research does not support a relationship between adoption and increased pregnancy rates. Clearly, not all couples referred for adoption have a 0% chance of pregnancy. It is likely, however, that a minority of couples who are given low probably of reproductive success and who continue to have unprotected appropriately timed intercourse will be able to get pregnant.

## Stopping or Starting Fertility Treatment as a Cause of Relaxation

Hypothesized to be the result of relief from the stress of fertility treatment (Hennelly, Harrison, Kelly, Jacob, & Barrett, 2000), spontaneous conception after the cessation of fertility treatment has been documented among patients with mild to severe infertility diagnoses (Kupka et al., 2003). Anecdotal stories of spontaneous conception following the cessation of unsuccessful fertility treatment offer patients hope that unsuccessful treatment is not the end to their family-building dream. However, research on spontaneous conception following cessation of fertility treatment does not appear to support the hypothesis that stopping treatment improves pregnancy chances.

For example, in a 5-year longitudinal study of Danish women referred for fertility treatment, less than 7% (54 of 817; 6.6%) of women had their first child after spontaneous conception. Overall, 18.2% (149 of 817) of the women had at least one birth after spontaneous conception, the majority of these women had their first child with the assistance of fertility treatment, and 11% of these women had changed partners at some time during the study period. Spontaneous conception was more common in women younger than 35 years with a diagnosis of male factor infertility, and a shorter duration of infertility (Pinborg et al., 2009). Multiple additional longitudinal studies of women who stopped IVF without achieving a live birth found an 11% to 24% rate of subsequent spontaneous conception and live birth. Again, younger age, shorter duration of infertility, and/ or less severe infertility diagnoses were generally associated with an increased chance of spontaneous conception (de La Rochebrochard et al., 2009; Kupka et al., 2003; Osmanagaoglu et al., 2002; Troude et al., 2012). Spontaneous conception has also been found after successful IVF, with 17% to 20.7% of women with spontaneous conception. Once again, younger age, shorter duration of infertility, and/or less severe fertility diagnoses were associated with increased chance of spontaneous conception (Hennelly et al., 2000; Shimizu et al., 1999; Troude et al., 2012). The large differences in rates of spontaneous conception have been attributed to studies with longer follow-up study periods and with younger patient populations, with most pregnancies occurring within 2 to 3 years after stopping fertility treatment (Osmanagaoglu et al., 2002).

Similar to the lack of support between stopping treatment and pregnancy, other studies have reported higher rates (e.g., 27% vs. 23%) of spontaneous conception in women who were randomly assigned to wait 6 months to begin fertility treatment as compared with women assigned to undergo IUI. The difference was small, however, and similar to other studies, there were no differences in overall rates of pregnancy found after 6 months of study (Snick, Collins, & Evers, 2008; Steures et al., 2006). These rates are higher than the 11% rate of spontaneous conception found among patients with a male factor infertility diagnosis who did not undergo fertility treatment (Osmanagaoglu et al., 2002). Furthermore, a recent meta-analysis of IUI as compared with timed intercourse or other control group found higher pregnancy rates in the IUI treatment group (Snick et al., 2008). Finally, another study of patients placed on a waiting list for IVF found higher rates of conception among patients who received treatment during the waiting period but also a spontaneous conception rate of 9% over a 12-month period for patients on the wait list; chance of spontaneous conception was associated with younger age, shorter duration of infertility, and having previously had a child (Eijkemans et al., 2008).

Overall, it appears that although some patients can conceive naturally while waiting for treatment and/or following the cessation of successful or unsuccessful treatment, more patients benefit from treatment than from waiting. Rates of spontaneous conception while not undergoing fertility treatment vary based on the patient population and duration of the study follow-up. It is not surprising that younger patients with less severe infertility diagnoses would get pregnant while waiting for or after stopping fertility treatment as patients undergoing fertility treatment are not given a 0% chance of pregnancy success (it would be unethical to provide fertility treatment to such a patient). It is unclear what role, if any, stress reduction plays in spontaneous pregnancy rates while either waiting for treatment or after cessation of treatment. It seems more likely that, given that these patients (particularly those who are younger with less severe diagnoses) continue to have appropriately timed unprotected intercourse over a number of months and ultimately have similar chances of pregnancy success as their non-infertile peers (though much lower monthly chance of conception if it is deemed that IVF is needed; less than 1% as compared with 25% in their fertile peers), it is the repeated appropriately timed intercourse that is the largest factor in achievement of spontaneous conception (Troude et al., 2012).

## SUMMARY

There does not appear to be solid evidence that supports the relationship between psychological stressors or psychological distress and reduced rates of pregnancy, other than perhaps in the context of functional hypothalamic amenorrhea or in couples wherein the frequency of appropriately timed sexual intercourse is limited due to emotional factors. At best, it appears that there may be a delay in the amount of time it takes for non-infertile couples to achieve pregnancy (TTP) but that if such a delay is attributable to stress, it is not clinically meaningful as it does not reduce overall chances of pregnancy. Furthermore, studies of pre-fertility treatment symptoms of anxiety and/or depression with nonsignificant differences in pregnancy rates suggest that if there is an effect of stress on infertility, it is likely overcome with medical intervention (Pasch et al., 2012; Zaig et al., 2012). Rates of spontaneous conception among couples either waiting for or following fertility treatment are likely indicative of the normal chances of pregnancy success based on infertility diagnosis and/or patients who were inappropriately referred for fertility treatment.

Inconsistent findings regarding the relationship among elevated stress hormones, subjective psychological survey measures, and psychological or CAM intervention on pregnancy rates do not provide a clear picture of the role of stress as a cause of infertility. Such a determination is likely not possible as this would require randomized controlled experiments that would unethically expose patients to stressful stimuli and then follow their rates of conception. Although correlational studies provide useful insight into stress during the course of family building, they cannot speak to any ultimate causative role of stress on reduced fertility. Anecdotally, many women and men report believing that stress is the cause of their infertility. It may be that patients and society at large, consciously or unconsciously, want stress to be a cause of infertility because we can theoretically control our stress levels to some degree; and perhaps our ability to control our stress levels will afford us greater (albeit illusory) control over our fertility.

## CONCLUSION

What is known is that patients often report experiencing a loss of control as well as symptoms of anxiety and depression as a result of an infertility diagnosis, infertility treatment, and treatment failure. Although the literature is inconsistent on the statistical significance of psychological intervention, including CAM, on the reduction of depressive and anxious symptomatology, patients view such treatment positively and often report a subjective improvement in well-being. Thus, the continued recommendation that patients receive emotional support during fertility treatment appears warranted. Finally, given the limited support for, at best, a small relationship between stress as a cause of infertility and the anecdotal data that many patients (particularly women) feel blamed for their infertility, it seems inappropriate to tell patients to "relax" in an effort to increase pregnancy chances and more appropriate to tell patients that "even miserable people get pregnant."

## REFERENCES

Agarwal, A., Durairajanayagam, D., Halabi, J., Peng, J., & Vazquez-Levin, M. (2014). Proteomics, oxidative stress and male infertility. *Reproductive Biomedicine Online, 29*(1), 32–58.

An, Y., Sun, Z., Li, L., Zhang, Y., & Ji, H. (2013). Relationship between psychological stress and reproductive outcome in women undergoing in vitro fertilization treatment: Psychological and neurohormonal assessment. *Journal of Assisted Reproduction and Genetics, 30*(1), 35–41.

Anderheim, L., Holter, H., Bergh, C., & Möller, A. (2005). Does psychological stress affect the outcome of in vitro fertilization? *Human Reproduction, 20*(10), 2969–2975.

Anderson, B., & Rosenthal, L. (2013). Acupuncture and in vitro fertilization: Critique of the evidence and application to clinical practice. *Complementary Therapies in Clinical Practice, 19*(1), 1–5.

Baldur-Felskov, B., Kjaer, S. K., Albieri, V., Steding-Jessen, M., Kjaer, T., Johansen, C., . . . Jensen, A. (2013). Psychiatric disorders in women with fertility problems: Results from a large Danish register-based cohort study. *Human Reproduction, 28*(3), 683–690.

Belachew, T., Hadley, C., Lindstrom, D., Getachew, Y., Duchateau, L., & Kolsteren, P. (2011). Food insecurity and age at menarche among adolescent girls in Jimma Zone Southwest Ethiopia: A longitudinal study. *Reproductive Biology and Endocrinology, 9*, 125.

Berghuis, J. P., & Stanton, A. L. (2002). Adjustment to a dyadic stressor: A longitudinal study of coping and depressive symptoms in infertile couples over an insemination attempt. *Journal of Consulting and Clinical Psychology, 70*(2), 433–438.

Bitler, M., & Schmidt, L. (2006). Health disparities and infertility: Impacts of state-level insurance mandates. *Fertility and Sterility, 85*(4), 858–865.

Bleil, M. E., Adler, N. E., Pasch, L. A., Sternfeld, B., Gregorich, S. E., Rosen, M. P., & Cedars, M. I. (2012). Psychological stress and reproductive aging among pre-menopausal women. *Human Reproduction, 27*(9), 2720–2728.

Boivin, J. (2003). A review of psychosocial interventions in infertility. *Social Science & Medicine (1982), 57*(12), 2325–2341.

Boivin, J., Griffiths, E., & Venetis, C. A. (2011). Emotional distress in infertile women and failure of assisted reproductive technologies: Meta-analysis of prospective psychosocial studies. *BMJ, 342*, d223.

Boivin, J., & Schmidt, L. (2005). Infertility-related stress in men and women predicts treatment outcome 1 year later. *Fertility and Sterility, 83*(6), 1745–1752.

Bouayed, J., Rammal, H., & Soulimani, R. (2009). Oxidative stress and anxiety: Relationship and cellular pathways. *Oxidative Medicine and Cellular Longevity, 2*(2), 63–67.

Brandes, M., van der Steen, J. O., Bokdam, S. B., Hamilton, C. J., de Bruin, J. P., Nelen, W. L., & Kremer, J. A. (2009). When and why do subfertile couples discontinue their fertility care? A longitudinal cohort study in a secondary care subfertility population. *Human Reproduction, 24*(12), 3127–3135.

Cannon, B. (1994). Walter Bradford Cannon: Reflections on the man and his contributions. *International Journal of Stress Management, 1*, 145–158. doi:10.1007/bf01857608

Clarke, R. N., Klock, S. C., Geoghegan, A., & Travassos, D. E. (1999). Relationship between psychological stress and semen quality among in-vitro fertilization patients. *Human Reproduction, 14*(3), 753–758.

Cousineau, T. M., & Domar, A. D. (2007). Psychological impact of infertility. *Best Practice & Research. Clinical Obstetrics & Gynaecology, 21*(2), 293–308.

Cousineau, T. M., Green, T. C., Corsini, E., Seibring, A., Showstack, M. T., Applegarth, L.,…Perloe, M. (2008). Online psychoeducational support for infertile women: A randomized controlled trial. *Human Reproduction, 23*(3), 554–566.

Custers, I. M., van Dessel, T. H., Flierman, P. A., Steures, P., van Wely, M., van der Veen, F., & Mol, B. W. (2013). Couples dropping out of a reimbursed intrauterine insemination program: What is their prognostic profile and why do they drop out? *Fertility and Sterility, 99*(5), 1294–1298.

de La Rochebrochard, E., Quelen, C., Peikrishvili, R., Guibert, J., & Bouyer, J. (2009). Long-term outcome of parenthood project during in vitro fertilization and after discontinuation of unsuccessful in vitro fertilization. *Fertility and Sterility, 92*(1), 149–156. doi:10.1016/j.fertnstert.2008.05.067

de Liz, T. M., & Strauss, B. (2005). Differential efficacy of group and individual/couple psychotherapy with infertile patients. *Human Reproduction, 20*(5), 1324–1332.

Demyttenaere, K., Bonte, L., Gheldof, M., Vervaeke, M., Meuleman, C., Vanderschuerem, D., & D'Hooghe, T. (1998). Coping style and depression level influence outcome in in vitro fertilization. *Fertility and Sterility, 69*(6), 1026–1033.

Domar, A. D. (2004). Impact of psychological factors on dropout rates in insured infertility patients. *Fertility and Sterility, 81*(2), 271–273.

Domar, A. D., Clapp, D., Slawsby, E. A., Dusek, J., Kessel, B., & Freizinger, M. (2000). Impact of group psychological interventions on pregnancy rates in infertile women. *Fertility and Sterility, 73*(4), 805–811.

Domar, A. D., Rooney, K. L., Wiegand, B., Orav, E. J., Alper, M. M., Berger, B. M., & Nikolovski, J. (2011). Impact of a group mind/body intervention on pregnancy rates in IVF patients. *Fertility and Sterility, 95*(7), 2269–2273.

Domar, A. D., Zuttermeister, P. C., & Friedman, R. (1993). The psychological impact of infertility: A comparison with patients with other medical conditions. *Journal of Psychosomatic Obstetrics and Gynaecology, 14*(Suppl), 45–52.

Downey, J., & McKinney, M. (1992). The psychiatric status of women presenting for infertility evaluation. *American Journal of Orthopsychiatry, 62*(2), 196–205.

Dyer, S., Lombard, C., & Van der Spuy, Z. (2009). Psychological distress among men suffering from couple infertility in South Africa: A quantitative assessment. *Human Reproduction, 24*(11), 2821–2826.

Dyer, S. J., Abrahams, N., Mokoena, N. E., Lombard, C. J., & van der Spuy, Z. M. (2005). Psychological distress among women suffering from couple infertility in South Africa: A quantitative assessment. *Human Reproduction, 20*(7), 1938–1943.

Ebbesen, S. M., Zachariae, R., Mehlsen, M. Y., Thomsen, D., Højgaard, A., Ottosen, L., ...Ingerslev, H. J. (2009). Stressful life events are associated with a poor in-vitro fertilization (IVF) outcome: A prospective study. *Human Reproduction, 24*(9), 2173–2182.

Eijkemans, M. J. C., Lintsen, A. M. E., Hunault, C. C., Bouwmans, C. A., Hakkaart, L., Braat, D. D. M., & Habbema, J. D. F. (2008). Pregnancy chances on an IVF/ICSI waiting list: A national prospective cohort study. *Human Reproduction, 23*, 1627–1632. doi:10.1093/humrep/den132

Farr, S. L., Anderson, J. E., Jamieson, D. J., Warner, L., & Macaluso, M. (2009). Predictors of pregnancy and discontinuation of infertility services among women who received medical help to become pregnant, National Survey of Family Growth, 2002. *Fertility and Sterility, 91*(4), 988–997.

Frederiksen, Y., Farver-Vestergaard, I., Skovgard, N. G., Ingerslev, H. J., & Zachariae, R. (2015). Efficacy of psychosocial interventions for psychological and pregnancy outcomes in infertile women and men: A systematic review and meta-analysis. *BMJ Open, 5*(1), e006592. doi:10.1136/bmjopen-2014-006592

Galatzer-Levy, I. R., Steenkamp, M. M., Brown, A. D., Qian, M., Inslicht, S., Henn-Haase, C., ...Marmar, C. R. (2014). Cortisol response to an experimental stress paradigm prospectively predicts long-term distress and resilience trajectories in response to active police service. *Journal of Psychiatric Research, 56*, 36–42.

Galhardo, A., Cunha, M., & Pinto-Gouveia, J. (2013). Mindfulness-Based Program for Infertility: Efficacy study. *Fertility and Sterility, 100*(4), 1059–1067.

Gameiro, S., Boivin, J., Peronace, L., & Verhaak, C. M. (2012). Why do patients discontinue fertility treatment? A systematic review of reasons and predictors of discontinuation in fertility treatment. *Human Reproduction Update, 18*(6), 652–669.

Garde, A. H., Persson, R., Hansen, A. M., Osterberg, K., Ørbaek, P., Eek, F., & Karlson, B. (2009). Effects of lifestyle factors on concentrations of salivary cortisol in healthy individuals. *Scandinavian Journal of Clinical and Laboratory Investigation, 69*(2), 242–250.

Gidwani, G. P. (1999). Amenorrhea in the athlete. *Adolescent Medicine, 10*(2), 275–290, vii.

Gleicher, N., & Barad, D. (2006). Unexplained infertility: Does it really exist? *Human Reproduction, 21*(8), 1951–1955.

Gleicher, N., Vanderlaan, B., Karande, V., Morris, R., Nadherney, K., & Pratt, D. (1996). Infertility treatment dropout and insurance coverage. *Obstetrics and Gynecology, 88*(2), 289–293.

Gollenberg, A. L., Liu, F., Brazil, C., Drobnis, E. Z., Guzick, D., Overstreet, J. W., ...Swan, S. H. (2010). Semen quality in fertile men in relation to psychosocial stress. *Fertility and Sterility, 93*(4), 1104–1111.

Gourounti, K., Anagnostopoulos, F., & Vaslamatzis, G. (2011). The relation of psychological stress to pregnancy outcome among women undergoing in-vitro fertilization and intracytoplasmic sperm injection. *Women & Health, 51*(4), 321–339.

Grases, G., Colom, M. A., Fernandez, R. A., Costa-Bauzá, A., & Grases, F. (2014). Evidence of higher oxidative status in depression and anxiety. *Oxidative Medicine and Cellular Longevity, 2014*, 1–5.

Greenberg, N., Carr, J. A., & Summers, C. H. (2002). Causes and consequences of stress. *Integrative and Comparative Biology, 42*(3), 508–516. doi: 10.1093/icb/42.3.508

Greil, A. L. (1997). Infertility and psychological distress: A critical review of the literature. *Social Science & Medicine (1982), 45*(11), 1679–1704.

Haemmerli, K., Znoj, H., & Berger, T. (2010). Internet-based support for infertile patients: A randomized controlled study. *Journal of Behavioral Medicine, 33*(2), 135–146.

Hakim, L. Z., Newton, C. R., MacLean-Brine, D., & Feyles, V. (2012). Evaluation of preparatory psychosocial counselling for medically assisted reproduction. *Human Reproduction, 27*(7), 2058–2066.

Hall, E., & Burt, V. K. (2012). Male fertility: Psychiatric considerations. *Fertility and Sterility, 97*(2), 434–439.

Hämmerli, K., Znoj, H., & Barth, J. (2009). The efficacy of psychological interventions for infertile patients: A meta-analysis examining mental health and pregnancy rate. *Human Reproduction Update, 15*(3), 279–295.

Hansell, P. L., Thorn, B. E., Prentice-Dunn, S., & Floyd, D. L. (1998). The relationships of primary appraisals of infertility and other gynecological stressors to coping. *Journal of Clinical Psychology in Medical Settings, 5*, 133–145.

Hargrove, M. B., Quick, J. C., Nelson, D. L., & Quick, J. D. (2011). The theory of preventative stress management: A 33-year review and evaluation. *Stress and Health, 27*, 182–193. doi:10.1002/smi.1417

Hennelly, B., Harrison, R. F., Kelly, J., Jacob, S., & Barrett, T. (2000). Spontaneous conception after a successful attempt at in vitro fertilization/intracytoplasmic sperm injection. *Fertility and Sterility, 73*(4), 774–778.

Hjollund, N. H., Bonde, J. P., Henriksen, T. B., Giwercman, A., & Olsen, J.; Danish First Pregnancy Planner Study Team. (2004). Reproductive effects of male psychologic stress. *Epidemiology, 15*(1), 21–27.

Hjollund, N. H., Kold Jensen, T., Bonde, J. P., Henriksen, T. B., Kolstad, H. A., Andersson, A. M., ... Olsen, J. (1998). Job strain and time to pregnancy. *Scandinavian Journal of Work, Environment & Health, 24*(5), 344–350.

Janevic, T., Kahn, L. G., Landsbergis, P., Cirillo, P. M., Cohn, B. A., Liu, X., & Factor-Litvak, P. (2014). Effects of work and life stress on semen quality. *Fertility and Sterility, 102*(2), 530–538.

Jordan, C., & Revenson, T. A. (1999). Gender differences in coping with infertility: A meta-analysis. *Journal of Behavioral Medicine, 22*(4), 341–358.

Kamath, M. S., & Bhattacharya, S. (2012). Demographics of infertility and management of unexplained infertility. *Best Practice & Research. Clinical Obstetrics & Gynaecology, 26*(6), 729–738.

Klock, S. C. (2006). Psychosocial evaluation of the infertile patient. In S. N. Covington & L. H. Burns (Eds.), *Infertility counseling. A comprehensive handbook for clinicians* (2nd ed., pp. 83–96). New York, NY: Cambridge University Press.

Ko, E. Y., Sabanegh, E. S., & Agarwal, A. (2014). Male infertility testing: Reactive oxygen species and antioxidant capacity. *Fertility and Sterility, 102*(6), 1518–1527.

Kupka, M. S., Dorn, C., Richter, O., Schmutzler, A., van der Ven, H., & Kulczycki, A. (2003). Stress relief after infertility treatment–spontaneous conception, adoption and psychological counselling. *European Journal of Obstetrics, Gynecology, and Reproductive Biology, 110*(2), 190–195.

Lawson, A. K., Klock, S. C., Pavone, M. E., Hirshfeld-Cytron, J., Smith, K. N., & Kazer, R. R. (2014). Prospective study of depression and anxiety in female fertility preservation and infertility patients. *Fertility and Sterility, 102*(5), 1377–1384.

Lazarus, R. S., & Folkman, S. (1984). *Stress, appraisal, and coping.* New York, NY: Springer.

Li, Y., Lin, H., Li, Y., & Cao, J. (2011). Association between socio-psycho-behavioral factors and male semen quality: Systematic review and meta-analyses. *Fertility and Sterility, 95*, 116–123. doi:10.1016/j.fertnstert.2010.06.031

Lintsen, A. M., Verhaak, C. M., Eijkemans, M. J., Smeenk, J. M., & Braat, D. D. (2009). Anxiety and depression have no influence on the cancellation and pregnancy rates of a first IVF or ICSI treatment. *Human Reproduction, 24*(5), 1092–1098.

ML

Louis, G. M., Lum, K. J., Sundaram, R., Chen, Z., Kim, S., Lynch, C. D.,…Pyper, C. (2011). Stress reduces conception probabilities across the fertile window: Evidence in support of relaxation. *Fertility and Sterility, 95*(7), 2184–2189.

Lynch, C. D., Sundaram, R., Buck Louis, G. M., Lum, K. J., & Pyper, C. (2012). Are increased levels of self-reported psychosocial stress, anxiety, and depression associated with fecundity? *Fertility and Sterility, 98*(2), 453–458.

Lynch, C. D., Sundaram, R., Maisog, J. M., Sweeney, A. M., & Buck Louis, G. M. (2014). Preconception stress increases the risk of infertility: Results from a couple-based prospective cohort study—the LIFE study. *Human Reproduction, 29*(5), 1067–1075.

Maeda, K., Ohkura, S., Uenoyama, Y., Wakabayashi, Y., Oka, Y., Tsukamura, H., & Okamura, H. (2010). Neurobiological mechanisms underlying GnRH pulse generation by the hypothalamus. *Brain Research, 1364*, 103–115.

Magarelli, P. C., Cridennda, D. K., & Cohen, M. (2009). Changes in serum cortisol and prolactin associated with acupuncture during controlled ovarian hyperstimulation in women undergoing in vitro fertilization-embryo transfer treatment. *Fertility and Sterility, 92*(6), 1870–1879.

Mai, F. M. (1971). Conception after adoption: An open question. *Psychosomatic Medicine, 33*(6), 509–514.

Matthiesen, S. M., Frederiksen, Y., Ingerslev, H. J., & Zachariae, R. (2011). Stress, distress and outcome of assisted reproductive technology (ART): A meta-analysis. *Human Reproduction, 26*(10), 2763–2776.

McCorry, L. K. (2007). Physiology of the autonomic nervous system. *American Journal of Pharmaceutical Education, 71*(4), 78.

Meldrum, D. R., Fisher, A. R., Butts, S. F., Su, H. I., & Sammel, M. D. (2013). Acupuncture—help, harm, or placebo? *Fertility and Sterility, 99*(7), 1821–1824.

Miles, L. M., Keitel, M., Jackson, M., Harris, A., & Licciardi, F. (2009). Predictors of distress in women being treated for infertility. *Journal of Reproductive and Infant Psychology, 27*, 238–257. doi:10.1080/02646830802350880

Moy, I., Milad, M. P., Barnes, R., Confino, E., Kazer, R. R., & Zhang, X. (2011). Randomized controlled trial: Effects of acupuncture on pregnancy rates in women undergoing in vitro fertilization. *Fertility and Sterility, 95*(2), 583–587.

Nater, U. M., & Rohleder, N. (2009). Salivary alpha-amylase as a non-invasive biomarker for the sympathetic nervous system: Current state of research. *Psychoneuroendocrinology, 34*(4), 486–496.

Nepomnaschy, P., & Salvante, K. (2012). The hypothalamo-pituitary-adrenal axis (HPAA) and the female hypothalamo-pituitary-gonadal axis (HPGA). Retrieved from www.sfu.ca/~pan2/current-research_PA-ROC.html

Nouri, K., Litschauer, B., Huber, J. C., Buerkle, B., Tiringer, D., & Tempfer, C. B. (2011). Saliva cortisol levels and subjective stress are not associated with number of oocytes after controlled ovarian hyperstimulation in patients undergoing in vitro fertilization. *Fertility and Sterility, 96*(1), 69–72.

Olivius, C., Friden, B., Borg, G., & Bergh, C. (2004). Why do couples discontinue in vitro fertilization treatment? A cohort study. *Fertility and Sterility, 81*, 258–261. doi:10.1016/j.fertnstert.2003.06.029

Osmanagaoglu, K., Collins, J., Kolibianakis, E., Tournaye, H., Camus, M., Van Steirteghem, A., & Devroey, P. (2002). Spontaneous pregnancies in couples who discontinued intracytoplasmic sperm injection treatment: A 5-year follow-up study. *Fertility and Sterility, 78*(3), 550–556.

Pasch, L. A., Gregorich, S. E., Katz, P. K., Millstein, S. G., Nachtigall, R. D., Bleil, M. E., & Adler, N. E. (2012). Psychological distress and in vitro fertilization outcome. *Fertility and Sterility, 98*(2), 459–464.

Peterson, B. D., Newton, C. R., Rosen, K. H., & Skaggs, G. E. (2006). Gender differences in how men and women who are referred for IVF cope with infertility stress. *Human Reproduction, 21*(9), 2443–2449.

Pinborg, A., Hougaard, C. O., Nyboe Andersen, A., Molbo, D., & Schmidt, L. (2009). Prospective longitudinal cohort study on cumulative 5-year delivery and adoption rates among 1338 couples initiating infertility treatment. *Human Reproduction, 24*(4), 991–999.

Pook, M., Tuschen-Caffier, B., Kubek, J., Schill, W. B., & Krause, W. (2005). Personality, coping and sperm count. *Andrologia, 37*(1), 29–35.

Quant, H. S., Zapantis, A., Nihsen, M., Bevilacqua, K., Jindal, S., & Pal, L. (2013). Reproductive implications of psychological distress for couples undergoing IVF. *Journal of Assisted Reproduction and Genetics, 30*(11), 1451–1458.

Ragni, G., & Caccamo, A. (1992). Negative effect of stress of in vitro fertilization program on quality of semen. *Acta Europaea Fertilitatis, 23*(1), 21–23.

Rajkhowa, M., McConnell, A., & Thomas, G. E. (2006). Reasons for discontinuation of IVF treatment: A questionnaire study. *Human Reproduction, 21*(2), 358–363.

Rohleder, N., & Nater, U. M. (2009). Determinants of salivary alpha-amylase in humans and methodological considerations. *Psychoneuroendocrinology, 34*(4), 469–485.

Rooney, K. L., & Domar, A. D. (2014). The impact of lifestyle behaviors on infertility treatment outcome. *Current Opinion in Obstetrics & Gynecology, 26*(3), 181–185.

Sandler, B. (1965). Conception after adoption: A comparison of conception rates. *Fertility and Sterility, 16*, 313–333.

Schweiger, U., Deuschle, M., Weber, B., Körner, A., Lammers, C. H., Schmider, J., ... Heuser, I. (1999). Testosterone, gonadotropin, and cortisol secretion in male patients with major depression. *Psychosomatic Medicine, 61*(3), 292–296.

Sejbaek, C. S., Hageman, I., Pinborg, A., Hougaard, C. O., & Schmidt, L. (2013). Incidence of depression and influence of depression on the number of treatment cycles and births in a national cohort of 42,880 women treated with ART. *Human Reproduction, 28*(4), 1100–1109.

Selye, H. (1955). Stress and disease. *Science, 122*(3171), 625–631.

Senior, J. (2015). *All joy and no fun: The paradox of modern parenthood.* New York, NY: Harper Collins Publishers.

Sheiner, E. K., Sheiner, E., Carel, R., Potashnik, G., & Shoham-Vardi, I. (2002). Potential association between male infertility and occupational psychological stress. *Journal of Occupational and Environmental Medicine, 44*, 1093–1099. doi:10.1097/00043764-200212000-00001

Shimizu, Y., Kodama, H., Fukuda, J., Murata, M., Kumagai, J., & Tanaka, T. (1999). Spontaneous conception after the birth of infants conceived through in vitro fertilization treatment. *Fertility and Sterility, 71*, 35–39. doi:10.1016/s0015-0282(98)00417-8

Showell, M. G., Brown, J., Clarke, J., & Hart, R. J. (2013). Antioxidants for female subfertility. *Cochrane Database Systematic Reviews, 8*, CD007807. doi:10.1002/14651858.CD007807.pub2

Showell, M. G., Mackenzie-Proctor, R., Brown, J., Yazdani, A., Stankiewicz, M. T., & Hart, R. J. (2014). Antioxidants for male subfertility. *Cochrane Database Systematic Reviews, 12*, CD007411. doi:10.1002/14651858.CD007411.pub3

Smeenk, J. M., Verhaak, C. M., Eugster, A., van Minnen, A., Zielhuis, G. A., & Braat, D. D. (2001). The effect of anxiety and depression on the outcome of in-vitro fertilization. *Human Reproduction, 16*, 1420–1423. doi:10.1093/humrep/16.7.1420

Smeenk, J. M., Verhaak, C. M., Vingerhoets, A. J., Sweep, C. G., Merkus, J. M. W. M., Willemsen, S. J., ... Braat, D. D. M. (2005). Stress and outcome success in IVF: The role of self-reports and endocrine variables. *Human Reproduction, 20*, 991–996. doi:10.1093/humrep/deh739

Smeenk, J. M. J., Verhaak, C. M., Stolwijk, A. M., Kremer, J. A. M., & Braat, D. D. (2004). Reasons for dropout in an in vitro fertilization/intracytoplasmic sperm injection program. *Fertility and Sterility, 81*, 262–268. doi:10.1016/j.fertnstert.2003.09.027

Snick, H. K., Collins, J. A., & Evers, J. L. H. (2008). What is the most valid comparison treatment in trials of intrauterine insemination, timed or uninfluenced intercourse? A systematic review and meta-analysis of indirect evidence. *Human Reproduction, 23*, 2239–2245. doi:10.1093/humrep/den214

Stegmann, B. J. (2011). Other nonstress influences can alter salivary alpha-amylase activity. *Fertility and Sterility, 95*, 2190–2191. doi:10.1016/j.fertnstert.2011.04.001

Steures, P., van der Steeg, J. W., Hompes, P. G., Habbema, J. D., Eijkemans, M. J., Broekmans, F. J.,...Collaborative Effort on the Clinical Evaluation in Reproductive, M. (2006). Intrauterine insemination with controlled ovarian hyperstimulation versus expectant management for couples with unexplained subfertility and an intermediate prognosis: A randomised clinical trial. *Lancet, 368*(9531), 216–221. doi:10.1016/S0140-6736(06)69042-9

Terry, D. J., & Hynes, G. J. (1998). Adjustment to a low-control situation: Reexamining the role of coping resources. *Journal of Personality and Social Psychology, 74*, 1078–1092. doi:10.1037/0022-3514.74.4.1078

Tiplady, S., Jones, G., Campbell, M., Johnson, S., & Ledger, W. (2013). Home ovulation tests and stress in women trying to conceive: A randomized controlled trial. *Human Reproduction, 28*, 138–151. doi:10.1093/humrep/des372

Troude, P., Bailly, E., Guibert, J., Bouyer, J., de la Rochebrochard, E., & Group, D. (2012). Spontaneous pregnancies among couples previously treated by in vitro fertilization. *Fertility and Sterility, 98*, 63–68. doi:10.1016/j.fertnstert.2012.03.058

Turner, K., Reynolds-May, M. F., Zitek, E. M., Tisdale, R. L., Carlisle, A. B., & Westphal, L. M. (2013). Stress and anxiety scores in first and repeat IVF cycles: A pilot study. *PloS One, 8*(5), e63743. doi:10.1371/journal.pone.0063743

Vahratian, A., Smith, Y. R., Dorman, M., & Flynn, H. A. (2011). Longitudinal depressive symptoms and state anxiety among women using assisted reproductive technology. *Fertility and Sterility, 95*, 1192–1194. doi:10.1016/j.fertnstert.2010.09.063

Valoriani, V., Lotti, F., Vanni, C., Noci, M. C., Fontanarosa, N., Ferrari, G.,...Noci, I. (2014). Hatha-yoga as a psychological adjuvant for women undergoing IVF: A pilot study. *European Journal of Obstetrics & Gynecology, and Reproductive Biology, 176*, 158–162. doi:10.1016/j.ejogrb.2014.02.007

Vammen, M. A., Mikkelsen, S., Hansen, A. M., Grynderup, M. B., Andersen, J. H., Bonde, J. P.,...Thomsen, J. F. (2014). Salivary cortisol and depression in public sector employees: Cross-sectional and short term follow-up findings. *Psychoneuroendocrinology, 41*, 63–74. doi:10.1016/j.psyneuen.2013.12.006

Vellani, E., Colasante, A., Mamazza, L., Minasi, M. G., Greco, E., & Bevilacqua, A. (2013). Association of state and trait anxiety to semen quality of in vitro fertilization patients: A controlled study. *Fertility and Sterility, 99*, 1565–1572. doi:10.1016/j.fertnstert.2013.01.098

Verberg, M. F. G., Eijkemans, M. J. C., Heijnen, E. M. E. W., Broekmans, F. J., de Klerk, C., Fauser, B. C. J. M., & Macklon, N. S. (2008). Why do couples drop-out from IVF treatment? A prospective cohort study. *Human Reproduction, 23*, 2050–2055. doi:10.1093/humrep/den219

Volgsten, H., Skoog Svanburg, A., Ekselius, L., Lundkvist, O., & Poromaa, I. S. (2010). Risk factors for psychiatric disorders in infertile women and men doing in vitro fertilization. *Fertility and Sterility, 93*, 1088–1096. doi:10.1016/j.fertnstert.2008.11.008

Warren, M. P., & Stiehl, A. L. (1999). Exercise and female adolescents: Effects on the reproductive and skeletal systems. *Journal of the American Medical Women's Association, 54*, 115–120, 138.

Whirledge, S., & Cidlowski, J. A. (2013). A role for glucocorticoids in stress-impaired reproduction: Beyond the hypothalamus and pituitary. *Endocrinology, 154*, 4450–4468. doi:10.1210/en.2013-1652

Williams, K. E., Marsh, W. K., & Rasgon, N. L. (2007). Mood disorders and fertility in women: A critical review of the literature and implications for future research. *Human Reproduction Update, 13,* 607–616. doi:10.1093/humupd/dmm019

Wischmann, T. H. (2003). Psychogenic infertility—Myths and facts. *Journal of Assisted Reproduction and Genetics, 20,* 485–494. doi:10.1023/b:jarg.0000013648.74404.9d

Wischmann, T. (2008). Implications of psychosocial support in infertility—A critical appraisal. *Journal of Psychosomatic Obstetrics & Gynaecology, 29,* 83–90. doi:10.1080/0167482070 1817870

Young, E. A., Midgley, A. R., Carlson, N. E., & Brown, M. B. (2000). Alteration in the hypo-thalamic-pituitary-ovarian axis in depressed women. *Archives of General Psychiatry, 57,* 1157–1162. doi:10.1001/archpsyc.57.12.1157

Zaig, I., Azem, F., Schreiber, S., Gottlieb-Litvin, Y., Meiboom, H., & Bloch, M. (2012). Women's psychological profile and psychiatric diagnoses and the outcome of in vitro fertiliza-tion: Is there an association? *Archives of Women's Mental Health, 15,* 353–359. doi:10.1007/s00737-012-0293-z

Zheng, C. H., Huang, G. Y., Zhang, M. M., & Wang, W. (2012). Effects of acupuncture on pregnancy rates in women undergoing in vitro fertilization: A systematic review and meta-analysis. *Fertility and Sterility, 97,* 599–611. doi:10.1016/j.fertnstert.2011.12.007

Zorn, B., Auger, J., Velikonja, V., Kolbezen, M., & Meden-Vrtovec, H. (2008). Psychological fac-tors in male partners of infertile couples: Relationship with semen quality and early miscar-riage. *International Journal of Andrology, 31,* 557–564. doi:10.1111/j.1365-2605.2007.00806.x

# CHAPTER 7

# THE ILLUSION OF NORMAL FERTILITY: WOMEN'S EXPERIENCES OF PREGNANCY AND BIRTH AFTER OOCYTE DONATION

*Astrid Indekeu and Ken Daniels*

Assisted reproductive technology (ART) with donor oocytes was introduced in 1984 to allow women with ovarian insufficiency to become pregnant (Lutjen et al., 1984). The success of the technique led to a broadening of the treatment's scope, after about one decade of use, to include indications of repeated in vitro fertilization (IVF) failure, advanced maternal age, or inheritable diseases (Rosenwaks, 1987). Pregnancy and birth rates after ART with donor oocytes are now among the highest of any infertility treatment, with successful pregnancies occurring in the United States in 56% of embryo transfers, compared with 37% to 46% for standard IVF treatment. What is also remarkable about this high success rate is that in women who are using their own eggs, the IVF success rate drops sharply with age after a woman passes the age of 42 years (Centers for Disease Control and Prevention [CDC], 2012). Similar trends are found in Belgian data regarding pregnancy and birth rates after IVF with donor oocytes (BELRAP, 2014). Despite these positive results, donor-oocyte pregnancies are associated with an increased risk of pregnancy-induced hypertension and first trimester vaginal bleeding (Stoop et al., 2012). Pregnancies with donor oocytes appear also to be associated with relatively high incidence of complications, including preeclampsia, gestational diabetes, preterm delivery, labor induction, and caesarean section. Yet, these complications do not seem significantly increased compared with intracytoplasmic sperm injection (ICSI) pregnancies with autologous (i.e., derived from the same individual) oocytes (Stoop et al., 2012).

Women prefer fertility treatment with donor oocytes to other options of family building, such as adoption, because of the opportunity to experience pregnancy itself, the ability to feel "normal," and the potential to nurture and establish a bond with the child during the prenatal period (Applegarth et al., 1995; Bartlett, 1991; Hershberger, 2007). Data suggest that donor-conceiving couples emphasize the similarities with couples conceiving with their own gametes, such as the presence of a gestational link and giving birth, while ignoring those aspects that are incongruous with traditional family structure, such as the absence of a genetic tie (Indekeu et al., 2013; Isaksson et al., 2011; van den Akker, 2001).

In alternative family forms, there has been an emphasis on appearing similar to traditional (i.e., genetically related) families. In couples conceiving with donor sperm, Grace, Daniels, and Gillett (2008) observed that emphasizing similarities to more traditional family forms supported the establishment of normative perceptions of "family" by donor sperm recipients. Donor-oocyte recipients' health care professionals (e.g., physicians, psychologists) highlighted the similarities of pregnancies with donated oocytes to pregnancies with autologous oocytes by presenting data that women who give birth to children created through oocyte donation are *in fact* [emphasis added] able to breastfeed (Applegarth et al., 1995; Söderström-Anttila, Sajaniemi, Tiitinen, & Hovatta, 1998). Breastfeeding is also promoted in other alternative family forms in which there is no biological connection between mother and child (e.g., adoptive mothers, see www.breastfeedingwithoutbirthing.com). Breastfeeding seems to be promoted by health professionals not only because it is healthy and beneficial to the child but also because it promotes good bonding and develops women's feeling of "being a good mother" (Marshall, Godfrey, & Renfrew, 2007). Although discourse emphasizes breastfeeding as best, women are exposed to a considerably more diverse set of values and influences from health professionals, their social networks, and the wider social and structural context of their lives (such as work) that will form their view on breastfeeding. For women, breastfeeding is generally equated with good mothering when the baby is seen as healthy and happy. However, when a baby is not seen as healthy or contented (either in terms of behavior or measurable outcomes, such as weight), this can undermine women's confidence and leave them open to the charge of bad mothering (Marshall et al., 2007).

Pregnancy with donor oocytes can seem to easily create the illusion of normal fertility and a normal pregnancy to the pregnant woman, her partner, and family as well as to those in her professional and social circles. Yet, IVF with donor oocytes represents a special case in the treatment of infertility in many ways. The pregnancy is unique, as it is achieved from an embryo that is immunologically foreign to the mother and the treatment involves a third party, an oocyte donor, which makes the treatment ethically and psychologically more complicated than traditional IVF with one's own oocytes (Söderström-Anttila, 2001). This contrast between "illusion of normalcy" and "uniqueness" of the treatment, and the resulting pitfalls thereof, can make it challenging for nurses and other health care professionals to offer the appropriate and necessary care to donor-oocyte recipients.

Hershberger's (2004) integrative review on the limited existing research on egg donation identified six focused areas of research: (a) motivation; (b) desired donor characteristics; (c) selection of a known versus an anonymous donor; (d) recipient's demographic, educational, and psychosocial profiles; (e) disclosure of the mode of conception to family, friends, and offspring; and (f) relationship between the recipient and her offspring. These foci were supported in other research (e.g., Greenfeld & Klock, 2004; Isaksson, Sydsjö, Skoog Svanberg, & Lampic, 2012; Lampic, Skoog Svanberg, & Sydsjö, 2014; Laruelle, Place, Demeestere, Englert, & Delbaere, 2011; Murray, MacCallum, & Golombok, 2006; Söderström-Anttila, Sälevaara, & Suikkari, 2010; Stuart-Smith, Smith, & Scott, 2012; Yee, Blyth, & Tsang, 2011). Although investigators have made some strides in the field, research regarding women's experience during an oocyte-donation pregnancy and their pre-, peri-, and postnatal experiences remains very limited (Guillou, Séjourné, & Chabrol, 2009; Hershberger, 2007; Hershberger, Klock, & Barnes, 2007). Nurses and other health care providers are left with little empirical evidence from which to guide clinical practice (Hershberger, 2007).

This chapter focuses on oocyte recipients' experiences of their pre-, peri-, and postnatal periods. These experiences can support and guide nurses and other health care professionals in their clinical practice.

## METHODS

An applied thematic analysis approach was used in this research. Applied thematic analysis is a rigorous, yet inductive, set of procedures designed to identify and examine themes from textual data in a way that is transparent and credible while presenting the stories and experiences voiced by study participants as accurately and comprehensively as possible (Guest, MacQueen, & Namey, 2012). Qualitative research involves an interpretive approach of the world (Denzin & Lincoln, 2008; Hennink, Hutter, & Bailey, 2011); it occupies with "the inside" perspective (of the participant), the intersubjective perspective (the participant in its often shared social, cultural, historical, or personal context) and, lastly, acknowledges that people's perception and experiences of reality are subjective. As a result, multiple perspectives on reality can exist rather than a single truth as in a positivist paradigm.

## Participants

This study was approved by the Commission for Medical Ethics of the University Hospitals Leuven, Leuven, Belgium. This chapter reports on a subset of participants of a larger (partly longitudinal) research project situated in Belgium which focused on heterosexual men and women using donor gametes (sperm or oocytes) to build their families. Participants were recruited at Leuven University Fertility Center and through advertisement in a women's magazine. For a full description of the sample and setting of the overall study see Indekeu (2013). The subset reported here consists of two women who were midwives themselves and one woman who was intensely supported by a midwife who was a close family member. This created the unique opportunity to gain "insiders' insight" and to collect information from infertile women with enhanced medical and professional knowledge, who could express their needs as patients and could reflect knowledgably on the received care and the care they would give as professionals to others. All of the women were treated in different clinics in Belgium. Infertility was due to idiopathic premature-ovarian failure in all cases. The women were all married and were 27 (participant #1), 33 (participant #2), and 40 (participant #3) years of age at the time of the birth of their donor-conceived child. At the time of the interviews, they were respectively 38, 40, and 41 years of age. Two women selected an anonymous oocyte donor and one woman selected a donor known to her. All women experienced complications during pregnancy such as hypertension, thrombosis, or multifoetal pregnancy with loss. Due to the focus of the study, no further medical data were collected.

## Context

In relation to the professional care oocyte recipients receive during treatment through birth, the following information was collected: no specific care pathways or guidelines are known to Belgian midwives/nurses regarding the (psychological) care of donor-oocyte pregnancies. Donor-oocyte pregnancies are treated "as other low/high risk pregnancies" (Flemish Organization for Midwives, personal communication, September 18, 2014). Information regarding the donor-conceived nature of the pregnancy is usually written down in the letter to the primary health care professionals (e.g., general practitioner, gynecologist) who will provide care for the woman during her pregnancy. Yet, in Belgium, the fertility specialists who carried out the donor-oocyte treatment can respect a woman's explicit request not to mention the donor-conceived nature of the pregnancy in the referral letter. As a result, it is not known for certain if the health care professionals who assume care for the pregnant woman at the maternity center are aware of the donor-conceived nature of the pregnancy. In Belgium, information regarding the medical file of a patient can be shared between physicians, but an independent midwife is not included in this information exchange. Another possibility is that, out of respect to the woman's privacy, some health care professionals assuming care for the pregnant women might decide not to share information about the donor conception with all members of the health care team, such as midwives/nurses (anonymous, Head of Department of Reproductive Medicine, personal communication, September 22, 2014).

## Data Collection and Analysis

A narrative in-depth interview style (Kvale & Brinkmann, 2008) was used asking participants to share their story. According to a narrative interview style, participants' responses dictated the course of the interview, yet an aide memoire (interview guide) existed containing broad topics to be discussed (see Table 7.1).

All interviews were semi-structured, audiotaped, and lasted 1.5 to 2 hours and were carried out by the first author (A.I.). To avoid dropout, home interviews were scheduled based on the belief that participants would invest more time and feel more at ease at home to openly discuss these topics. Interviews were scheduled during evening and weekend hours in an effort to maximize participation. The interviewer was introduced as a researcher with professional expertise in medical psychology and sexology, to demonstrate the researcher's familiarity with the topic. Participants often mentioned that this information helped them to discuss the topic. After each interview, observations were recorded as memos. A narrative interview was conducted by the researcher, asking the participants to tell about their infertility experience, the choice and experience of an IVF with donor gametes, their experience and perception of the donor, and the question regarding disclosure of the donor conception to the offspring and/or others. Although the interviewer did not probe systematically about received care by midwives, the interviewer did pursue questions about it when participants raised concerns related to midwifery or nursing care.

**TABLE 7.1 Aide Memoire of Interview Topics**

The interview started with the questions "Can you tell me your story about your infertility experience and choice for a treatment with donated eggs?"

Topics that needed to be covered during the interview were:

- Experience of choice for donated eggs

- Experience of pregnancy

- Experience of birth

- Bonding experience with the child and the emerging family bonds

- Reactions from their intimate and broader social contexts (e.g., what was the first reaction to the baby, experience of resemblance remarks)

- Experience and perception of the donor

- Disclosure question

Participants #1 and #2 participated in two interviews and were interviewed when their donor offspring were, respectively, 10 years and 8 years old. Participant #3 participated in three interviews that occurred during the last trimester of the pregnancy, 3 months after birth, and 1.5 years after birth. Interviews were audio-taped, transcribed verbatim, and checked for accuracy. After corrections were made, the interview data were analyzed using a thematic analysis approach (Braun & Clarke, 2006).

## RESULTS

Four major themes emerged from the women's narratives, which focused on the pre-, peri-, and postnatal care periods and are as follows: (a) experiencing of "forcing the boundaries of nature"; (b) the importance of "a birth to be proud of"; (c) "breastfeeding is not obvious"; and (d) the absence of a place where emotions other than happiness and thankfulness could be addressed. In the following, the four themes and exemplar quotes from the participants themselves are provided.

### The Experience of: "Forcing the Boundaries of Nature" and "This Pregnancy Is Not Natural"

Although a donor-oocyte pregnancy carried an illusion of normalcy, the pregnancy was perceived in a different way by these women. Complications caused the pregnancy to be experienced as "forcing the boundaries of nature" and consequently perceived as not obvious. This caused the pregnancy to be stressful and not enjoyable. Birth was seen as potentially a first moment of relief and joy.

The participants reported that treatment with donor oocytes was often presented to them as "a makeable and successful solution" ("we can solve your problem, we have a solution") and resembling procreation with own gametes ("normal" procreation). Although the resulting birth was personally perceived as reaching their goal of having a child, the complications they were faced with during pregnancy (e.g., hypertension, preterm birth) were experienced as reminders that this pregnancy was not like normal pregnancies and could not be taken for granted. The participants also interpreted the experienced complications as tokens of "forcing the boundaries of nature": a sign "that I was not meant to be pregnant," and/or a reminder that this pregnancy was different from normal pregnancies. The distinctiveness mostly referred to the pregnancy not being natural because it was manipulated ("It's manipulated, it's because of all this medication you have to take, the pregnancy was heavily directed by medication"—participant #3) and not inherent to the body ("It's nature saying this is actually something foreign to the body and the body wants to reject it a bit"—participant #2).

Participant #3, who as a midwife was familiar and knowledgeable about fertility treatments, explicitly stated that the pregnancy had been mentally and physically "heavier" than expected, mainly referring to the fact that the pregnancy was so intensely and medically controlled. She had also been confronted with reactions from family, friends, and colleagues that corresponded with and supported her initial expectations of carrying a seemingly normal pregnancy. Some family members and friends had taken the pregnancy for granted. When complications arose, she described being struck by the fact that family members and friends had forgotten about her infertility. During the pregnancy, she had the impression that the health care professionals approached her pregnancy as normal and had forgotten that it was a highly technological complex pregnancy. As a midwife, she was well aware of the risks and she had expected to be able to share this with her professional colleagues, yet she felt left unrecognized and unsupported in her worries and feelings: "You are pregnant, problem solved. What are you still worrying about? Well, there are some side effects." Later on, the staff had admitted that they felt worried as well but had not expressed these concerns to her during the pregnancy:

> In retrospect the doctor and colleagues admitted that they had been walking on the tips of their toes the whole time. That they had hoped the end of the pregnancy would come as soon as possible and that it all would end well, because everyone was aware of the complications and their implications. (Participant #3)

The complications during pregnancy made them fearful and anxious about the outcome of the pregnancy ("'It's so fragile,' 'this will not end well,' 'what's next?'"—participant #2) and the implications of it for the yet unborn child. For participant #1, the complications she experienced and her perceived risk made her give up her desire for a second child.

Moreover, these women expressed feeling responsible for the possible consequences because making the decision to fulfill their desire for a child in this manner was their own personal decision.

> Did I make the right decision to force my body anyway? Because nature didn't grant me to be pregnant. Maybe I should have listened to my

body. I was getting confused by it. Are we doing well? Aren't we taking too many risks? (Participant #3)

Furthermore, the characteristics of the treatment process when using an oocyte donor, such as the shortage of donors and the resulting long waiting list to start treatment, enhanced the level of pressure: "This is our diamond, our 'once in a life-time.' Someone else can say 'I'll give it another go.' That's not possible for us." Consequently, pregnancy was more colored by fear than joy ("9 months of stress," "a nightmare"), which disabled them to enjoy the pregnancy and this could prolong until childbirth:

> I wasn't tired of being pregnant, I was worried. That's something totally different. It was a relief I could give birth, although I remained cautious during labor, but at least it started and afterwards we could begin to enjoy it. (participant #3)

When it was clear that the baby was healthy, the mothers expressed relief to have reassurance their baby was healthy. Participant #3 had noticed the relief of her supporting health care team as well: "Everyone was relieved, when he uttered his first breath, everyone sighed 'it's okay.' Everyone said it was quite a long 9 months."

## The Importance of: "A Birth You Can Be Proud of"

After experiencing an infertility diagnosis and a pregnancy with complications, the women expressed high expectations of the delivery. Birth could offer opportunities to repair some of the previous feelings of failure and a sense of regaining control. Yet, simultaneously birth could entail specific challenges. Just as the pregnancy had not been obvious and was strongly medically managed rather than experienced as a natural process, concerns existed whether giving birth would be so obvious. For example, participant #3 said,

> Because I can't be pregnant spontaneously, the next question is "can I deliver spontaneously?" My body might not be able to or needs to be forced to. It's not natural because you don't have the hormones needed for labor. They needed to give me a lot of medication before my body would go into labor.

All the women wished for a "natural" delivery, a "good" birth, a birth they "could be proud of": Participant #3 stated, "This I can do. I myself put him on to the world and I'm proud of it. That I managed to do." Being able to give birth was for some experienced as an opportunity to regain some of the self-confidence as woman and mother that was lost during the diagnosis of infertility and diffi-cult pregnancy ("I even can't carry a child properly"—participant #1). Even when the expectations of a "natural, good" birth could not be met (e.g., an epidural treatment was required), remarks from midwives could help them to see positive contributions they made and could support their self-confidence. Participant #1 described: "I wasn't proud of the epidural. That was a shame, I felt really bad. The only thing I liked was the midwife saying 'Oh my, you haven't panicked at any time!' That was nice."

Being able to play an active role felt important in the context of feeling like a mother. Being in some way active in the conceiving process made them feel necessary in the procreation process and seemed to create the feeling they were entitled to be called mother. Participant #3 said, "Birth itself directly gave me a mommy feeling—without me this wouldn't have been successful—I was not just the packaging for my child but I played my part in putting him into the world." Participant #2, who had to undergo a nonelective cesarean section, emphasized her contribution to the conceiving process by highlighting the necessity of her body during the pregnancy: "We always thought 'this happens in my body, it's because of me that he is born. If my body didn't cause him to grow, he would have never been here.'" Moreover, she described how she coped with a culture in which a caesarean birth is perceived to cause less bonding with your child: "I had a cesarean section but I had an immediate bond with my child. I've never been afraid of that." Evidence that she had carried him and therefore had played a role in his conception ("I still have a scar from the cesarean." "Each month we took pictures of my belly") seemed to highlight the importance of feeling part of the procreation process in some way.

Participants felt the need to not only regain self-confidence but also to regain control over their life. IVF was experienced as taking control over the procreation process as well as parts of their life due to treatment protocols.

> My biggest fear was a cesarean cause then I had to give the care of my
> child out of my hands. It was important to me that I could do it myself.
> That I was not too dependent on other people. (participant #3)

## "When You Become a Mother It Is Obvious That You Breastfeed" Yet "Breastfeeding Is Not Obvious"

All women presented conflicting experiences regarding breastfeeding: on the one hand, they faced physical difficulties with breastfeeding; on the other hand, they were confronted by cultural and personal expectations in which breastfeeding was the norm. Not reaching this norm was felt to be very stressful and there seemed few opportunities available to discuss their feelings.

Similar to their experience with carrying a pregnancy and giving birth, breast-feeding was perceived as something people take for granted ("When you become a mother it's obvious that you will breastfeed"—participant #1). Only participant #3 was cautioned by her gynecologist that breastfeeding might be physically difficult. Her previous experiences of body processes that failed and deviated from the norm made her realize that breastfeeding was no certainty: "No one knows how a body works … so in terms of breastfeeding we had to wait and see if it would it work or not." Despite the caution, she felt very disappointed when breastfeeding turned out extremely difficult. Participants #1 and #2 had not received such cautions by their gynecologist or nursing/midwifery professionals and had high expectations regarding breastfeeding. Not being able to achieve the "obvious" and to meet up to their own and/or others' expectations ("They all expect you will succeed," "I wanted to succeed as woman"—participant #1) created feelings of failure and sadness. These feelings could come on top of the previous failure experiences during pregnancy and childbirth. "Because the pregnancy was disappointing I had hoped that this part would turn out better, that I succeeded at least in something, I failed already in so many things" (participant #1).

The existing (in Belgium) cultural context in which breastfeeding is strongly promoted enhanced the pressure to succeed and the feeling of failure in case of nonsuccess. Being a midwife herself, participant #3 felt especially pressured to breastfeed because she was convinced of the benefits of breastfeeding herself as a professional and she knew colleagues would question her about it.

Yet, even with good intentions, endurance, and effort, continuation of the breastfeeding just seemed not feasible. Negative emotions would influence the mother–child bond ("In the end, I'd just been very unhappy toward my child cause I didn't succeed") or the child itself ("He just deteriorated and was so skinny") and a decision to stop had to be considered.

This decision to stop breastfeeding and accept their limits was experienced by all women as extremely difficult for several reasons. Participant #3 described herself as a "down-to-earth" midwife, stating that she as a professional was aware and accepting that sometimes breastfeeding was just not feasible. Despite her attitude, she stated that it was extremely difficult to keep thinking rationally during the postnatal period: "All these hormones make you more emotional and make you act different than you normally would do." Participant #1 described how difficult it was to be clear-sighted during that time: "When I look back at the pictures I'm ashamed, he was so skinny! When you're in the middle of it, you just don't see it!" Pressure from colleagues inquiring if she was still breastfeeding ("You do still offer breastfeeding? You aren't giving up yet, are you?") or a family-member midwife described as "Very well intended but a breastfeeding-freak. She said 'you need to give it time, don't give additional bottle milk because then it won't get going!'" was also mentioned as hindering the decision-making process and respecting their own limits. Both women felt torn between their colleagues/family member midwives' advice and their own personal experiences. Due to this, participant #3 not only felt very insecure and lonely in her decision process, she also felt she had to justify her decision to stop the breastfeeding and felt not recognized in all her attempts to continue breastfeeding. She felt inquiries about the breastfeeding could have been formulated more sensitively with less pressure to continue. This made her sad and she felt disappointed in her colleague's reaction and lack of empathy. Participant #1 described how she perceived advice from a professional organization as an approval to change her mode of feeding. By following this professional advice she felt "a good mother taking good care of her child": "Child and Family [governmental postnatal care service] came along. They insisted that I would offer bottles of infant formula! That was so comforting. I was allowed to give bottle milk! He started gaining weight and became healthy."

Another reason that hindered the decision was related to Belgian labor laws. Options to enjoy paid breastfeeding leave exist. To receive this benefit, the mother has to provide proof that she breastfeeds her baby. Participant #3, who wanted to breastfeed but who was physically unable to, felt enhanced pressure, as she would have to resume work sooner and thus be separated from her child sooner:

> I experienced a lot of pressure from my department heads. I was on breastfeeding leave so it's obvious that you breastfeed. For me that was important so I could stay longer at home with my child. So I would do anything to breastfeed.

Notwithstanding all the emotions aroused by the breastfeeding concerns, there seemed to be little space to express feelings other than positive ones. Participant #3 described how she felt she had to fit into the views on breastfeeding and there seemed just no other view available:

> Breastfeeding that's the greatest time of your life! That bond between mother and child. When you open up the books, every woman should experience that, it's so wonderful! Sorry, I am pro-breastfeeding but that was not the greatest time of my life. Now I enjoy my child much more. But I dare not to say that out loud! Definitely not to midwives who think that way about breastfeeding.

## "You Had to Toe the Line, There Was No Room for Something Else"

Some of the aforementioned emotions are the opposite of the emotions that are expected or perceived appropriate considering the whole context of oocyte donation such as thankfulness and happiness. The absence of a place where emotions other than happiness and thankfulness could be addressed left these women in a conflicted position and little other discourse to call on. Participant #3 stated: "You had to toe the line [stay positive and be thankful], … they just wouldn't listen, there was no room for something else."

Several elements unique to the practice of conceiving by means of an oocyte donor seemed to influence this: Thankfulness seemed appropriate toward all the efforts that the donor had made and the unique chance they were given by her donation ("Without the donor he wouldn't been here, I would not have had a chance. We may regard ourselves lucky"—participant #2). It became even more difficult when the donor was a friend. Participant #1 described how she did not dare to tell the donor/her friend that she felt unhappy at the onset when she was still struggling to accept her infertility and the fact that this child was not genetically related to her. This would have seemed an insult to her friend.

Moreover, the efforts and challenges these women had endured to fulfill their desire for a child left little room for feelings of doubts, concerns, or sadness ("You have what you have been waiting for so long, now you need to be happy and feel good"— participant #1). Likewise, all three women referred to several incidents in their daily life in which they were confronted with remarks treating their donor conception as normal conception. People (e.g., family, friends, and professionals) seemed unaware of some of the unique implications donor conception has. Participant #3 stated that although all her colleagues/midwives were informed about the donor conception and the treatment procedure, she still received remarks like "with a second child everything will go smoother." In this case, the remarks were experienced as rude, insensitive, and thoughtless regarding the fact that conceiving with donor oocytes is not self-evident. On another occasion, participant #2 witnessed a colleague/midwife commenting to an oocyte-recipient mother that her child did not look like either mother or father: "That must have hurt that lady so much. She made so much effort and then my colleague says 'it doesn't resemble one of you!' That poor lady being so proud of her baby." Being approached as "a pregnancy with autologous oocytes" could be experienced positive ("They accept us and see as normal") or negative ("Your grief about the infertility and efforts are not being recognized"). The women themselves felt ambivalent about what reactions they preferred and it seemed to depend on how they felt at that particular time. Yet, feeling there was no room to express negative feelings was experienced by all as unhelpful. Above all, the expectation existed that at least colleagues, midwives/nurses in the field, would respond positively (or at least neutral) to donor-conceiving patients due to their expected knowledge about it, and feeling in general familiar and less awkward with the theme of infertility as family and friends might feel. This expectation did lead to additional disappointments when these expectations were not met.

## DISCUSSION

Most of the scientific literature on donor-oocyte recipients involves research into the successes of the treatment (e.g., high success rates, healthy babies) and its similarity with "natural/normal" procreation (i.e., carrying pregnancy, giving birth, and breastfeeding). Oocyte-recipient treatment is indeed successful (BELRAP, 2014; CDC, 2012) and as it does help women to carry a desired pregnancy and to fulfill their desire for a child. However, our findings indicate that the biological success of donor-oocyte treatment is not sufficient for oocyte-recipient women to experience the treatment also as a psychological success. Despite the reintroduction of "normality" through establishing pregnancy, our findings support prior work delineating the need to acknowledge the pain and psychological injury due to the infertility and the contribution of a third person in the conception (Guillou et al., 2009; Hershberger et al., 2007).

Literature on the experiences of pregnancy, birth, and breastfeeding of oocyte-recipient women is almost nonexistent (Hershberger, 2004). Some of our findings are in line with women conceiving with their own oocytes, such as the participant's experiences regarding breastfeeding in which normative, cultural frameworks on breastfeeding leave women with limited options for articulating and defining their subjective position. The most notable, "the good mother" and the "breast is best," discourses, as expounded in antenatal classes, set women up to expect to breastfeed without difficulty (Ryan, Bissell, & Alexander, 2010). The problem is that when this is not a woman's experience, she has few other discourses to call upon but the one who says "I failed, I feel guilty, I've let them down"; this causes a crisis in her sense of self. Ryan et al. (2010) have identified ways in which women are able to mentally rewrite the script they have of themselves from an uncomfortable position ("I fail") to one that they felt or expect to feel more comfortable or socially acceptable ("I succeed/do well"). Yet, for these women to succeed a culture of openness is necessary to develop new subjective positions around infant feeding practices (Ryan et al., 2010). Listening to women's narratives of their breastfeeding experiences may open up a way of thinking that leads to new ways of communicating about breastfeeding than solely in terms of success or failure (Ryan et al., 2010). Moreover, very little literature on breastfeeding after donor-oocyte pregnancies could be located and only emphasized that oocyte recipients were in fact being able to breastfeed (Applegarth et al., 1995; Söderström-Anttila et al., 1998). Specific meaning of breastfeeding following donor-oocyte pregnancies and its possible difficulties were not addressed. Finally, the assumptions on a positive role of breastfeeding on the mother–infant relationship are not supported by empirical evidence. Recommendations of breastfeeding should solely be based on its well-documented positive effects on infant and maternal health (Jansen, De Weerth, & Riksen-Walraven, 2008).

Women in this study were often dealing with loneliness and incomprehension and a need for more psychological support was expressed throughout the pre-, peri-, and postnatal periods, such as that reported by Guillou et al. (2009). Yet, in line with Sachs and Hammer Burns (2006), this chapter demonstrates that donor-oocyte treatments entail opportunities to restore self-esteem and self-image and to regain self-confidence and control among donor-oocyte-recipient women. Simultaneously, perceptions and interpretations of the infertility and subsequent treatment could be undermining forces, sometimes persisting throughout the process of pregnancy and after birth (Sachs & Hammer Burns, 2006). Women in this study provide additional understanding on how experiences regarding pregnancy, birth, and breastfeeding—beyond the experience of infertility and the treatment—entail opportunities to regain self-confidence and self-control.

Although biologically comparable to a normal pregnancy (pregnancy with autologous oocytes), the participants' experiences convey four themes in which the events of pregnancy, birth, and breastfeeding are given unique psychological meanings as a result of the infertility and subsequent treatment with donor oocytes. Approaching a donor-oocyte pregnancy as a normal pregnancy will cause these specific meanings to be overseen, even when the biological higher risks associated with donor-oocyte pregnancy are pointed out (Stoop et al., 2012) and the donor-oocyte pregnancy is approached according to a protocol for high-risk pregnancies. When these experiences are not addressed adequately, they risk the development of failure experience on top of the previously felt failure experiences. Reasons for overlooking these experiences seemed partly due to "the illusion of normal fertility," the presence of normative views (regarding mode of delivery, breastfeeding), and the organization of the health care in which care for a patient can be divided over different professional teams (fertility clinic and maternity). Information about the fertility history is needed to approach the patient in an appropriate and adapted manner, yet might not always be available or given the necessary attention. Transfer of this information might be hindered between the various professionals (e.g., physicians, midwives, nurses) due to nondisclosure of the mode of conception by the woman herself or other health care professionals. Being focused on one specific event (e.g., pregnancy, birth, breastfeeding) can cause thinking about the history of the conception or the long-term consequences to be challenging. Finally, knowledge about the meaning and impact of infertility and donor-oocyte conception on the experience of pregnancy, childbirth, and breastfeeding might be lacking.

Although the number of participants is small, the homogeneity of the group and its uniqueness ("insiders position") result in unprecedented in-depth insight into the experiences of donor-oocyte-recipient women's experiences. Two of the participants were interviewed 8 to 10 years after donor-egg conception and their recall about their experiences may have been limited or modified. However, Quigley, Hockley, and Davidson (2007) have shown that women's recall about significant life events is highly reliable and that being familiar with perinatal events and terminology, as these participants were, enhanced the reliability. We do provide a novel in-depth description of oocyte-recipient women's experiences of pregnancy, birth, and breast-feeding. Further research regarding the psychological effects of pregnancy complications and the experience of breastfeeding after oocyte donation is necessary.

## IMPLICATIONS FOR PRACTICE

Since the first report of a live birth from oocyte donation in 1984, the request for treatment with donor oocytes has increased worldwide. In the United States, the number of oocyte-recipient pregnancies represents almost 12% of all ARTs (CDC, 2012). Nurses are confronted with oocyte-recipient women in different health care settings, including fertility clinics, prenatal, maternity, and pediatric centers. Nurses caring for oocyte-recipient women need to be informed about the unique psychological aspect of oocyte donor conception. Moreover, nurses and other health care providers should be aware of the significant role that they play in supporting oocyte-recipient women to cope with their infertility and to regain confidence and restore self-esteem. Nurses can improve clinical care by anticipating the needs of donor-oocyte recipients as they move through pregnancy, birth, and into the post-partum period. Collaboration with other professionals, including mental health professionals pointing out the psychological specificities of a donor-oocyte pregnancy, may also improve care, especially when formulating guidelines or models of care for oocyte-recipient women.

Continuous awareness, self-reflection, and sensitivity to the pitfall of the illusion of normality and the presence of normative views (e.g., view on breastfeeding) are needed to be able to support the patient in her management of her infertility and the development of a confident concept of motherhood. Team supervision can address the impact of normative frameworks, their suitability for oocyte pregnancies, and openness to different views.

## CONCLUSION

Limited research has been done regarding the experience of pregnancy, birth, and breastfeeding of oocyte-recipient women. The results of this study provide a beginning and understanding of the specific psychological processes that take place during the pre-, peri-, and postnatal periods of oocyte-recipient women. The experiences presented in this chapter raise the issue of a special care pathway for pregnancies after oocyte donation is recommended to foster the development of a confident maternal identity. Greater awareness and understanding of the distinctive psychological qualities of oocyte-recipient pregnancies and the cultural expectations regarding breastfeeding and oocyte-recipient treatment are needed during the pre-, peri-, and postnatal periods to provide appropriate care.

## ACKNOWLEDGMENTS

We are grateful to the couples who generously shared their stories. The data were collected during the doctoral research of Dr. Indekeu at the University of Leuven (Belgium). At present, Dr. Indekeu is a fellow at the University of Leuven (Belgium) and a postdoctoral researcher at the Karolinska Institutet (Sweden). This research has been made possible with the support of the Research Foundation-Flanders (FWO; Project Grant No. G.0594.09). There are no competing interests.

## REFERENCES

Applegarth, L., Goldberg, N. C., Cholst, I., McGoff, N., Fantini, D., Zellers, N.,...Rosenwaks, Z. (1995). Families created through ovum donation: A preliminary investigation of obstetrical outcome and psychosocial adjustment. *Journal of Assisted Reproduction and Genetics, 12*(9), 574–580.

Bartlett, J. A. (1991). Psychiatric issues in non-anonymous oocyte donation. Motivations and expectations of women donors and recipients. *Psychosomatics, 32*(4), 433–437.

BELRAP. (2014). *Report of the college of physicians of assisted reproductive therapy, Belgium 2011.* Retrieved from http://www.belrap.be/Documents/Reports/Global/FinalReportV2_IVF11_10JAN14.pdf

Braun, V., & Clarke, V. (2006). Using thematic analysis in psychology. *Qualitative Research in Psychology, 3*, 77–101. doi:10.1191/1478088706qp063oa

Centers for Disease Control and Prevention (CDC). (2012). *Assisted reproductive technology (ART) report: 2012 national summary.* Retrieved from http://nccd.cdc.gov/DRH_ART/Apps/NationalSummaryReport.aspx

Denzin, N. K., & Lincoln, Y. S. (Eds.). (2008). *The landscape of qualitative research.* Thousand Oaks, CA: Sage.

Grace, V. M., Daniels, K. R., & Gillett, W. (2008). The donor, the father, and the imaginary constitution of the family: Parents' constructions in the case of donor insemination. *Social Science & Medicine (1982), 66*(2), 301–314.

Greenfeld, D. A., & Klock, S. C. (2004). Disclosure decisions among known and anonymous oocyte donation recipients. *Fertility and Sterility, 81*(6), 1565–1571.

Guest, G., MacQueen, K. M., & Namey, E. E. (2012). *Applied thematic analysis.* London, UK: Sage.

Guillou, J., Séjourné, N., & Chabrol, H. (2009). Appréhensionetvécud'unegrossesseobtenue après un don d'ovocyteanonyme [Pregnancy following anonymous oocyte donation: Experience and feelings]. *GynécologieObstétriqueFertilité, 37*(5), 410–414. doi:10.1016/j.gyobfe.2008.10.009

Hennink, M., Hutter, I., & Bailey, A. (2011). *Qualitative research methods.* London, UK: Sage.

Hershberger, P. (2004). Recipients of oocyte donation: An integrative review. *Journal of Obstetric, Gynecologic, and Neonatal Nursing, 33*(5), 610–621.

Hershberger, P. E. (2007). Pregnant, donor oocyte recipient women describe their lived experience of establishing the "family lexicon." *Journal of Obstetric, Gynecologic, and Neonatal Nursing, 36*(2), 161–167.

Hershberger, P., Klock, S. C., & Barnes, R. B. (2007). Disclosure decisions among pregnant women who received donor oocytes: A phenomenological study. *Fertility and Sterility, 87*(2), 288–296.

Indekeu, A. (2013). *Parenthood by donor conception. Exploring (intended) parents' experiences and disclosure behaviour* (Doctoral dissertation). Retrieved from lirias.kuleuven.be/handle/123456789/416072

Indekeu, A., Rober, P., Schotsmans, P., Daniels, K. R., Dierickx, K., & D'Hooghe, T. (2013). How couples' experiences prior to the start of infertility treatment with donor gametes influence the disclosure decision. *Gynecologic and Obstetric Investigation, 76*(2), 125–132.

Isaksson, S., Skoog Svanberg, A., Sydsjö, G., Thurin-Kjellberg, A., Karlström, P. O., Solensten, N. G., & Lampic, C. (2011). Two decades after legislation on identifiable donors in Sweden: Are recipient couples ready to be open about using gamete donation? *Human Reproduction, 26*(4), 853–860.

Isaksson, S., Sydsjö, G., Skoog Svanberg, A., & Lampic, C. (2012). Disclosure behaviour and intentions among 111 couples following treatment with oocytes or sperm from identity-release donors: Follow-up at offspring age 1–4 years. *Human Reproduction, 27*(10), 2998–3007.

Jansen, J., De Weerth, C., & Riksen-Walraven, J. M. (2008). Breastfeeding and the mother-infant relationship—A review. *Developmental Review, 28*, 503–521. doi:10.1016/j.dr.2008.07.001

Kvale, S., & Brinkmann, S. (2008). *InterViews: Learning the craft of qualitative research interviewing*. Thousand Oaks, CA: Sage.

Lampic, C., Skoog Svanberg, A., & Sydsjö, G. (2014). Attitudes towards disclosure and relationship to donor offspring among a national cohort of identity-release oocyte and sperm donors. *Human Reproduction, 29*(9), 1978–1986.

Laruelle, C., Place, I., Demeestere, I., Englert, Y., & Delbaere, A. (2011). Anonymity and secrecy options of recipient couples and donors, and ethnic origin influence in three types of oocyte donation. *Human Reproduction, 26*(2), 382–390.

Lutjen, P., Trounson, A., Leeton, J., Findlay, J., Wood, C., & Renou, P. (1984). The establishment and maintenance of pregnancy using in vitro fertilization and embryo donation in a patient with primary ovarian failure. *Nature, 307*(5947), 174–175.

Marshall, J. L., Godfrey, M., & Renfrew, M. J. (2007). Being a "good mother": Managing breastfeeding and merging identities. *Social Science & Medicine (1982), 65*(10), 2147–2159.

Murray, C., MacCallum, F., & Golombok, S. (2006). Egg donation parents and their children: Follow-up at age 12 years. *Fertility and Sterility, 85*(3), 610–618.

Quigley, M. A., Hockley, C., & Davidson, L. L. (2007). Agreement between hospital records and maternal recall of mode of delivery: Evidence from 12 391 deliveries in the UK Millennium Cohort Study. *BJOG: An International Journal of Obstetrics and Gynaecology, 114*(2), 195–200.

Rosenwaks, Z. (1987). Donor eggs: Their application in modern reproductive technologies. *Fertility and Sterility, 47*(6), 895–909.

Ryan, K., Bissell, P., & Alexander, J. (2010). Moral work in women's narratives of breastfeeding. *Social Science & Medicine (1982), 70*(6), 951–958.

Sachs, P. L., & Hammer Burns, L. (2006). Recipient counseling for oocyte donation. In S. N. Covington & L. H. Hammer Burns (Eds.), *Infertility counseling: A comprehensive handbook for clinicians* (2nd ed., pp. 319–338). New York, NY: Cambridge University Press.

Söderström-Anttila, V. (2001). Pregnancy and child outcome after oocyte donation. *Human Reproduction Update, 7*(1), 28–32.

Söderström-Anttila, V., Sajaniemi, N., Tiitinen, A., & Hovatta, O. (1998). Health and development of children born after oocyte donation compared with that of those born after in-vitro fertilization, and parents' attitudes regarding secrecy. *Human Reproduction, 13*(7), 2009–2015.

Söderström-Anttila, V., Sälevaara, M., & Suikkari, A. M. (2010). Increasing openness in oocyte donation families regarding disclosure over 15 years. *Human Reproduction, 25*(10), 2535–2542.

Stoop, D., Baumgarten, M., Haentjens, P., Polyzos, N. P., De Vos, M., Verheyen, G.,…Devroey, P. (2012). Obstetric outcome in donor oocyte pregnancies: A matched-pair analysis. *Reproductive Biology and Endocrinology, 10*, 42.

Stuart-Smith, S. J., Smith, J. A., & Scott, E. J. (2012). To know or not to know? Dilemmas for women receiving unknown oocyte donation. *Human Reproduction, 27*(7), 2067–2075.

Yee, S., Blyth, E., & Tsang, A. K. (2011). Views of donors and recipients regarding disclosure to children following altruistic known oocyte donation. *Reproductive Biomedicine Online, 23*(7), 851–859.

van den Akker, O. (2001). The acceptable face of parenthood: The relative status of biological and cultural interpretations of offspring in infertility treatment. *Psychology, Evolution & Gender, 3*, 137–153. doi:10.1080/14616660110067366

# CHAPTER 8

# INDIVIDUAL AND FAMILY OUTCOMES OF FIRST-TIME PARENTS OLDER THAN 40 YEARS: IMPLICATIONS OF LATER-LIFE PARENTING

*Julia T. Woodward and Katherine E. MacDuffie*

Numerous studies point to the consequences of embarking on parenthood too early in life (Mirowsky & Ross, 2002; Spence, 2008; Williams, McGee, Olaman, & Knight, 1997), but the implications of conceiving at a significantly older age are just beginning to receive systematic study. With the advent of assisted reproductive technologies (ART) and the use of donor oocytes, women can now pursue parenthood into their 40s or even 50s. Couples working with an oocyte donor and a gestational carrier are no longer bound to a reproductive "biological clock" and can theoretically pursue parenthood at any age. Characterizing the medical and psychosocial implications of choosing to pursue first-time parenthood in one's 40s, 50s, and beyond is the aim of this chapter.

The number of women choosing later-life parenthood has increased substantially in the past three decades, largely due to both societal changes and increased use of ARTs. In 1970, one out of every 100 first births in the United States was to a woman aged 35 years or older; by 2006, that number had grown to one out of every 12 first births (Matthews & Hamilton, 2009). From 1996 to 2008, although the overall United States birth rate increased by only 9%, the number of births among women aged 40 to 44 years increased by 48% and the number of births among women aged 45 to 49 years increased by 133% (Martin et al., 2010; Zweifel, Covington, & Applegarth, 2012). Although the absolute number remained relatively low, birth to women 50 to 54 years old increased by 276% in the same period. Later-life fatherhood has also increased, though more gradually; in 1970, the birth rate for men aged 45 to 49 years was 6.1 births per 1,000, compared with 8.8 in 2013 (Matthews & Hamilton, 2009).

Although it is clear that becoming a parent at a later-life stage is increasingly prevalent, review of this literature reveals a variety of terms and an even greater variety of definitions. Researchers use terms such as *delayed child bearing, late-life parenthood, older motherhood, advanced maternal age* (first-time motherhood at age 35 years or older), and even *extreme advanced maternal age* (defined as first-time motherhood at age 45 years or older; Yogev et al., 2010). Depending on the era when the data were collected and the particular hypotheses investigated, authors alternatively classify a parent as being "older" anywhere from 30 to 55 years of age. Many studies designed to investigate the experience of teen motherhood applied the label "older mother" to their comparison group of women in their 20s and 30s. This lack of clarity about when an individual becomes an "older" parent confounds the data and makes comparisons across studies more difficult. In this chapter, we conduct a careful review of the extant literature on parenting at an older age. Given their rapidly growing numbers and potential for unique medical and psychosocial sequelae, we are particularly interested in individuals who become parents at 40 years and beyond and make special note of studies referring to this population. Given the ways in which Western culture celebrates youth and disparages older age in order to minimize stigma, we have chosen the term *"later-life" parent* to refer to parenting at a more mature, nontraditional stage.

## MEDICAL IMPLICATIONS OF LATER-LIFE PARENTING

It is well known that female fertility declines with age. This decline is caused by a diminishing number of oocytes, decreased quality of those oocytes, and an altered hormonal environment that can interfere with ovulation (Rowe, 2006). Although the exact timing of these biological declines differs among individuals, on average fertility begins to decline significantly at age 32 years and precipitously at age 37 years (The American College of Obstetricians and Gynecologists Committee on Gynecologic Practice & the Practice Committee of the American Society for Reproductive Medicine, 2014). Thus, women who choose to become mothers later in life may face significant challenges as they start building their families. Both historical epidemiological and current clinical data have shown that spontaneous pregnancy after age 45 years is rare and is virtually nonexistent after age 50 years (Matthews & Hamilton, 2009). The inverse relationship between age and fertility also holds for men, though the association is not as strong. Sperm volume and motility have been shown to decrease with age (Frattarelli, Miller, Miller, Elkind-Hirsch, & Scott, 2008), and the average time to pregnancy increases with the age of the male partner, even after controlling for female age (Ford et al., 2000).

As a woman ages, her egg quality decreases and her offspring faces a higher risk of birth defects and genetic disorders (American College of Obstetricians and Gynecologists Committee on Gynecologic Practice & the Practice Committee of the American Society for Reproductive Medicine, 2014). This may be due to dysfunction in the final stage of cell division in aging oocytes, specifically, in the formation of the meiotic spindle (Battaglia, Goodwin, Klein, & Soules, 1996). If this process is disrupted, it can lead to aneuploidy, a condition in which the resulting embryo has either too many or too few chromosomes. Aneuploidy is thought to be responsible for a large proportion of spontaneous abortions or miscarriages experienced during later-life pregnancy, as the abnormal chromosome count can make a fetus nonviable (Mills & Lavender, 2011). Aneuploidy can also lead to chromosomal disorders such as Down syndrome, caused by an extra 21st chromosome. The increased risk of Down syndrome with advanced maternal age has led to the recommendation that all women older than 35 years have genetic testing for the disorder.

The older age of both female and male gametes can contribute to increased risk of birth defects and disease. The effects of paternal age on fertility and pregnancy outcomes are less well studied and are often difficult to dissociate from the confounding effects of maternal age. Some of the best data come from studies of couples undergoing donor egg cycles, in which the sperm of an older male is combined with eggs from a young donor. These studies have shown that paternal age greater than 50 years is associated with an increase in pregnancy loss and decreased rates of blastocyst formation and live birth (Frattarelli et al., 2008). These effects may be a consequence of the fact that, unlike female germ cells, male germ cells continue to replicate throughout adulthood. For comparison, the total lifetime number of cell divisions for an egg is 24, whereas the average number of divisions for a male germ cell is 380 by the age of 30 years and 840 by the age of 50 years (Crow, 2000). The result of these repeated cell divisions is an increased rate of de novo mutations, or new mutations, that occur either due to errors in copying of genetic material or errors in cell division. These mutations can have a variety of consequences for the offspring. For example, new mutations can lead to the expression of rare birth defects or to chromosomal disorders such as Down syndrome or Kleinfelter syndrome (McIntosh, Olshan, & Baird, 1995). The high mutation rate may also explain the link between increased paternal age and higher long-term risk for psychiatric disorders such as schizophrenia (Wohl & Gorwood, 2007) and bipolar disorder (Frans et al., 2008) in adult offspring of older fathers. Similarly, both paternal and maternal age have been shown to be independently related to an increased risk for autism (Durkin et al., 2008). These comparative recent discoveries have led to the recommendation that males older than 40 years be counseled about the relative increased risks for their offspring (Toriello & Meck, 2008).

## Pregnancy Risks Associated With Advanced Maternal Age

ART allows for pregnancy to be achieved beyond a woman's natural reproductive life cycle. A woman whose own ovarian reserve is poor, either due to natural aging or premature menopause, can use eggs from a younger donor, thus serving to reset the risk profile for the resulting fetus. However, whether a woman conceives with her own eggs or those of a donor, there are risks associated with carrying a pregnancy later in life. First, it is more likely that a woman in her 40s or 50s will have a preexisting medical condition, such as hypertension or obesity, which makes pregnancy more risky (Gilbert, Young, & Danielsen, 2007). Even if a woman enters a pregnancy in excellent health, later-life mothers are at higher risk for developing pregnancy complications such as pregnancy-related hypertension and preeclampsia (Mills & Lavender, 2011). Increased maternal age is also implicated in higher risks for gestational diabetes, placenta previa, and multiple gestation (Beemsterboer et al., 2006; Jacobsson, Ladfors, & Milsom, 2004). Due in part to these pregnancy complications, there is a greatly increased incidence of cesarean deliveries in mothers older than 40 years (Cleary-Goldman et al., 2005; Mills & Lavender, 2011). Recent evidence suggests that cesarean delivery may compromise the development of an infant's immune system, due to lack of exposure to bacteria in the birth canal and lack of fetal stress response that occurs during vaginal delivery (Cho & Norman, 2013). Elective cesareans have been associated with immature lung development and higher respiratory morbidity in newborns (Hansen, Wisborg, Uldbjerg, & Henriksen, 2008) and are chosen as an alternative to vaginal delivery more often for women of advanced maternal age (Ecker, Chen, Cohen, Riley, & Lieberman, 2001). Preterm birth is also more likely to occur for women older than 40 years (Cleary-Goldman et al., 2005; Jacobsson et al., 2004); preterm and near-term infants have consistently poorer outcomes compared with those who are carried to full term (Wang, Dorer, Fleming, & Catlin, 2004).

Perhaps the most sobering data related to pregnancy at an advanced maternal age reflect the increased rates of stillbirth and maternal death—complications that are rare but catastrophic. Advanced maternal age (and perhaps advanced paternal age, though the data are less clear; Slama et al., 2005) is related to increased risk of spontaneous abortion and stillbirth (Jacobsson et al., 2004; Whitcomb et al., 2011). Although an uncommon event, risk of maternal death of a woman older than 40 years is five times that of a woman aged 25 to 29 years (9 vs. 45 per 100,000 live births; Chang et al., 2003). Because of these risks associated with later-life pregnancies, the American Society for Reproductive Medicine (ASRM) Ethics Committee developed guidelines for the use of donor eggs in women of advanced maternal age (Ethics Committee of the ASRM, 2013). The committee recommends that egg donation to women between the ages of 50 and 54 years should be allowed only if the woman is healthy and unaffected by any preexisting medical conditions that could increase her risks during pregnancy. Given the increased incidence of spontaneous twinning that can occur with in vitro fertilization (IVF; Vitthala, Gelbaya, Brison, Fitzgerald, & Nardo, 2009) and the greater health risk associated with multiple gestations, single-embryo transfer is strongly recommended for this age group. The committee further recommends that pretreatment consultation for women older than 50 years should include input from a physician who specializes in high-risk obstetrics, and the woman (and her partner, if applicable) should be counseled about the increased risks associated with carrying a later-life pregnancy. Finally, the committee discourages egg donation to women older than 55 years, even in the absence of any preexisting health conditions.

## Later-Life Parenthood and Health Outcomes

There is some evidence that becoming a parent later in life actually improves parental health (Mirowsky, 2002), perhaps because later-life parents are more motivated to engage in positive health behaviors that foster keeping up with young children. Indeed, compared with teenage parents, later-life mothers are more likely to take good care of themselves during pregnancy, avoid substance use, take prenatal vitamins, and attend prenatal check-up appointments (Mills & Lavender, 2011). However, because maternal age is often correlated with years of education, greater education rather than maternal age may be the key variable explaining the increased frequency of these health behaviors (Mirowsky, 2002). The positive health behaviors of later-life parents may also have an impact on their children's health outcomes. One study found that children of older mothers had fewer unintentional injuries and hospital admissions and higher rates of immunization (Sutcliffe, Barnes, Belsky, Gardiner, & Melhuish, 2012). Conflicting evidence suggests that there are long-term negative health implications of becoming a parent later in life. For example, Alonzo

(2002) found that women giving birth after the age of 35 years were more likely to have a clinician rate their mobility at age 50 years or beyond as "less than good."

Somewhat surprisingly, there may also be negative long-term health consequences for children born to later-life parents. Liu, Zhi, and Li (2011) found that advanced parental age was linked to shortened life expectancy for their children. Although the mechanism for this effect is not well understood, it has been suggested that the child's reduced life span may be a consequence of poor gamete quality. Myrskylä, Elo, Kohler, and Martikainen (2014) also found a link between older parental age and shorter life span for children. Analyzing epidemiological data, the authors found that children of older parents were more likely to experience parental death before they reached the age of 35 years, and those who had experienced parental loss before age 35 years had a shortened life expectancy. If the child's parents were still alive when the child reached the age of 35 years, no association between older parental age and earlier child death was found.

These findings are interesting to consider from the perspective of the psychological literature about the impacts of early life trauma. The death of one's parent during childhood is a traumatic event and is placed in the same category with physical or sexual abuse in studies of posttraumatic stress disorder in children. Indeed, exposure to the death of a parent during childhood is associated with the development of psychiatric disorders later in life (Agid et al., 1999), perhaps due to enduring changes in the neurobiological systems that regulate the stress response. Exposure to early traumatic stress is an alternate explanation to reduced gamete quality that may explicate the link between older parental age and shorter life span for their offspring.

## PSYCHOSOCIAL IMPLICATIONS OF LATER-LIFE PARENTING

Although medical data on the health outcomes of later-life parents are largely negative as compared with their younger peers, health care providers do not make stark recommendations against pursuing parenthood at an age above 40 years. With careful informed consent discussions, clinicians support later-life fathers as they pass on their genes. With careful informed consent discussions and medical management, physicians can assist the majority of later-life mothers through pregnancy and delivery with generally good outcomes. However, delivering a baby places a parent at the starting line of the parenthood journey, a journey that continues in varying intensities for the rest of one's life. In this next section, we turn to the data on the psychosocial implications of delayed parenthood for both parents and their children.

### Advantages and Positive Outcomes

MacDougall, Beyene, and Nachtigall (2012) conducted interviews with 117 parents who had conceived using IVF at age 40 years or older. Like the majority of individuals who are able to pursue this type of advanced fertility treatment, these IVF parents were primarily Caucasian, highly educated, and had a median income three to four times the national average. Of note, the median age of children in this study was 3.5 years, thus only providing insights into early adaptation to parenthood. When queried about their experience of later-life parenting, respondents described many benefits. Exemplifying the maternal maturity hypothesis (Hofferth, 1987) that proposes older mothers' greater life experience promotes a richer family environment, participants described feeling more mature, emotionally ready to parent, and financially secure than they were at an earlier life stage. Parents reported being involved in a strong co-parenting relationship, which allowed each partner to share childcare responsibilities and develop an individual relationship with the child. Parents reported that having children later in life made them feel young longer and motivated them to stay physically fit (MacDougall et al., 2012). Further, participants reported that already having established their careers and solidifying their professional reputations allowed them greater flexibility in juggling work and family. They reported that because they already had achieved many of their personal and professional life goals, it was easier to "re-orient their priorities to spend time and energy with their families" (MacDougall et al., 2012, p. 1060). Overall, they reported having fewer regrets about the sacrifices required by parenting than they likely would have had at an earlier life stage.

In a study assessing parenting satisfaction and behaviors of mothers aged 16 to 38 years whose children were infants, Ragozin et al. (1982) found that compared with mothers in their teens and early 20s, older maternal age was significantly related to greater parenting satisfaction, greater time commitment to the role of parenting, and a more engaged parenting style. Reflecting the "hard to achieve pregnancy" hypothesis (van Balen, 1998), older mothers conceiving children with fertility treatment have reported less parenting stress (Abbey, Andrews, & Halman, 1994) and have demonstrated a warmer, more interactive parenting style (Golombok et al., 1996) as compared with their naturally conceiving peers.

Looking at parental outcomes up to 6 months after the birth of a first child, Guedes and Canavarro (2014) reported few differences in the psychosocial adjustment of a group of mothers 35 years and older (mean age = 37 years [standard deviation, SD = 2.3]) as compared with mothers aged 20 to 34 years. In a study by Boivin et al. (2009), first-time mothers older than 38 years reported no significant differences in levels of anxiety and physical stress as compared with their younger peers. From a methodological perspective, it is important to note that these studies largely focus on mothers still in their 30s with children who are infants or young children.

## Disadvantages and Negative Outcomes

The parents older than 40 years interviewed by MacDougall et al. (2012) also reported a number of disadvantages of parenting later in life. Participants reported that their decision to delay pursuit of parenthood resulted in difficulty conceiving resolved only through expensive, stressful IVF treatment. Women who delay pursuit of motherhood are more likely to face a diagnosis of diminished ovarian reserve, requiring use of donor eggs from a younger woman in order to conceive (ESHRE Capri Workshop Group, 2005). Donor oocyte recipients frequently describe experiencing a mourning process when relinquishing their long-held dream of a genetically related child. Later-life parents fortunate enough to conceive with their own gametes still may experience disappointment at having a smaller family size than originally desired (MacDougall et al., 2012). Once becoming parents, MacDougall et al. report that almost 40% of the mothers and a quarter of the fathers in their sample struggled with a lack of physical energy and reported feeling depleted by the demands of parenthood. One mother stated: "I wish I was 10 years younger...then I would have more energy to keep up with my daughter, but I'm tired" (MacDougall et al., 2012, p. 1062). Counter to the perception that having children later in life would motivate them to stay physically fit, many of these older parents reported a decrease in their own personal exercise routines due to the demands of childcare.

Other studies of delayed conception serve to elucidate the unique social and marital context associated with later-life parenting. Boivin et al. (2009) reported that, compared with their younger peers, individuals who became parents at age 38 years and older expressed and received significantly less warmth in their marital relationship. Pursuing parenthood later in life can trigger a negative response from one's social network, from less peer support to frank social sanctions, resulting in more isolation for older parents (Carlson, 2011). Conducting interviews with 79 couples who conceived using donor oocytes at an average age of 41 years, Friese, Becker, and Nachtigall (2008) found that "the age of the mother worked to mark the family as different from others" (Friese et al., 2008, p. 68). Later-life parents in this sample reported experiencing stigmatizing interactions on the playground or at school, feeling out of place in social situations, finding it more difficult to fit in to the community of mothers, and feeling marginalized at times. Respondents described discomfort at being misidentified as their child's grandmother or at having their use of donor oocytes guessed at by strangers based on their older physical appearance. Parents older than 40 years also report concern that their children will experience social stigma as a result of having older parents (Friese et al., 2008; MacDougall et al., 2012).

From a methodological perspective, it is noteworthy that these parents hailed from Northern California, a demographic region that may be viewed as more progressive and supportive of later-life parenting. It is likely that older parents may feel even more different and experience even more stigma in more traditional or conservative areas where later-life parenting is less common. It will be important to replicate this study to better understand societal attitudes and stigma toward later-life parents in other geographic regions.

With regard to the long-term implications of the choice to pursue parenthood after 40 years, MacDougall et al. (2012) found that 31% of later-life mothers and 19% of later-life fathers reported an increased awareness of the earlier onset of their own "old age" and concerns about having fewer years of life left to spend with their child. Parents reported regret that they might miss important milestones in their child's life, like getting married or having children of their own (Friese et al., 2008). Of note, these parents' concerns about the risks of their own illness and death emerged only *after* the birth of their child. It may be that making risk calculations about the consequences of later-life parenting is difficult to do while in the throes of yearning for a baby and pursuing fertility treatment. Despite a generally positive experience of later-life parenting of young children, two thirds of both later-life fathers and mothers concluded that the optimal age for becoming parents was in the early to mid-30s and 90% believed that individuals should pursue parenthood before age 40 years (MacDougall et al., 2012). Overall, participants in the

MacDougall et al. (2012) study believed that being older made them better parents. However, literature in this area suggests that although becoming a parent too early is associated with poorer outcomes, there are no additional benefits or rising health impacts to becoming a parent beyond age 30 years (Bewley, Davies, & Braude, 2005; Boivin et al., 2009; Mirowsky, 2002; Mirowsky & Ross, 2002).

Turning to the impact of later-life parenting on maternal mood, there have been a number of studies linking older maternal age at first birth to an increased risk of depressive symptoms. Analyzing data from the National Longitudinal Survey of Mature Women, a nationally representative cohort study of 967 U.S. women aged 30 to 44 years, Spence (2008) found a robust association between childbearing after 35 years and depressive symptoms, even after controlling for race, age, and cohort effects. Mirowsky and Ross (2002) identified a curvilinear relationship between depressive symptoms and age at first birth whereby mothers younger than 23 years and older than 36 years showed the highest levels of depressive symptoms. Impact of later-life motherhood on one's physical health was the strongest correlate of depressive symptoms for older mothers.

Carlson (2011) replicated this curvilinear relationship between maternal age and depressive symptoms, but found that the impact of having a child later than one had expected (called a mistimed or nonnormative birth experience) was a better predictor of depressive symptoms than physical health problems. Using self-discrepancy theory and normative life course perspective theory, the author argues that discrepancies between one's expected and one's actual identity can create "negative feelings about one's current and future self" (Carlson, 2011, p. 496). When a woman's life story, especially her timing of becoming a mother, deviates substantially from the path she imagined or desired earlier in life, depressive symptoms can result.

Boivin et al. (2009) also found a relationship between older maternal age and greater depressive symptomatology, which remained significant after controlling for income and education. Interestingly, this relationship became nonsignificant after use of donor oocytes was entered into the multivariate model. The authors hypothesize that onset of menopause, which is associated with both the need for donor oocytes and increased risk of depression, may be the actual mechanism linking advanced maternal age and depression. An alternate hypothesis is that the onset of menopause triggers the need for donor oocytes, which in turn triggers greater long-term depressive symptomatology. It will be important to understand whether later-life mothers conceiving with donor oocytes continue to struggle with the loss of a genetic connection over time.

Unlike many studies described thus far that categorize a woman still in her 30s as "older," Steiner and Paulson (2007) conducted one of the few existing studies on the psychosocial aspects of postmenopausal parenting. The authors recruited 49 patients undergoing IVF age 50 years or older, as well as two matched control groups: women who had undergone IVF in their 30s or 40s, respectively. The authors found no significant between-group differences in mothers' mental functioning, physical functioning, or reported level of parenting stress and, therefore, argued that concerns about extreme advanced maternal age are misguided. Several methodological limitations should be considered when interpreting these data, however. First, the study had a very small sample size, with data available for only 15 mothers in the older-than-50-years group. Second, data were entirely self-reported, raising questions about social desirability and biased reporting. Third, the mean age of the children in the study was 3 years. Ongoing, longitudinal follow-up of these families would provide helpful information about family functioning and outcomes when children are teenagers and parents are in their 60s or 70s.

## Psychosocial Implications for the Children of Later-Life Parents

### Advantages and Positive Outcomes

Rigorous, long-term study of children of parents older than 40 years has not yet been conducted. Studies of delayed conception conclude that waiting until a more mature developmental stage to pursue parenting is associated with a wide range of benefits for children. Specifically, when compared with mothers in their teens or early 20s, mothers aged 30 years or older are more likely to provide a more nurturing, stable home environment, which may produce their children's superior neurocognitive scores and reduced risks of educational underachievement or mental health problems (Fergusson & Woodward, 1999; Saha et al., 2009). It is clearly better for children to have parents who are beyond adolescence and ready to invest themselves in nurturing a child. In contrast to concerns about the implications of later-life motherhood on child outcomes, Boivin et al. (2009) found no significant differences in child well-being in early to middle childhood when comparing first-time mothers aged 38 years and older to younger first-time mothers.

Two older books provide the most detailed and rich qualitative data gathered on the perspectives of children born to later-life parents (Morris, 1988; Yarrow, 1991). The authors conducted interviews with almost 100 adult children born to parents aged 35 years and older. These children reported numerous positive aspects of having older parents, characterizing their parents as devoted to them and to their parenting role. They perceived their parents as having high levels of patience and wisdom. Mirroring the perception of later-life parents themselves, the children felt that their older parents approached childrearing from a place of emotional and financial security.

### Disadvantages and Negative Outcomes

However, these adult children also reported a number of disadvantages of having older parents (Morris, 1988; Yarrow, 1991). Children reported being afraid that their parents would die when they were still young. They described feelings of social stigma and feeling different from their friends with younger parents. Their later-life parents were more likely to be unable to have additional children and themselves have very old parents. As a result, the children reported feelings of loss at having fewer siblings and less connection with very elderly or already deceased grandparents.

Compared with children with younger parents, these children may also face different realities related to the declining health of their later-life parent. Using data from the National Center for Health Statistics, Zweifel et al. (2012) highlight that although a 65-year-old woman may be predicted to have an additional 19 years of life, approximately 30% of those years are likely to involve declining health, increased medical intervention, and diminishing quality of life. These decrements in vitality and functioning may interfere with older parents' ability to meet the daily demands of parenting. In turn, children of later-life parents report having greater caregiving responsibility than their peers (Morris, 1988; Yarrow, 1991). Spence (2008) found that a greater proportion of later-life mothers were likely to have at least one child who lived nearby and assisted with personal, household, or medical care. And as a result of this increased caregiving responsibility, children of later-life parents reported having to make accommodations in their own educational, career, and/or relationship plans (Morris, 1988; Yarrow, 1991). It was harder to go backpacking across Europe or apply for graduate school in another state when one's older parent needed frequent help.

Independent of whether one's parent is vital and active at 70 years or in assisted living, there is one universal consequence of having older parents: the risk of earlier parental death. Using actuarial predictions based on life expectancy data from the National Vital Statistics Reports, Zweifel et al. (2012) estimated that a woman who becomes a mother at the age of 50 years has a 15% chance of death by the child's 20th birthday and is likely to be deceased by the time her child reaches the age of 32 years. Compared with a woman delivering at age 35 years, a woman delivering at 55 years is five times more likely to die by the time her child reaches adolescence (Zweifel, 2015). A man who becomes a father at age 50 years has a 22% chance of death by the child's 20th birthday and is likely to be deceased by the time his child reaches the age of 29 years. Compared with a man who becomes a father at the age of 35 years, a man becoming a father at 55 years is four times more likely to die by the time his child reaches adolescence (Zweifel, 2015). Additionally, the same health conditions that prevented a woman from carrying her pregnancy and created the need for a gestational carrier may in turn contribute to an earlier death once she becomes a parent (Ethics Committee of the ASRM, 2013). These data raise a difficult ethical question for fertility centers: How many anticipated years of life should be considered "enough" for an individual to receive ARTs?

Although parents of any age are not guaranteed the chance to parent their children to adulthood, data on the significant, long-term impact on children resulting from the early death of a parent (particularly death of a mother) must be acknowledged (Howarth, 2011; Rostila & Saarela, 2011; Zweifel, 2015). Children whose parents die at an earlier developmental stage are at increased risk of social problems such as withdrawal from peers and social skill deficits, emotional problems such as depression and low self-confidence, and face higher risks of health problems into adulthood (Biank & Werner-Lin, 2011; Rostila & Saarela, 2011; Zweifel, 2015). Being nurtured through childhood by one's parent and primary caregiver does more than provide a foundation for a child to flourish—it also protects the child from exposure to a traumatic experience that has long-term negative effects. As a result of their experiences growing up, adult children of older parents frequently concluded that they would not follow their parents' example of later-life parenthood and wanted to start their families sooner (Morris, 1988; Yarrow, 1991).

## THE IMPACT OF ELECTIVE OOCYTE CRYOPRESERVATION ON THE PREVALENCE OF LATER-LIFE PARENTING

The advent of elective oocyte cryopreservation (or social egg freezing) may lead to even greater prevalence of later-life parenting. Reclassified as nonexperimental by the American Society for Reproductive Medicine (ASRM) in 2013 (Practice Committee of the ASRM & Practice Committee of the Society for Assisted Reproductive Technology, 2013), this procedure allows women to freeze their eggs to preserve their fertility and postpone parenthood. The procedure has been celebrated as a "great equalizer," allowing women to pursue their career and relationship goals free from the pressure of their biological clocks (Bennett, 2014). Women who elect to freeze their eggs for fertility preservation describe the experience as "empowering" (Hodes-Wertz, Druckenmiller, Smith, & Noyes, 2013) and report that it "takes the pressure off" finding a partner by removing the time limits imposed by the biological clock (Gold, Copperman, Witkin, Jones, & Copperman, 2006). Several high-profile companies (including Apple, Facebook, and Microsoft) now offer employee coverage for fertility preservation. Private egg-freezing companies encourage and help finance elective freezing, even holding promotional "egg-freezing parties" in major cities to recruit eligible women.

Despite the growing public enthusiasm for egg-freezing technology, there is currently no research on the efficacy of social egg freezing for fertility preservation. One study of egg freezing in the context of IVF found that women aged 30 to 36 years required 12.1 frozen eggs to achieve one live birth; for women age 37 to 39 years, the rate was 29.6 frozen eggs per one live birth (Chang et al., 2013). These statistics are sobering considering the average age at which women currently elect to freeze their eggs is 38 (Hodes-Wertz et al., 2013). Keeping in mind that eggs frozen at age 38 years may not be thawed until much later, the rates for successful live birth may be even lower.

Women should be educated about elective cryopreservation as a reproductive option, preferably in their 20s. However, informed consent discussions must include a careful review of risks and costs as well as a realistic assessment of the likely success rates. Furthermore, a woman who chooses elective oocyte cryopreservation must be well informed about the data on later-life parenting. If the medical community gives a young woman the opportunity to freeze her eggs in her 20s or 30s with no understanding of the risks of waiting to thaw them until her 40s or 50s, we have done her a disservice.

## RESEARCH NEEDS

In reviewing the literature thus far, one could point to data suggesting that later-life parents and their children have better outcomes, similar outcomes, and worse outcomes. The problems resulting from the lack of definitional clarity thus become quite clear. One way to make sense of these conflicting conclusions is to hypothesize a curvilinear relationship between parental age and family outcomes. The curvilinear relationship Mirowsky and Ross (2002) have identified between maternal age and depression and health outcomes is likely to be a model that applies to other outcome data. Specifically, if an individual becomes a parent too young, the experience for both parent and child is worse. Worse outcomes are also more likely if an individual becomes a parent too late. Identifying the window associated with optimal parent and child outcomes will require additional systematic and longitudinal research. Furthermore, informing young adults of these data and supporting them in pursuing parenthood in a way that balances biological and societal forces will be vitally important.

Although social scientists have begun to characterize the experiences of later-life parents and their children, additional well-designed studies in this area are critical. First, we need data on the experience of parents beyond their 30s. This age cohort is not typically considered "older" in fertility centers today, where patients in their 40s and 50s comprise a significant proportion of the patient population. Second, we need prospective, longitudinal studies to better elucidate the long-term outcomes associated with later-life parenting. Most studies report data on later-life parenting immediately after birth. The longest follow-up period in the existing literature assessed families with children who were on average only 7 years old (Boivin et al., 2009). It is vitally important to understand the middle childhood and adolescent experiences of these families with later-life parents. For example, how do older adults in their 60s and 70s who are parenting a teenager fare with regard to physical health, depressive symptoms, social support, and parenting stress? How do the teens describe their experiences with older parents? Third, we need to move beyond reliance on self-report measures, which are prone to social desirability and bias, and incorporate observational measures and multiple raters. Fourth, although we have made an effort to include data on outcomes associated with later-life fatherhood, the current data are skewed toward study of older mothers. Inclusion of older fathers will be a critical component of well-designed future research in this area.

Finally, we need to better understand the factors that influence individuals in their 40s and 50s to make the bold choice to begin the journey of parenthood. Rather than continuing to focus on personal fulfillment or professional challenge, what motivates a middle-aged person to pursue a pregnancy? Are motivations similar to those of younger parents or do concerns such as permanently being different from the majority of one's peers or having a caregiver during old age play a more significant role? How well do later-life parents appreciate their increased risk profile and subsequently prepare themselves for this experience? A review of the nascent literature on motivations of older parents is beyond the scope of this chapter, but much work remains to be done to better understand the choices of individuals seeking parenthood later in life.

## RECOMMENDATIONS FOR CLINICIANS AND CARE PROVIDERS

Given that later-life parenthood has been associated with negative as well as positive outcomes for both parents and children, individuals deferring parenthood will need guidance in evaluating the data and applying it to their personal situation. Health care providers should initiate conversations about interest in parenthood and age-related fertility declines during annual well-visit exams, particularly with patients in their mid- to late 20s who likely have more time to adjust the course. Young women interested in elective egg freezing should be informed about the optimal time to both freeze *and thaw* oocytes and given data on emotional and financial costs as well as success rates.

We must inform women about the actual success rates of IVF, especially after age 40 years. Overall, more than 70% of women pursuing IVF do not deliver a healthy baby conceived with their own eggs and this number climbs to 90% when the woman is older than 40 years (Bewley et al., 2005). The authors warn that "the availability of IVF may lull women into infertility while they wait for a suitable partner and concentrate on their careers and achieving security and a comfortable living standard" (Bewley et al., 2005, p. 588). In our experience, it is common for well-educated, professional women to be aware of age-related declines in fertility and to have assumed that fertility treatment, even IVF, would be necessary to help them become parents. However, data about the limits of IVF often come as a shock. Patients subsequently recommended to donor eggs commonly report experiencing a significant grief reaction at the loss of the genetic tie to their child. Women who value maintaining a genetic connection to their child should be aware that a decision to delay motherhood could significantly increase her odds of having to relinquish that connection. We do patients a disservice by having these conversations for the first time only after a diagnosis of diminished ovarian reserve, when timelines and options are already limited.

Health care providers should counsel patients about the high costs of IVF and IVF with donor oocytes, which typically run in the tens of thousands of dollars. Furthermore, patients should be informed about the requirement in many fertility centers to pass a medical evaluation before receiving treatment at age 45 years or older (Bewley et al., 2005; Heffner, 2004). In a review for the *New England Journal of Medicine*, Heffner (2004) writes, "Perimenopausal and postmenopausal pregnancy remains an option for those women who are lucky enough to find themselves healthy and sufficiently wealthy to pursue it" (p. 1929).

For individuals medically and financially able to become later-life parents, Zweifel et al. (2012) outline a series of topics that should be discussed to assist prospective parents in creating a preparedness plan. This consultation, optimally conducted by a mental health professional, should include a review of social supports, plans for coping with sandwich generation issues, and legal guardianship in the event of parental death. It should provide education about how to communicate with one's child about the unique social and emotional aspects of having later-life parents as well as how to disclose use of donor oocytes. It should highlight the difference between number of additional years of life and number of additional years of *healthy* life and resultant importance of regular exercise, medical checkups, and self-care (Zweifel et al., 2012).

Finally, fertility centers should be supported in developing written guidelines regarding age limits for initiating fertility treatment (Zweifel, 2015). As noted previously, the Ethics Committee of the ASRM (2013) concluded that it is permissible to decline treatment to women older than 50 years and that treatment of women older than 55 years should be discouraged. Importantly, however, because these ethics guidelines are focused on minimizing the medical risks of carrying a pregnancy in women of extremely advanced maternal age, they make no mention of age limits for fathers or for couples using both an oocyte donor and gestational carrier. Zweifel et al. (2012) propose that fertility centers offer treatment only if there is a reasonable presumption that the parents will live for at least 20 years. Other centers use combined parental age of 100 years as a cutoff for fertility treatment. Regardless of the actual age limits adopted, fostering discussion among the care providers who work with later-life parents will better serve the unique needs of this expanding population.

## CONCLUSION

A review of the literature on parenting at a later-life stage reveals a mix of both positive and negative outcomes and thus is neither entirely reassuring nor wholly alarming. Individuals who wait to have children until they are adults themselves clearly have better outcomes, as do their children. However, waiting until middle age to parent when one's personal, social, and financial circumstances are more ideal is associated with significant risks for both later-life parents and their children. Although we may circumvent the reproductive biological clock through the use of ARTs and elective oocyte cryopreservation, we have not similarly increased our life expectancy in the past 50 years. Life remains finite, even if reproductive capacity is now less so. It is likely that parental age and family outcomes follow a curvilinear pattern and that there is an optimal window with a finite end point for embarking on parenthood. Additional comprehensive study is needed to delineate this optimal window and elucidate the relative weight of the myriad advantages and disadvantages of later-life parenthood.

## REFERENCES

Abbey, A., Andrews, F. M., & Halman, L. J. (1994). Infertility and parenthood: Does becoming a parent increase well-being? *Journal of Consulting and Clinical Psychology, 62*, 398–403. doi:10.1037/0022–006X.62.2.398

Agid, O., Shapira, B., Zislin, J., Ritsner, M., Hanin, B., Murad, H.,... Lerer, B. (1999). Environment and vulnerability to major psychiatric illness: A case control study of early parental loss in major depression, bipolar disorder and schizophrenia. *Molecular Psychiatry, 4*, 163–172. doi:10.1038/sj.mp.4000473

Alonzo, A. A. (2002). Long-term health consequences of delayed childbirth: NHANES III. *Women's Health Issues, 12*, 37–45. doi:10.1016/S1049–3867(01)00135–9

American College of Obstetricians and Gynecologists Committee on Gynecologic Practice, & the Practice Committee of the American Society for Reproductive Medicine. (2014). Female age-related fertility decline [Committee opinion No. 589]. *Fertility and Sterility, 101*, 633–634. doi:10.1016/j.fertnstert.2013.12.032

Battaglia, D. E., Goodwin, P., Klein, N. A., & Soules, M. R. (1996). Fertilization and early embryology: Influence of maternal age on meiotic spindle assembly oocytes from naturally cycling women. *Human Reproduction, 11*, 2217–2222. doi:10.1093/oxfordjournals.humrep.a019080

Beemsterboer, S. N., Homburg, R., Gorter, N. A., Schats, R., Hompes, P. G. A., & Lambalk, C. B. (2006). The paradox of declining fertility but increasing twinning rates with advancing maternal age. *Human Reproduction, 21*, 1531–1532. doi:10.1093/humrep/del009

Bennett, J. (2014, October 15). Company-paid egg freezing will be the great equalizer. *Time Magazine.* Retrieved from http://time.com

Bewley, S., Davies, M., & Braude, P. (2005). Which career first? *British Medical Journal, 331*, 588–589. doi:10.1136/bmj.331.7517.588

Biank, N. M., & Werner-Lin, A. (2011). Growing up with grief: Revisiting the death of a parent over the life course. *Omega, 63*, 271–290. doi:10.2190/om.63.3.e

Boivin, J., Rice, F., Hay, D., Harold, G., Lewis, A., van den Bree, M. M. B., & Thapar, A. (2009). Associations between maternal older age, family environment and parent and child wellbeing in families using assisted reproductive techniques to conceive. *Social Science & Medicine, 68*, 1948–1955. doi:10.1016/j.socscimed.2009.02.036

Carlson, D. L. (2011). Explaining the curvilinear relationship between age at first birth and depression among women. *Social Science & Medicine, 72*, 494–503. doi:10.1016/j.socscimed.2010.12.001

Chang, C.-C., Elliott, T. A., Wright, G., Shapiro, D. B., Toledo, A. A., & Nagy, Z. P. (2013). Prospective controlled study to evaluate laboratory and clinical outcomes of oocyte vitrification obtained in in vitro fertilization patients aged 30 to 39 years. *Fertility and Sterility, 99*, 1891–1897. doi:10.1016/j.fertnstert.2013.02.008

Chang, J., Elam-Evans, L. D., Berg, C. J., Herndon, J., Flowers, L., Seed, K. A., & Syverson, C. J. (2003). *Pregnancy-related mortality surveillance—United States, 1991–1999* (No. SS-2). Retrieved from http://www.cdc.gov/mmwr/PDF/ss/ss5202.pdf

Cho, C. E., & Norman, M. (2013). Cesarean section and development of the immune system in the offspring. *American Journal of Obstetrics and Gynecology, 208*, 249–254. doi:10.1016/j.ajog.2012.08.009

Cleary-Goldman, J., Malone, F. D., Vidaver, J., Ball, R. H., Nyberg, D. A., Comstock, C. H., . . . D'Alton, M. (2005). Impact of maternal age on obstetric outcome. *Obstetrics & Gynecology, 105*, 983–990. doi:10.1097/01.AOG.0000158118.75532.51

Crow, J. F. (2000). The origins, patterns and implications of human spontaneous mutation. *Nature Reviews Genetics, 1*, 40–47. doi:10.1038/35049558

Durkin, M. S., Maenner, M. J., Newschaffer, C. J., Lee, L.-C., Cunniff, C. M., Daniels, J. L., . . . Schieve, L. A. (2008). Advanced parental age and the risk of autism spectrum disorder. *American Journal of Epidemiology, 168*, 1268–1276. doi:10.1093/aje/kwn250

Ecker, J. L., Chen, K. T., Cohen, A. P., Riley, L. E., & Lieberman, E. S. (2001). Increased risk of cesarean delivery with advancing maternal age: Indications and associated factors in nulliparous women. *American Journal of Obstetrics and Gynecology, 185*, 883–887. doi:10.1067/mob.2001.117364

ESHRE Capri Workshop Group. (2005). Fertility and ageing. *Human Reproduction Update, 11*, 261–276. doi:10.1093/humupd/dmi006

Ethics Committee of the American Society for Reproductive Medicine. (2013). Oocyte or embryo donation to women of advanced age: A committee opinion. *Fertility and Sterility, 100*, 337–340. doi:10.1016/j.fertnstert.2013.02.030

Fergusson, D. M., & Woodward, L. J. (1999). Maternal age and educational and psychosocial outcomes in early adulthood. *Journal of Child Psychology and Psychiatry, 40*, 479–489. doi:10.1111/1469-7610.00464

Ford, W. C. L., North, K., Taylor, H., Farrow, A., Hull, M. G. R., & Golding, J. (2000). Increasing paternal age is associated with delayed conception in a large population of fertile couples: Evidence for declining fecundity in older men. *Human Reproduction, 15*, 1703–1708. doi:10.1093/humrep/15.8.1703

Frans, E. M., Sandin, S., Reichenberg, A., Lichtenstein, P., Långström, N., & Hultman, C. M. (2008). Advancing paternal age and bipolar disorder. *Archives of General Psychiatry, 65*, 1034–1040. doi:10.1001/archpsyc.65.9.1034

Frattarelli, J. L., Miller, K. A., Miller, B. T., Elkind-Hirsch, K., & Scott, R. T., Jr. (2008). Male age negatively impacts embryo development and reproductive outcome in donor oocyte assisted reproductive technology cycles. *Fertility and Sterility, 90*, 97–103. doi:10.1016/j.fertnstert.2007.06.009

Friese, C., Becker, G., & Nachtigall, R. D. (2008). Older motherhood and the changing life course in the era of reproductive technologies. *Journal of Aging Studies, 22*, 65–73. doi:10.1016/j.jaging.2007.05.009

Gilbert, W. M., Young, A. L., & Danielsen, B. (2007). Pregnancy outcomes in women with chronic hypertension: A population-based study. *The Journal of Reproductive Medicine, 52*, 1046–1051.

Gold, E., Copperman, K., Witkin, G., Jones, C., & Copperman, A. B. (2006). P-187: A motivational assessment of women undergoing elective egg freezing for fertility preservation [Supplemental material]. *Fertility and Sterility, 86,* S201. doi:10.1016/j.fertnstert.2006.07.537

Golombok, S., Brewaeys, A., Cook, R., Giavazzi, M. T., Guerra, D., Mantovani, A., . . . Dexeus, S. (1996). The European study of assisted reproduction families: Family functioning and child development. *Human Reproduction, 11,* 2324–2331. doi:10.1093/oxfordjournals .humrep.a019098

Guedes, M., & Canavarro, M. C. (2014). Psychosocial adjustment of couples to first-time parenthood at advanced maternal age: An exploratory longitudinal study. *Journal of Reproductive and Infant Psychology, 32,* 425–440. doi:10.1080/02646838.2014.962015

Hansen, A. K., Wisborg, K., Uldbjerg, N., & Henriksen, T. B. (2008). Risk of respiratory morbidity in term infants delivered by elective caesarean section: Cohort study. *BMJ, 336,* 85–87. doi:10.1136/bmj.39405.539282.BE

Heffner, L. J. (2004). Advanced maternal age—How old is too old? *New England Journal of Medicine, 351*(19), 1927–1929. doi:10.1056/NEJMp048087

Hodes-Wertz, B., Druckenmiller, S., Smith, M., & Noyes, N. (2013). What do reproductive-age women who undergo oocyte cryopreservation think about the process as a means to preserve fertility? *Fertility and Sterility, 100,* 1343–1349. doi:10.1016/j.fertnstert.2013.07.201

Hofferth, S. L. (1987). The children of teen childbearers. In S. L. Hofferth & C. D. Hayes (Eds.), *Risking the future: Adolescent sexuality, pregnancy, and childbearing: Volume II Working papers* (pp. 174–206). Washington, DC: National Academies Press.

Howarth, R. A. (2011). Promoting the adjustment of parentally bereaved children. *Journal of Mental Health Counseling, 33,* 21–32. doi:10.17744/mehc.33.1.a2m06x0835352741

Jacobsson, B., Ladfors, L., & Milsom, I. (2004). Advanced maternal age and adverse perinatal outcome. *Obstetrics & Gynecology, 104,* 727–733. doi:10.1097/01.AOG.0000140682.63746.be

Liu, Y., Zhi, M., & Li, X. (2011). Parental age and characteristics of the offspring. *Ageing Research Reviews, 10,* 115–123. doi:10.1016/j.arr.2010.09.004

MacDougall, K., Beyene, Y., & Nachtigall, R. D. (2012). "Inconvenient biology": Advantages and disadvantages of first-time parenting after age 40 using *in vitro* fertilization. *Human Reproduction, 27,* 1058–1065. doi:10.1093/humrep/des007

Martin, J. A., Hamilton, B. E., Sutton, P. D., Ventura, S. J., Mathews, T. J., & Osterman, M. J. K. (2010). *Births: Final data for 2008* (National Vital Statistics Reports Vol. 59, No. 1). Retrieved from http://www.cdc.gov/nchs/data/nvsr/nvsr59/nvsr59_01.pdf

Matthews, T. J., & Hamilton, B. E. (2009). *Delayed childbearing: More women are having their first child later in life* (NCHS Data Brief No. 21). Retrieved from http://www.cdc.gov/nchs/ data/databriefs/db21.pdf

McIntosh, G. C., Olshan, A. F., & Baird, P. A. (1995). Paternal age and the risk of birth defects in offspring. *Epidemiology, 6,* 282–288. doi:10.1097/00001648-199505000-00016

Mills, T. A., & Lavender, T. (2011). Advanced maternal age. *Obstetrics, Gynaecology and Reproductive Medicine, 21,* 107–111. doi:10.1016/j.ogrm.2010.12.003

Mirowsky, J. (2002). Parenthood and health: The pivotal and optimal age at first birth. *Social Forces, 81,* 315–349. doi:10.1353/sof.2002.0055

Mirowsky, J., & Ross, C. E. (2002). Depression, parenthood, and age at first birth. *Social Science & Medicine, 54,* 1281–1298. doi:10.1016/S0277-9536(01)00096-X

Morris, M. (1988). *Last-chance children: Growing up with older parents.* New York, NY: Columbia University Press.

Myrskylä, M., Elo, I. T., Kohler, I. V., & Martikainen, P. (2014). The association between advanced maternal and paternal ages and increased adult mortality is explained by early parental loss. *Social Science & Medicine, 119,* 215–223. doi:10.1016/j.socscimed.2014.06.008

Practice Committee of the American Society for Reproductive Medicine, & Practice Committee of the Society for Assisted Reproductive Technology. (2013). Mature oocyte cryopreservation: A guideline. *Fertility and Sterility, 99,* 37–43. doi:10.1016/j .fertnstert.2012.09.028

Ragozin, A. S., Basham, R. B., Crnic, K. A., Greenberg, M. T., & Robinson, N. M. (1982). Effects of maternal age on parenting role. *Developmental Psychology, 18*, 627–634. doi:10.1037/0012-1649.18.4.627

Rostila, M., & Saarela, J. M. (2011). Time does not heal all wounds: Mortality following the death of a parent. *Journal of Marriage and Family, 73*, 236–249. doi:10.1111/j.1741-3737.2010.00801.x

Rowe, T. (2006). Fertility and a woman's age. *The Journal of Reproductive Medicine, 51*, 157–163.

Saha, S., Barnett, A. G., Foldi, C., Burne, T. H., Eyles, D. W., Buka, S. L., & McGrath, J. J. (2009). Advanced paternal age is associated with impaired neurocognitive outcomes during infancy and childhood. *PLoS Medicine, 6*(3), e1000040. doi:10.1371/journal.pmed.1000040

Slama, R., Bouyer, J., Windham, G., Fenster, L., Werwatz, A., & Swan, S. H. (2005). Influence of paternal age on the risk of spontaneous abortion. *American Journal of Epidemiology, 161*, 816–823. doi:10.1093/aje/kwi097

Spence, N. J. (2008). The long-term consequences of childbearing: Physical and psychological well-being of mothers in later life. *Research on Aging, 30*, 722–751. doi:10.1177/0164027508322575

Steiner, A. Z., & Paulson, R. J. (2007). Motherhood after age 50: An evaluation of parenting stress and physical functioning. *Fertility and Sterility, 87*, 1327–1332. doi:10.1016/j.fertnstert.2006.11.074

Sutcliffe, A., Barnes, J., Belsky, J., Gardiner, J., & Melhuish, E. (2012). Health of children born to older mothers in the UK. *Archives of Disease in Childhood, 97*(Suppl. 1), A98–A99. doi:10.1136/archdischild-2012-301885.233

Toriello, H. V., & Meck, J. M. (2008). Statement on guidance for genetic counseling in advanced paternal age. *Genetics in Medicine, 10*, 457–460. doi:10.1097/GIM.0b013e318176fabb

van Balen, F. (1998). Development of IVF children. *Developmental Review, 18*, 30–46. doi:10.1006/drev.1997.0446

Vitthala, S., Gelbaya, T. A., Brison, D. R., Fitzgerald, C. T., & Nardo, L. G. (2009). The risk of monozygotic twins after assisted reproductive technology: A systematic review and meta-analysis. *Human Reproduction Update, 15*, 45–55. doi:10.1093/humupd/dmn045

Wang, M. L., Dorer, D. J., Fleming, M. P., & Catlin, E. A. (2004). Clinical outcomes of near-term infants. *Pediatrics, 114*, 372–376. doi:10.1542/peds.114.2.372

Whitcomb, B. W., Turzanski-Fortner, R., Richter, K. S., Kipersztok, S., Stillman, R. J., Levy, M. J., & Levens, E. D. (2011). Contribution of male age to outcomes in assisted reproductive technologies. *Fertility and Sterility, 95*, 147–151. doi:10.1016/j.fertnstert.2010.06.039

Williams, S., McGee, R., Olaman, S., & Knight, R. (1997). Level of education, age of bearing children and mental health of women. *Social Science & Medicine, 45*, 827–836. doi:10.1016/S0277-9536(96)00423-6

Wohl, M., & Gorwood, P. (2007). Paternal ages below or above 35 years old are associated with a different risk of schizophrenia in the offspring. *European Psychiatry, 22*, 22–26. doi:10.1016/j.eurpsy.2006.08.007

Yarrow, A. L. (1991). *Latecomers: Children of parents over 35*. New York, NY: Free Press.

Yogev, Y., Melamed, N., Bardin, R., Tenenbaum-Gavish, K., Ben-Shitrit, G., & Ben-Haroush, A. (2010). Pregnancy outcome at extremely advanced maternal age. *American Journal of Obstetrics & Gynecology, 203*(6), 558.e1–e7. doi:10.1016/j.ajog.2010.07.039

Zweifel, J. E. (2015). Last chance or too late? Counseling prospective older parents. In S. N. Covington (Ed.), *Fertility counseling: Clinical guide and case studies* (pp. 150–165). Cambridge, England: Cambridge University Press.

Zweifel, J. E., Covington, S. N., & Applegarth, L. D. (2012). "Last-chance kids": A good deal for older parents—But what about the children? *Sexuality, Reproduction and Menopause, 10*(2), 4–12.

# CHAPTER 9

# UNDERSTANDING THE IMPACT OF DELAYED PARENTING: GENDER, PAID WORK, AND WORK–FAMILY STRATEGIES

*Tiffany Romain and Robert D. Nachtigall*

In order to understand men's and women's changing experiences with work and family, scholars have frequently employed gender as an analytic lens that reveals a dynamic set of social relations in which hierarchies and power inequalities are practiced, produced, resisted, and performed by individuals, institutions, and societies (see Ferree, 2010, for a review). Prior to the mid-20th century, industrial societies were largely, although not exclusively, organized around divisions between public and private spheres, with men assigned to the former through paid work and public participation, and women the latter through caring for the family and home (Potuchek, 1997). Discourses about how men and women ought to spend their time permeated these divisions (Daly, 1996), such that by the 1950s, the male breadwinner earning a "family salary" was the ideological norm, at least among the White middle class in the United States (Bernard, 1981). The past half-century has witnessed social, cultural, economic, and demographic changes that have challenged and disrupted notions of how men and women should engage in and experience paid work. Nevertheless, even as ideologies of gender and labor transform, structures of employment have remained stubbornly predicated on workers choosing either the workplace or family as if the two domains were not intrinsically interrelated (Christensen & Schneider, 2011).

The resurgence of the women's movement and the enforcement of equal employment laws in the late 1960s and early 1970s marked a period of change in cultural understandings of and social attitudes toward women's participation in previously male-dominated occupations and supported an historical shift in women's opportunities in the workplace (Potuchek, 1997). Even so, studies of working women in the 1970s and 1980s demonstrate that women employed full time also performed a "second shift" of domestic work so that the total quantity of work women performed—paid and unpaid—surpassed that of men (Brines, 1994; Hochschild & Machung, 2003). Since then, men have increased their time spent on housework and parenting (Bianchi, Robinson, & Milkie, 2006; Parker & Wang, 2013), particularly among highly educated men (Craig & Mullen, 2010), and over time, men and women have increasingly sought more egalitarian marriages or partnerships

(Blair-Loy, 2001; Gerson, 2002, 2009). Nevertheless, when men and women become parents in the United States, women are more likely to reduce paid work hours and increase participation in unpaid housework and caregiving, whereas men are more likely to increase paid work hours, resulting in an employment gender gap that is more pronounced among parents than nonparents (Craig & Mullen, 2010; Pew Research Center, 2013). Yet, mothers continue to spend more time on all work combined than do fathers, despite trends toward greater equity (Sayer, 2005; Yavorsky, Kamp Dush, & Schoppe-Sullivan, 2015).

Since the 1950s, the percentage of American family households in which all adults work has increased due to rising rates of divorce, increasing rates of single motherhood among the poor and nonpoor, and a steady growth in dual-earner families (Bianchi et al., 2006). This has resulted in more women and men carrying responsibility for both earning an income and caring for children (Gerson & Jacobs, 2004). At the same time, changes in the workplace have often been in conflict with the needs of families; for example, employees in the United States are rarely paid enough to support a family on a single salary, and thus the former normative ideal of a single-earner household has become less attainable (Gerson, 2002). Employment trends are also moving away from the legal standard of 40 hours per week, such that full-time workers are spending more time at work and part-time workers are not getting as much work as they need (Negrey, 2012). Both sides of this trend are putting increased pressure on those who must also care for children (Gerson & Jacobs, 2004; Negrey, 2012). Studies have also shown that women are less likely than men to experience flexible work hours, which poses significant challenges for working mothers in particular (Peterson & Wiens-Tuers, 2014), and working parents of young children, both men and women, are experiencing a sense of always being rushed and pressed for time (Craig & Mullen, 2009; Parker & Wang, 2013).

Even though women's participation in the workforce has risen, their earnings still fall below those of men (Getz, 2010; National Partnership for Women and Families, 2011). Furthermore, research comparing women with children to those without demonstrates that mothers across all income and education levels in the United States are subject to a lifelong wage penalty that has been estimated at 5% in earnings for each child (Correll, Benard, & Paik, 2007). This "motherhood penalty" begins with the birth of their first child (Budig & Hodges, 2010) and is especially pronounced for lower income women (Correll et al., 2007). While women are penalized for their parental status, fathers tend to work more hours than men without children (Parker & Wang, 2013), and often see greater career advancement than their childless male coworkers (Correll et al., 2007; Glauber, 2008; Mason & Goulden, 2002).

A demographic shift toward later parenthood, particularly among highly educated women, has taken place in the United States and Europe over the past several decades (Billari, Kohler, Andersson, & Lundström, 2007). One out of every five American women is now having her first child after the age of 35 years, an eightfold increase over the previous generation (Martin et al., 2009). This demographic trend has been linked to a variety of factors including the availability and use of contraception and abortion, increasing educational opportunities for women, women's expanding presence in the workforce, changing notions of family and marriage, insufficient institutional support for working parents, shifting models of adulthood, and the availability of advanced reproductive technology to achieve pregnancy later in life (Franklin & McKinnon, 2001; Fry & Cohn, 2010; Furstenberg, 2010; Leridon & Slama, 2008; Wu & MacNeill, 2002).

This chapter focuses on the intersection of delayed parenting, gender, and work among men and women who became parents when the woman was 40 years of age or older and who required in vitro fertilization (IVF) in order to conceive. Many of the challenges associated with parenting small children while in the early stages of career building have been well described (Hewlett, 2004; Mason & Goulden, 2002), and the economic benefits of delaying motherhood have been established (Buckles, 2008; Miller, 2010). This chapter contributes to the recent literature on work and family (see Bianchi & Milkie, 2010) by examining the experiences of men and women who delayed parenthood to the outer boundary of a woman's reproductive life. Based on qualitative data, it offers insight into how "late-parents" understand and negotiate work environments, caregiving, and gendered expectations about forms of labor. It also describes an increasing dependence on advanced reproductive technology amid demographic shifts toward delayed first-time parenthood.

## METHOD

This chapter draws on exploratory qualitative research conducted in 2009 to 2011 on the experiences of later-life parenting after IVF. We recruited respondents for this study through two large fertility centers in Northern California that sent letters on our behalf to former patients who had conceived their first child with IVF when the woman was at least 40 years of age. Partners' ages were not specified. All participants were interviewed twice, with approximately 3 months between interviews. For couples in which both members agreed to participate, the initial interview was conducted with both partners together and the second interview was conducted with each separately in order to collect data on how couples jointly perceived their parenting experiences and to allow individuals to discuss differences privately. The interviews were conducted in person, with the exception of those with families that had moved out of the metropolitan area, which were conducted by phone. The interviews were semi-structured with open-ended questions. Each interview lasted 1 to 2 hours and was audio-recorded and transcribed. The attrition rate between the first and second interview was 2%.

Using qualitative data analysis methods (Mays & Pope, 2000), the research team engaged in a systematic process of coding interview transcripts in order to identify and compare themes, both those about which we asked direct questions and those that were unanticipated but emerged from our data. The research team conducted successive phases of trial coding until coders reached a high level of agreement (Pope, Ziebland, & Mays, 2000). Then, the entire dataset was coded using Atlas.ti (Muhr, 1993–2011).

The findings in this chapter are derived from an analysis of participants' responses to, and any ad hoc discussion of, questions about how parenting roles and responsibilities were divided; how parenting responsibilities were balanced with other aspects of life; how parenting affected career and career trajectory; if and how career influenced timing of parenthood; what effects, if any, parenting had on changes in identity; and what, if any, policy recommendations could be made to support first-time parents in their 40s or that would affect the timing of parenthood. We looked for patterns in how participants thought about, understood, and interpreted their decisions and practices. These patterns and emergent themes were then analyzed for gender relationships.

The "Career" and "Parenting Roles" codes were also analyzed in conjunction with demographic information collected outlining individual occupation, amount of time spent in paid work at the time of the interview (i.e., full time, part time, none), and the total income of the household. Using the Nam–Boyd Occupational Status Scale (Nam & Boyd, 2004), we interpreted the status of each participant's occupation based on self-reported occupation in combination with interview material that further described previous and current employment. We then compared the occupational status of each participant with that of his or her partner to determine which member of a couple, if any, had the higher status occupation. Finally, we examined relationships between the relative occupational status of each member of a couple and which member, if any, reduced paid employment after the birth of their child.

The 61 families included in the study were composed of 51 heterosexual couples, four lesbian couples, and six single women. The median age of participants at the birth of the IVF-conceived child was 42 years for women and 43 years for men. In seven families, male partners had older children from previous relationships that ranged in age from 9 to 36 years. The women in our study were highly educated with 35% holding college degrees and 58% holding postgraduate degrees. The men were also highly educated, but less so than the women: 47% held college degrees and 35% held postgraduate degrees. Prior to having children, all of our participants engaged in paid work full time, but at the time of our interviews, 80% of the men were employed full time, 16% part time, and 4% were not employed, whereas 52% of the women were employed full time, 23% part time, and 25% were not employed. The majority of participants were Caucasian, employed, married, identified as a member of a religious group, and reported median family incomes of $150,000 to $199,000. Most families had one child via IVF, the median age of which was 3.5 years. The median age of participants at the time of interview was 46 for women and 45 for men (ranges: 41–51 for women and 38–71 for men). The demographic description of our participants is detailed in Table 9.1.

## FINDINGS

We identified four overarching themes related to the impact of late parenting on paid work. First, although participants had previously ranked their education and experiences in the workplace as the main focus in their day-to-day lives, after they had children, they prioritized parenthood over paid work and found parenting to have greater meaning. Second, participants believed that their dedication of many years to education and career had resulted in job mastery, work seniority, trust, and respect among colleagues, and the development of strong professional networks. This in turn allowed them to implement a variety of strategies to balance the demands of work and family life including reducing work hours, placing

TABLE 9.1 Study Demographics

|  |  | NO. | %[a] |
|---|---|---|---|
| Participants | Total | 107 | 100 |
|  | Men | 42 | 39 |
|  | Women | 65 | 61 |
| Partnership | Heterosexual couples | 51 | 80 |
|  | Lesbian couples | 4 | 7 |
|  | Single women | 6 | 10 |
| Children | Median number of children per family[b] | 1 (1–3) | |
|  | Median age of first child[b] | 3.5 (>1–0)[c] | |
| Median age at birth of first child | Men[b] | 43 (35–67)[c] | |
|  | Women | 42 (40–46)[c] | |
| Ethnicity[d] | Caucasian | 96 | 83 |
|  | African American | 2 | 2 |
|  | Pacific Islander | 1 | 1 |
|  | Asian | 6 | 5 |
|  | Middle Eastern | 5 | 4 |
| Household income | $50,000–74,999 | 1 | 2 |
|  | $75,000–99,999 | 4 | 7 |
|  | $100,000–149,999 | 11 | 18 |
|  | $150,000–199,999 | 17 | 28 |
|  | $200,000–249,999 | 8 | 13 |
|  | More than $250,000 | 19 | 31 |
|  | Not reported | 1 | 2 |
| Education: men[e] | High school | 1 | 2 |
|  | Some college | 8 | 16 |
|  | College | 24 | 47 |
|  | Postgraduate | 18 | 35 |
| Education: women | High school | – | 0 |
|  | Some college | 4 | 6 |
|  | College | 23 | 35 |
|  | Postgraduate | 38 | 58 |

(continued)

TABLE 9.1  Study Demographics  (*continued*)

|  |  | NO. | %[a] |
|---|---|---|---|
| Employment: men[e] | No paid work | 2 | 4 |
|  | Part-time employment | 8 | 16 |
|  | Full-time employment | 41 | 80 |
| Employment: total women | No paid work | 16 | 25 |
|  | Part-time employment | 15 | 23 |
|  | Full-time employment | 34 | 52 |
| Employment: heterosexual, coupled women | No paid work | 15 | 29 |
|  | Part-time employment | 14 | 27 |
|  | Full-time employment | 22 | 43 |
| Employment: lesbian, coupled women | No paid work | 1 | 12.5 |
|  | Part-time employment | 1 | 12.5 |
|  | Full-time employment | 6 | 75 |
| Employment: single women | No paid work | – | 0 |
|  | Part-time employment | – | 0 |
|  | Full-time employment | 6 | 100 |

[a]Not all category percentages sum up to 100%.
[b]Excluding children from men's previous relationships.
[c]Reporting as median age not as number.
[d]Including all adult members of each of the 61 family units.
[e]Counting 51 men total, including 42 men who were interviewed and 10 men who declined to participate directly but whose partners were interviewed.

limits on work-related commitments, and implementing flexible work scheduling. Third, although couples believed in the principles of gender equality and equity in marriage, women reduced their paid employment more than men, despite their higher educational achievements and regardless of their relative occupational status. Finally, both men and women identified a tension between the demands of the workplace and those of caregiving and recommended family-friendly workplace policies such as "meaningful" part-time work, job sharing, protected maternity/paternity/leave policies, and on-site childcare.

## Parenting Expectations, the Value of Parenting, and Career

Prior to giving birth to their first child, all of our participants engaged in paid work. The majority of men and women in our study worked in middle- and upper level management, law, marketing, biomedicine, software engineering, or sales (real estate, cars, insurance, and software), but participants also included artists, carpenters, chefs, courier personnel, editors, finance workers, firefighters, researchers, executive recruiters, military personnel, pilots, police officers, professors, scientists, steelworkers, teachers, and writers. Notably, the vast majority of both men and women described their current or former paid work as a "career" rather than as a "job." These participants explained that throughout their 20s and 30s, their work life had been both the primary focus of their time and energy as well as the underpinning of their social and personal identity. For example, a 42-year-old mother and former health care manager said, "I realize now how so much of my identity came from working and all of that." Similarly, a 41-year-old single mother with an executive-level position self-consciously referred to her transgression of traditional gender roles saying, "I'm very manlike in that much of my ego is caught up in what I do and my job."

Yet almost all participants in our study explained that once they became parents, children and family became their new "top priority" and the focal point of their time, energy, and sense of self. This shift in priorities was related not only to a reallocation of the activities that took up their time but also which daily activities they found meaningful. Although prioritizing children is by no means unique to this cohort, our participants often described an enhanced sense of pleasure and even enchantment that they attributed to having become parents at a late age. For example, a female full-time judge, aged 51 years, said

> We become skeptical and cynical by this age if there's not a child
> around. When he comes down at Christmas and sees the tree for
> the first time and there's that just unabashed wonder, that's just
> incredible.... It's just absolute delight.

Participants claimed that parenting made them happier and fostered new kinds of reflection on themselves and the world. Some parents expressed that having a child transformed them through the experience of unconditional love. They often explained that having a career helped develop self-assuredness, but parenting helped develop compassion for others.

Many participants described their strong desire to be active caregivers, and wondered if their wish to be actively involved was related to having delayed parenthood. For example, this 47-year-old mother and part-time product manager stated:

> I waited so long to have her,... other than my own family, I'm not
> letting anybody else raise her. My father-in-law says, "For your
> present, here's a check. Go hire a night nurse for a month." And I said,
> "No.... It's part of being a parent. Why do you let somebody else do
> it?" ... Whereas our neighbor, who's younger, had a baby and they had
> a night nurse. I just felt that at my age I wanted a child so badly that
> I wanted to be a mom. I didn't want to outsource. I'd rather give up on
> other things than to give up the experience.

Many participants utilized outside resources such as family members, nannies, day cares, and preschools for help with childcare, but the desire to immerse oneself in the experiences of parenting was typical of the entire study population.

The fathers in our study also expressed the desire to be "hands-on," involved parents, which they frequently attributed to their emotional maturity and career flexibility. This was especially evident among the seven fathers in our study who had children from earlier relationships. These men compared their current and previous parenting experiences as being quite different emotionally and behaviorally, such as this 53-year-old physician:

> I enjoy it more this time.... It's just a different time in my life.... With my older kids,... I was more busy working, and... their mother and a younger sister who lived with us did most of the caring. And with [young son], it's more shared evenly and I'm much more directly involved in the day-to-day, which I like. So I guess my priorities are different now. So I feel like I'm really making the most of it, not missing anything this time.

Indeed, all of the second-time fathers described being far more involved with their younger children and cited less intense work demands, more egalitarian marital dynamics, a new perspective on life, and the desire for new experiences.

Our participants expressed some concerns about being older parents. They often felt fatigued, which they attributed to their age. They also expressed a heightened sense of mortality and felt saddened by the perception of having less of their lifetime to spend with their children with the possibility of not living to see their grandchildren. Aside from these concerns, however, both men and women in our study felt distinctly well prepared, emotionally and financially, to devote time, energy, and resources to parenting because of their accumulated life experience.

## Strategies to Manage Work and Family Time

We identified three primary strategies that participants used to manage or combine paid work with caregiving. The predominant strategy was to significantly reduce the amount of total time the household devoted to paid work. In approximately three quarters of couples, one partner reduced paid work from full time to part time or no work. This strategy is addressed in greater detail in a later section (Gender, Reductions in Paid Work, and Structural Inequality). We observed two additional strategies among full-time working participants: placing limits on work-related commitments and implementing flexible work scheduling.

### Placing Limits on Work-Related Commitments

Men and women who were employed full time described reducing the extra effort that they had previously devoted to work in order to redirect their time, energy, and mental focus to their family life. Sometimes these limits were thought to be temporary, until children were in school, and other times they were described as a permanent change in attitude toward work. Placing limits was exemplified by reducing travel, refusing long commutes, minimizing overtime hours, taking on fewer extra work responsibilities, foregoing promotions, and carving out circumscribed time for caregiving. Those who described setting limits almost always described the change in work-related behavior as welcome and positive. For example, a lawyer who has a retired, stay-at-home husband said, "I've...very voluntarily cut back on a lot of the extra things I used to do. The benefit of being an older parent is that...I don't feel like I'm damaging my career."

All of the single women in our study remained in full-time work, but they set limits nevertheless, such as this executive, age 41 years:

> I have my son on my calendar from 6:30 p.m. to 7:30 p.m. So I say, I can take calls at 8:00 p.m. I can take calls at 9:00 p.m. I can take calls at 10:00 p.m. I don't care. I'm happy to talk to Singapore at 11 o'clock at night but I will not answer the phone from 6:30 p.m. to 7:30 p.m. So everyone knows that.... [These are] hard lines that I never drew before. I don't get to the office until 8:15, 8:30 in the morning now.

The single women were in the position of having to remain in full-time work to make financial ends meet, and yet, because they were also sole caregivers, they felt they had to place limits on paid work wherever possible.

The full-time working participants who did not report placing limits on work-related commitments all had spouses who worked only part time or not at all. Moreover, participants with stay-at-home spouses were less likely to report placing limits at work. In addition, these participants were more likely to report that their career ambition was just as strong as it had been before becoming a parent. In other words, those with spouses dedicated to childcare had the time and energy to continue working at full tilt and the freedom to remain ambitious, if they chose to.

## Flexible Work Scheduling

Like the mother taking calls late into the night, a large number of full-time working participants reported taking advantage of flexible work hours in order to create more family time. Implementing flexible scheduling was exemplified by working from home after the children were asleep and/or shifting work hours to earlier or later in the day to accommodate mealtimes, bedtimes, or taking a child to school. In a typical example, a 44-year-old full-time market researcher working from home described how flexible hours allowed her to divide her time and to shape her work schedule around the needs of others in her household:

> Sometimes I haven't finished work and I stop at 5:00 when the nanny goes home, and I come out and I hang out with my son, feed him, give him a bath, whatever....And then sometimes I have dinner with my husband and go back to work or get up really early and work. So I just have to figure out how to portion my time so everybody gets some.

Despite the intrusion on home life that flexible work hours can produce, working parents identified that having scheduling flexibility was not only a valuable benefit, but was perceived to be a privilege available only to those who were self-employed or those whose work histories had established a high level of trust by their employer.

We also found that when one partner's work schedule was flexible, the other partner could devote more concentrated time to their work. For example, this 44-year-old production director's work life changed very little with the birth of her son because of her husband's flexible and part-time schedule: "I do think I can balance it all right now....I think with him being a little more flexible in his job, it allows me to perhaps excel a little bit more."

An adjunct to implementing flexible hours was multitasking, an effort to parent while working. For example, one father, a 47-year-old scientist and consultant, said, "I like to drive the kids to school, and I like to pick them up whenever I can, and so inevitably I'll have a conference call that'll start, and I'll be on it. I'll get the kids in the car, be on it, drive them to school, drop them off, and I'll be on it the whole time." Similarly, one mother described sending work e-mails while playing with her toddler. These particular parents viewed multitasking to be a productive extension of both family and work time. In contrast, other parents, such as the mother who scheduled an hour every evening to be with her son, deliberately turned off their cell phones or put aside their work during family time.

Our participants believed that the potential negative effect on their work life of each of these strategies was minimized because successful career building had preceded parenting in their life course. Both men and women explained how being established professionally before having children enabled them to shift their personal priorities from work to family. Participants explained that the time they had invested in career development in their 20s and 30s had earned them mastery over their job, some level of seniority at work, trust and respect among colleagues, and professional networks that would ensure future employment. These workplace advancements contributed not only to job satisfaction but also to concrete benefits that helped to support family life such as financial security, job stability, accumulated sick/vacation days, and leverage to negotiate for flexible or reduced hours.

Almost all of our participants felt that these strategies for managing work and family played out very differently for themselves than for younger parents, not only because older parents were in the unique position of not having to split their attention between establishing a career and taking care of a family, but because this position enabled and supported a shifting of personal priorities. For example, a part-time orthodontist, now 48 years, who spent her early adulthood in college, graduate school, and establishing her private practice, said, "When you have your family more toward the end of your life or the end of your career, you've already done your career and it's not going to be your top priority." Participants also believed they were sacrificing less in professional development and income and had more time for parenting because of career stability than younger parents. Nevertheless, some full-time working participants who were placing limits on work-related commitments or using flexible work hours were still concerned about damaging future career prospects. These participants were willing to sacrifice further career advancement because of what they had already achieved and because they desired to be involved parents, but they were also disappointed that future opportunities depended on continual devotion to the workplace, even after two decades of career development.

## Gender, Reductions in Paid Work, and Structural Inequality

The most common strategy for managing paid work and family was for one or both parents to reduce the number of hours of paid work. In approximately three quarters of couples, one parent reduced their workload from full time to either part time or no work. Aside from the couples in which one partner was laid off or ready to retire, couples reported that they made the pragmatic decision that the higher earner would maintain full-time work in order to maximize the household's earnings. Ultimately, however, the reductions were far from gender neutral. Only 52% of women were working full time at the time of our interviews, whereas 80% of men worked full time. These differences are especially pronounced when comparing the 51 men in our study to their partners: of the coupled, heterosexual women, only 43% worked full time. That is, almost three times as many coupled, heterosexual women reduced their work than did their partners. In contrast, all six single mothers remained in full-time occupations, and the four lesbian couples were more fully employed than the heterosexual coupled women: six remained fully employed, one reduced to part time, and one stopped working to stay home with her child.

When comparing the occupational status of people within couples, we found that the parent in the lower status job reduced paid work except when the higher occupational status partner was looking for a "life change" or when the partner with the lower status job had high enough earnings to support the family. We found evidence of structural inequality in that the men in our study were often in higher paying and higher status occupations than their partners, despite the women's greater educational achievements. As a result of their lower income, women were more likely to reduce paid work. However, pragmatism alone did not dictate which partner reduced paid work. We found cases in which the person in the higher status job reduced paid work rather than his or her partner, and of these, the women were roughly twice as likely as the men to have reduced their workload. Strikingly, of the 21 couples in which men and women had equal status occupations—about 40% of the heterosexual couples—eight women reduced paid work, but only one man did. Yet, both men and women in our study firmly supported equal opportunities for women.

Despite evidence of surface-level pragmatic decision making, women in our study described internal conflict and external pressure in negotiating the amount of paid work to maintain. Many women experienced ambivalence when facing the prospect of giving up a fulfilling career, such as this 42-year-old health care manager:

> It's so hard to figure out what the right next step is for me
> professionally. . . . Do I take a career job or do I take like a stepdown job
> because that's not my priority right now. . . . I'll take more of a stepdown
> job because I can work less hours . . . but it's hard to imagine actually
> doing that professionally.

Even as women felt confident that they were in a better position to temporarily leave the workforce than younger, less experienced workers, many expressed frustration that making this choice could potentially have negative long-term consequences on their future career prospects. One 45-year-old stay-at-home mother who planned to return to her job as a physician said, "It [having kids and taking time away from my career] doesn't really feel like a sacrifice to me at all, but I know it is, people keep telling me. That's just the reality of the current culture we live in." Women who reduced their paid work hours to part time or who left the workforce temporarily expressed more concerns about future career prospects than those who stayed in full-time jobs and implemented other strategies for family and work balance.

Women also expressed far more awareness than men about how they are perceived in the workplace. Some women downplayed their parental status in order to maintain their colleagues' respect and avoid what several participants referred to as "mommy tracking." For example, a university professor, aged 46 years, working full time, said:

> I made a very conscious decision…to not talk about the kids at work,
> to never say, if I had to miss a meeting, that it was because of kids.…
> I see the men in my department sort of play the exact opposite game.
> They're always bringing up the kids and going on and on about what
> great dads they are.

In contrast, other mothers embraced the "mommy track" in an effort to set limits on extra work-related commitments.

We also found that some men felt pressure to inhabit the traditionally masculine role of the breadwinner. One woman described her husband's behavior this way:

> [My husband] was on a 2-and-a-half-year sabbatical. When I got pregnant,
> he decided, "I'd better get a job." Because…"I don't want to tell my child
> I don't work." And I thought, "Why not?" And he goes, "Because it would
> send the wrong message in her school." I said, "Who cares?".

Several participants expressed surprise that they were enacting traditional gender roles in spite of their belief in gender equality. For example, this 41-year-old father working full time in customer support said:

> When we had our son…it was very 50/50, we did everything.
> We switched off, very natural. … But when she lost her job, we started to
> fall more and more into a pattern, where it's traditional, and I thought
> how funny this is.…I'm the bread winner. I go to work. I come home.
> I eat. I have my routine. I give my son a bath. She puts him to sleep.
> He wakes up at night (if he does), she goes and deals with him because
> I have to work in the morning.

Many of the women who had stopped working and assumed full-time parenting responsibilities were aware that they were modeling traditional gender expectations for their children who had never witnessed their mother's role as a breadwinner. For example, this 45-year-old mother and part-time web strategist said:

> Actually, I was thinking the other day that we were creating a very
> traditional view for [our daughter] because I do all the cooking. I do most
> of the laundry … When I was working, the first 2 years…every Saturday

my husband had our daughter all day, morning till she went to bed.
She doesn't remember that time anymore....I don't want her to have a
totally traditional view of this is the way the world is, mommies do this and
daddies do that, but yet, there we are! But I think it'll change....Something
will change and she'll see other options as she gets older.

In some cases, women voiced the intention to return to work explicitly so that
they could model opportunity for their daughters.

A minority of participants reversed traditional gender roles in their households,
although in a modified form. Typically stay-at-home dads relied on nannies, family
help, or day care more than stay-at-home moms. Nevertheless, these fathers enthusi-
astically assumed their caregiver role. Some of these fathers perceived the transition
from being a full-time worker to a caregiver as a new kind of career. This 48-year-
old semiretired, former technology industry worker stated: "I really embrace the
role I have of being the parent....I love jumping into that as kind of a career move,
I've sort of adopted that as my job, and I love it."

With few exceptions, our participants ascribed to a philosophy of gender egali-
tarianism within marriage, believing that marriage should be characterized by egalitarian partnership and teamwork. In most coupled households, the division of total
labor—paid work and parenting duties combined—was voluntarily self-reported
by both men and women to be fairly equal between the members. For example, this
stay-at-home mom, 43 years old, said:

> There's just always stuff for both of us to do even though we just have
> one child. It's like he might be doing yard work; I have to clean the
> house....I'll do laundry and he's whatever, cleaning the fishbowl, and
> it just seems like we're always doing work. He'll go to the grocery.
> We just really share, which honestly was important to me.

A minority of women felt that they did more total work than their husbands,
even when the couple aimed for equity. We also found that women were far more
often identified as the household organizer, regardless of whether they were a stay-
at-home mother or working full time. As the web strategist quoted above put it:
"I'm the one who worries about doctor appointments and dentist appointments,
and buys her clothes." Indeed, women more often kept track of their children's
medical appointments, play dates, and weekend schedules, and more often managed what their children eat and wear, even when the majority of day-to-day caregiving work was carried out by the father.

## Workplace Policy

When asked to reflect on their parenting experiences, participants often reported
that the biggest challenge, aside from sleeplessness, was the demands of the workplace. For example, an attorney and a single mother, aged 45 years, said:

> [Being a lawyer is] very stressful and everything's based on the billable
> hour versus efficiency, and there's a demand for more and more and

> more hours and more and more and more 24/7 availability. I think all
> of those things are bad just for human beings, generally. I think they're
> lousy for parenting.

They indicated that the perceived incompatibility of paid work and parenting played a significant role in having delayed parenthood.

When asked what potential policies participants thought would be helpful to support older parents, both men and women suggested a variety of public policies and changes to the workplace that would support parents of all ages. These suggestions include guaranteed maternity leave, sanctioned paternity leave, family leave, flexible work hours, limits on overtime requirements, stimulating part-time jobs, job sharing, on-site childcare, and affordable childcare. Participants frequently compared American workplace culture to that in Sweden, Norway, France, Germany, and other European countries and argued that American workplaces should adopt similar maternity and paternity leave policies and family-friendly workplace culture.

The strategies our participants used to manage paid work and caregiving were often conceptualized as a necessary response to a lack of such policies in the United States. For example, this 46-year-old mother working part time as a consultant reported:

> Flexible scheduling and ability to take time off, I think those are things
> that are really important for families with small children. And we've
> [my husband and I] worked it out, but it hasn't been because of that
> much help from a supportive environment or society. We just arranged
> our life that way.

Indeed, both this participant and her husband created consulting positions for themselves in order to have the flexibility to care for their children. Despite the almost universally expressed desire for more family-friendly workplaces, participants were also resigned to the demands of the American workplace, which they perceived to be particularly entrenched.

## DISCUSSION

Women's fertility begins to decline significantly after age 35 years (Billari et al., 2007). Therefore, women who seek professional careers and also hope to have children face a dilemma because their most fertile years are those in which they must complete their education and establish their career trajectory, a period that generally requires an intensive, uninterrupted time commitment (Hewlett, 2004; Mason & Goulden, 2002). Although our participants ultimately succeeded in having both careers and families, their experience highlights the broader social problem of a direct conflict between women's window of fertility and the demands of the workplace.

By having their first child after age 40 years, the women in our study pushed the limits of their fertility to the extent that they required IVF in order to conceive. In fact, even after utilizing this expensive and invasive biomedical procedure, they were fortunate to become parents at all, as most women who wait until age 40 years are unable to conceive children, even with IVF (Billari et al., 2007). Our participants' ability to become parents at such a late age depended on the availability of IVF, their geographic and financial access to it, and their favorable responses to treatment. After undergoing treatment—often multiple cycles—our participants did not take their parenthood for granted, and, indeed, felt quite lucky.

The women in our participant group were born between 1959 and 1969, a generation that followed the baby boomers and had access to significant financial and educational resources. They also grew up during the women's movement of the 1960s and 1970s and came of age after the movement had significantly transformed the landscape of opportunities for women. Our participants reported that, while growing up, their parents encouraged them to pursue education and career before family to take full advantage of the opportunities available to them. Their access to safe and legal contraception and abortion may have also contributed to their assumption that conception did not require much effort. Many had little or no awareness of the realities of age-related infertility until they were in their late 30s or older, often not until after they sought out fertility treatment. Although our participants anticipated that they would become parents at some point in their lives, the time required to become educated, build job stability, establish financial security, and, in many cases, find an appropriate partner—in combination with their lack of awareness of age-related infertility—led them to delay conception attempts, intentionality or not.

Scholars have documented ways that the structures of paid work in the United States are often in conflict with the needs of parents of young children (Becker & Moen, 1999; Blair-Loy, 2001; Hewlett, 2004; Potuchek, 1997) and are often biased against mothers in particular (Correll et al., 2007). Specifically, in recent decades, families are increasingly dependent on two incomes, childcare remains expensive, and workplaces are expecting longer workweeks from their higher paid, full-time employees and are offering fewer hours to their lower paid, part-time workers; at the same time women—and increasingly men as well—are encouraged to dedicate large amounts of time to parenting (Becker & Moen, 1999; Bianchi, Sayer, Milkie, & Robinson, 2012; Bianchi et al., 2006; Jacobs & Gerson, 2001). By waiting to have children, our participants first established financial security and career achievement, which allowed them more time and flexibility for subsequent child rearing. Nevertheless, it did not lead to women and men having equal participation in the workforce nor in the home.

The women in our study were confined by structural inequalities in the workplace prior to having children. Overall, they earned less than the men, even though they had more education and had dedicated equal amounts of time to paid work. This income inequality has been attributed to a gender bias in promotion structures and career opportunities as well as pay disparities in typically gendered professions (Getz, 2010). In turn, when couples used pragmatic decision making to decide which parent, if either, would reduce paid work, women reduced more often than men due to their lower income. Significantly, we can assume that because these women reduced their paid work, their future earning potential and job opportunities are likely to be greatly diminished (Budig & Hodges, 2010; Correll et al., 2007), further accentuating gendered income disparities.

Furthermore, despite the fact that 40% of heterosexual couples in our study were made up of men and women with equal status occupations, among these equal status couples, women were much more likely to reduce their paid work than men. In these couples, either parent could reduce paid work to the same net financial effect, yet women assumed a much greater share of parenting responsibilities. Thus, despite their expressed dedication to gender equality and equity within marriages, most couples divided labor along traditional gender expectations. In part this was due to biological constraints such as breastfeeding or having already reduced paid work because of pregnancy complications requiring bed rest. Several women also reported that they were seeking a life change from full-time work. Nevertheless, this enactment of traditional gender roles was surprising to many of our participants who had anticipated greater gender equality. Women in particular were cognizant of their position as role models for their children and expressed ambivalence at reducing their participation in paid work in comparison with their male partners.

Sayer finds that between 1965 and 1998, women's paid work time increased, while men's decreased slightly, and women's unpaid work decreased, while men's increased slightly, hinting at a gradual progression toward gender equity in the combined total (paid and domestic) time spent in work (Sayer, 2005). Studies of men's and women's allocation of the combined time dedicated to paid and unpaid work indicate that in the United States and Australia, mothers are still working more than fathers, and parents are working more than childless adults (Bittman, England, Sayer, Folbre, & Matheson, 2003; Craig & Mullen, 2010; Parker & Wang, 2013; Sayer, 2005; Yavorsky et al., 2015). Furthermore, mothers have significantly less uninterrupted leisure time than fathers or childless people (Bittman & Wajcman, 2000). These large-scale time use studies provide a useful backdrop to the gendered experiences of our participants. The men and women in our study reported that they tried to equalize the total amount of time that each partner was dedicating to some form of labor, regardless of whether both partners worked outside the home or worked full time. Nevertheless, some women felt they were doing more work than their partners, but no men felt they were working more than their partners.

We find it useful to apply Blair-Loy's concept of competing and overlapping devotional schemas—the "family schema" and "occupational schema"—to better understand "how people can simultaneously conform to and challenge gendered social structures" (Blair-Loy, 2001, p. 706). In her study of highly successful women in finance, Blair-Loy finds that her participants adopted an occupational devotion schema in order to advance in their careers, but they adopted it alongside a family devotion schema, which informed how they approached marriage and parenthood. Her three cohorts of women each came of age at a slightly different time in relationship to the women's movement on college campuses—one just before, one during, and one just after. Blair-Loy shows that each cohort grappled with the family devotion schema differently—not marrying, not having children, divorcing, delaying marriage, having smaller families, and hiring help—but never dismantled it, only defining oneself and one's decisions in relationship to it. Our participants came of age slightly later than the last of Blair-Loy's cohorts, had greater access to education and more career opportunities, and would have been childless without the use of IVF, all of which are factors that contributed to them engaging with occupational and family devotion differently still. Like the youngest of Blair-Loy's cohort, our participants delayed parenting (and often marriage) and utilized hired help, but our participants often resented the occupational devotion schema and its apparent incompatibility with devotion to family, and they longed to not have to choose between one and the other. Those who remained in paid work often made use of flexible work hours and multitasking, strategies that are enacted where the occupational devotion schema and the family devotion schema overlap and coexist. Flexible work hours and multitasking also represent an erosion of separate work and family spheres and contribute to the potential expansion of the work day to include virtually all waking hours (Bianchi et al., 2006).

Becker and Moen's (1999) study of middle-class dual-earner couples shows that couples often act as a pragmatic decision-making unit and employ a wide range of strategies in order to accomplish both domestic and paid work. These strategies are all variants of "scaling back," and include "placing limits," transitioning from career to job, and "trading off" (Becker & Moen, 1999). Their life course study focuses on a wide age range and on both parents and nonparents, and the parents in their study had children during the intensive, building phase of career development. Despite the differences between Becker and Moen's participant group and ours, the results of our study similarly show that dual-earner families employ various strategies, almost all of which involve reducing paid work, whether limiting overtime commitments, transitioning to part-time work, or leaving the workforce for a period of time. In both study populations, couples acted as a decision-making unit and found that reducing the couple's combined time spent on paid work was necessary for caring for children. Our participant group, like that of Becker and Moen, believed that marriage should be characterized by partnership, teamwork, and fairness and they believed in gender equality. Nevertheless, like Becker and Moen, we found that men's careers were privileged and that women performed more domestic work.

Although our participants employed strategies similar to those described by Becker and Moen, our participants' scaling back was experienced and understood through having significantly delayed parenting until well after their careers were established. For example, our participants' understanding of what it means to quit a career for a period of time relied on their beliefs that certain career goals had already been met and that a long work history would help to ensure a future career. Yet women in particular continued to experience uncertainty and ambivalence about their future opportunities. Were we to describe delayed parenting as one additional "strategy" for negotiating the demands of work and caregiving, it is significant that this strategy would have left our participants childless if not for IVF. Yet, our participants had access to IVF due to their financial success and/or the comprehensive health insurance that was a prequisite of their employment.

It is significant that our participants scaled back their work primarily because they wanted to spend time with their children, which is different from other families that may have to scale back because of the prohibitive cost of childcare or the inaccessibility of childcare. Scholars have discussed the rising expectations placed onto mothers, particularly in industrialized nations (Arendell, 2001; Bianchi et al., 2006). In the United States, "modern mothering" is shaped by an ideology of "intensive mothering" in which mothers are expected to be "child-centered, emotionally involved and attentive, and active managers of their children's lives, intervening in and directing children's time and activities" (Arendell, 2001, p. 168). Men are also increasing their participation in parenting in the United States, and expectations about their participation are mounting as well (Bianchi et al., 2006, 2012). Most of the women and men in our study maximized the time they could spend with their children, thus adopting a family devotion schema and intensive parenting ideology. Although intensive mothering (and parenting) is an important theoretical construct for understanding how ideologies of being a "good" mother influence everyday labor practices, we also suggest that participants' desires to be hands-on with their children, to the extent that they sometimes quit their paid work, represents more than a structuring ideology. In fact, both men and women expressed great personal gratification and growth from their experiences of parenting, which they valued especially because parenting came late and was hard to achieve.

## CONCLUSION

There are many well-described obstacles to having both meaningful paid work and time to care for children, particularly in the United States (Becker & Moen, 1999; Blair-Loy, 2001; Hewlett, 2004; Potuchek, 1997). Our participants were highly educated and had built successful careers. In turn, they delayed parenting until the last possible moment, disregarding the biological reality of age-related infertility, and in so doing, they enacted one approach to negotiating these obstacles. Our findings show that first-time parents in their 40s have distinct experiences incorporating both paid work and childcare into their lives. Our participants embraced parenting as a significant life change for which they believed themselves to be financially and emotionally well prepared, in part because they had already secured their careers by working for almost two decades. They sequenced career building followed by parenthood, which allowed them to focus their energy on one and then the other. In this way, they can also be seen as having sequenced caring: first they cared for themselves by building career and gaining financial stability—which they considered necessary for successful parenthood—and then they cared for their children. Moreover, they claimed that caring for their children was an enriching experience for themselves, thus collapsing a dichotomy of care. Their cumulative financial security and career stability allowed them flexibility in caregiving, yet it jeopardized their ability to conceive without reproductive technology. Nevertheless, women reduced their paid employment far more than men, leading us to conclude that ideologies of gendered forms of labor and structural obstacles to achieving work–family balance persist, even for these individuals who seek gender equality.

This is a qualitative study not meant to generalize, but to shed light on the experiences of first-time parents after 40 years of age and the intersection of late parenting, work, caregiving, and gender expectations. Although our participants were much more likely to be highly educated, Caucasian, and financially secure than national population norms, their sociodemographic makeup is typical of those who utilize IVF in the United States, particularly in states without mandated insurance coverage of fertility treatment.

Even among this economically privileged group, our findings indicate that more effort should be put into modifying workplace policy and workplace culture in the United States in order to ease the obstacles for working parents and to enable people to have children earlier, when they are most fertile, without compromising their income or potential in the workplace. In addition, not only women, but society at large needs to be educated about the realities of age-related infertility. Our findings are also in agreement with other scholars (e.g., Christensen & Schneider, 2011; Gerson, 2004; Mason & Goulden, 2002) who have recommended changes to the structures of the American workplace in order to better accommodate working caregivers, including reducing the American workweek across professions, providing stimulating and protected part-time jobs, providing benefits to those in part-time positions, providing high-quality, affordable childcare and on-site childcare, protecting maternity and paternity leave, and ceasing to discriminate against those who have gaps in their resumes due to caregiving.

## ACKNOWLEDGMENT

The study was funded by the National Institute of Child and Human Development, RO1-HD056202.

## REFERENCES

Arendell, T. (2001). The new care work of middle class mothers: Managing childrearing, employment and time. In K. J. Daly (Ed.), *Minding the time in family experience: Emerging perspectives and issues* (pp. 163–204). Bingley, England: Emerald Group Publishing.

Becker, P. E., & Moen, P. (1999). Scaling back: Dual-earner couples' work-family strategies. *Journal of Marriage and Family, 61*, 995–1007. doi:10.2307/354019

Bernard, J. (1981). The good-provider role: Its rise and fall. *American Psychologist, 36*, 1–12. doi:10.1037/0003–066X.36.1.1

Bianchi, S. M., & Milkie, M. A. (2010). Work and family research in the first decade of the 21st century. *Journal of Marriage and Family, 72*, 705–725.

Bianchi, S. M., Robinson, J. P., & Milkie, M. A. (2006). *Changing rhythms of American family life.* New York, NY: Russell Sage Foundation.

Bianchi, S. M., Sayer, L. C., Milkie, M. A., & Robinson, J. P. (2012). Housework: Who did, does or will do it, and how much does it matter? *Social Forces, 91*, 55–63. doi:10.1093/sf/sos120

Billari, F. C., Kohler, H.-P., Andersson, G., & Lundström, H. (2007). Approaching the limit: Long-term trends in late and very late fertility. *Population and Development Review, 33*, 149–170. doi:10.1111/j.1728–4457.2007.00162.x

Bittman, M., England, P., Sayer, L. C., Folbre, N., & Matheson, G. (2003). When does gender trump money? Bargaining and time in household work. *American Journal of Sociology, 109*, 186–214. doi:10.1086/378341

Bittman, M., & Wajcman, J. (2000). The rush hour: The character of leisure time and gender equity. *Social Forces, 79*, 165–189. doi:10.1093/sf/79.1.165

Blair-Loy, M. (2001). Cultural constructions of family schemas: The case of women finance executives. *Gender & Society, 15*, 687–709. doi:10.1177/089124301015005004

Brines, J. (1994). Economic dependency, gender, and the division of labor at home. *American Journal of Sociology, 100*, 652–688. doi:10.1086/230577

Buckles, K. (2008). Understanding the returns to delayed childbearing for working women. *American Economic Review, 98*, 403–407. doi:10.1257/aer.98.2.403

Budig, M. J., & Hodges, M. J. (2010). Differences in disadvantage: Variation in the motherhood penalty across White women's earnings distribution. *American Sociological Review, 75*, 705–728. doi:10.1177/0003122410381593

Christensen, K., & Schneider, B. (2011). Making a case for workplace flexibility. *The Annals of the American Academy of Political and Social Science, 638*, 6–20. doi:10.1177/0002716211417245

Correll, S. J., Benard, S., & Paik, I. (2007). Getting a job: Is there a motherhood penalty? *American Journal of Sociology, 112,* 1297–1338. doi:10.1086/511799

Craig, L., & Mullen, K. (2009). "The policeman and the part-time sales assistant": Household labour supply, family time and subjective time pressure in Australia 1997–2006. *Journal of Comparative Family Studies, 40,* 547–561. Retrieved from http://www.jstor.org/stable/41604550

Craig, L., & Mullen, K. (2010). Parenthood, gender and work-family time in the United States, Australia, Italy, France, and Denmark. *Journal of Marriage and Family, 72,* 1344–1361. doi:10.1111/j.1741–3737.2010.00769.x

Daly, K. J. (1996). Spending time with the kids: Meanings of family time for fathers. *Family Relations, 45,* 466–476. doi:10.2307/585177

Ferree, M. M. (2010). Filling the glass: Gender perspectives on families. *Journal of Marriage and Family, 72,* 420–439. doi:10.1111/j.1741–3737.2010.00711.x

Franklin, S., & McKinnon, S. (2001). *Relative values: Reconfiguring kinship studies.* Durham, NC: Duke University Press.

Fry, R., & Cohn, D. (2010). Women, men and the new economics of marriage. Retrieved from http://www.pewsocialtrends.org/2010/01/19/women-men-and-the-new-economics-of-marriage

Furstenberg, F. F., Jr. (2010). On a new schedule: Transitions to adulthood and family change. *The Future of Children, 20*(1), 67–87. doi:10.1353/foc.0.0038

Gerson, K. (2002). Moral dilemmas, moral strategies, and the transformation of gender. *Gender & Society, 16,* 8–28. doi:10.1177/0891243202016001002

Gerson, K. (2004). Understanding work and family through a gender lens. *Community, Work & Family, 7,* 163–178. doi:10.1080/1366880042000245452

Gerson, K. (2009). Changing lives, resistant institutions: A new generation negotiates gender, work, and family change. *Sociological Forum, 24,* 735–753. doi:10.1111/j.1573–7861.2009.01134.x

Gerson, K., & Jacobs, J. A. (2004). The work-home crunch. *Contexts, 3*(4), 29–37. doi:10.1525/ctx.2004.3.4.29

Getz, D. M. (2010). Men's and women's earnings for states and metropolitan statistical areas: 2009 [Report No. ACSBR/09–3]. Retrieved from www.census.gov/prod/2010pubs/acsbr09-3.pdf

Glauber, R. (2008). Race and gender in families and at work: The fatherhood wage premium. *Gender & Society, 22,* 8–30. doi:10.1177/0891243207311593

Hewlett, S. A. (2004). Fast-track women and the quest for children. *Sexuality, Reproduction and Menopause, 2,* 15–18. doi:10.1016/j.sram.2004.02.004

Hochschild, A. R., & Machung, A. (2003). *The second shift.* New York, NY: Penguin Books.

Jacobs, J. A., & Gerson, K. (2001). Overworked individuals or overworked families? Explaining trends in work, leisure, and family time. *Work and Occupations, 28,* 40–63. doi:10.1177/0730888401028001004

Leridon, H., & Slama, R. (2008). The impact of a decline in fecundity and of pregnancy postponement on final number of children and demand for assisted reproduction technology. *Human Reproduction, 23,* 1312–1319. doi:10.1093/humrep/den106

Martin, J. A., Hamilton, B. E., Sutton, P. D., Ventura, S. J., Menacker, F., Kirmeyer, S., & Mathews, T. J. (2009). *Births: Final data for 2006* (National Vital Statistics Reports Vol. 57, No. 7). Retrieved from http://www.cdc.gov/nchs/data/nvsr/nvsr57/nvsr57_07.pdf

Mason, M. A., & Goulden, M. (2002). Do babies matter? The effect of family formation on the lifelong careers of academic men and women. *Academe, 88*(6), 21. doi:10.2307/40252436

Mays, N., & Pope, C. (2000). Assessing quality in qualitative research. *BMJ, 320,* 50–52. doi:10.1136/bmj.320.7226.50

Miller, A. R. (2010). The effects of motherhood timing on career path. *Journal of Population Economics, 24,* 1071–1100. doi:10.1007/s00148–009-0296-x

Muhr, T. (1993–2011). *Atlas.ti* (Version 6.2.19) [Computer software]. Berlin, Germany: Scientific Software Development GmbH.

Nam, C. B., & Boyd, M. (2004). Occupational status in 2000; over a century of census-based measurement. *Population Research and Policy Review*, 23, 327–358. doi:10.1023/B:POPU.0000040045.51228.34

National Partnership for Women and Families. (2011). On equal pay day, new data show that wage gap costs America's working women hundreds of billions in critical income each year [Press release]. Retrieved from http://www.nationalpartnership.org/news-room/press-releases/on-equal-pay-day-new-data.html and http://www.nationalpartnership.org/site/News2?page=NewsArticle&id=28306&security=2141&news_iv_ctrl=2181

Negrey, C. L. (2012). *Work time: Conflict, control, and change*. Malden, MA: Polity Press.

Parker, K., & Wang, W. (2013). Modern parenthood: Roles of moms and dads converge as they balance work and family. Retrieved from www.pewsocialtrends.org/2013/03/14/modern-parenthood-roles-of-moms-and-dads-converge-as-they-balance-work-and-family

Peterson, J., & Wiens-Tuers, B. (2014). Work time, gender, and inequality: The conundrums of flexibility. *Journal of Economic Issues*, 48, 387–394. doi:10.2753/JEI0021–3624480212

Pew Research Center. (2013). *On pay gap, millennial women near parity—For now, despite gains, many see roadblocks ahead*. Retrieved from http://www.pewsocialtrends.org/2013/12/11/chapter-1-trends-from-government-data

Pope, C., Ziebland, S., & Mays, N. (2000). Analysing qualitative data. *BMJ*, 320, 114–116. doi:10.1136/bmj.320.7227.114

Potuchek, J. L. (1997). *Who supports the family? Gender and breadwinning in dual-earner marriages*. Stanford, CA: Stanford University Press.

Sayer, L. C. (2005). Gender, time and inequality: Trends in women's and men's paid work, unpaid work and free time. *Social Forces*, 84, 285–303. doi:10.1353/sof.2005.0126

Wu, Z., & MacNeill, L. (2002). Education, work, and childbearing after age 30. *Journal of Comparative Family Studies*, 33, 191–213. Retrieved from http://www.jstor.org/stable/41603810

Yavorsky, J. E., Kamp Dush, C. M., & Schoppe-Sullivan, S. J. (2015). The production of inequality: The gender division of labor across the transition to parenthood. *Journal of Marriage and Family*, 77, 662–679. doi:10.1111/jomf.12189

# CHAPTER 10

# YOUNG WOMEN'S REASONS REGARDING WHETHER TO UNDERGO FERTILITY PRESERVATION TREATMENT WHEN FACING A CANCER DIAGNOSIS: A LITERATURE REVIEW

*Patricia E. Hershberger*

In the United States, current birth rates for teens (15–19 years) and women in their 20s declined to record low levels; however, birth rates for women in their 30s and 40s increased by 1% to 7% (Hamilton, Martin, Osterman, & Curtin, 2014). At the same time, survival rates after cancer therapy have increased and resulted in an expanded focus of cancer care that includes improving the quality of cancer survivors' lives in all areas (American Cancer Society, 2014). These concurrent developments have led to an increasing number of young women who are diagnosed with cancer and find themselves neither having begun nor completed their families. To meet the reproductive needs of these young women, many of whom are at risk for fertility loss as a result of their cancer therapy, advances in reproductive science have resulted in a wave of fertility treatment including egg, embryo, and ovarian tissue freezing (De Vos, Smitz, & Woodruff, 2014; Practice Committees of the American Society for Reproductive Medicine and the Society for Assisted Reproductive Technology, 2013; Trudgen & Ayensu-Coker, 2014). Indeed, the worldwide number of fertility centers that offer fertility preservation treatment (i.e., egg, embryo, ovarian tissue freezing) to young women with cancer continues to increase (Ory et al., 2014). However, the decision to undergo fertility preservation treatment is complex and can be challenging for many young women with cancer (Connell, Patterson, & Newman, 2006; Hershberger, Finnegan, Pierce, & Scoccia, 2013).

This chapter provides a review of the literature about young women's decisions to undergo or not undergo fertility preservation treatment. Specifically, the focus is on furthering understanding about young women's underlying reasons for their preference-based decision, with an eye toward the young women's perspective. Because there is little known about how individuals form preferences and develop values in order to make informed decisions (Epstein & Peters, 2009), understanding young women's underlying reasons provides a critical step in advancing knowledge about what drives young women's fertility decisions when facing a life-threatening illness. Clinicians and others who are aware of young women's reasons for their decisions can better support young women in their decision-making processes regarding fertility treatment.

## EARLY RESEARCH EXAMINES NATURAL PREGNANCY POST-CANCER

The science about decision making surrounding fertility preservation for young women diagnosed with cancer began to gain momentum in the early 1990s when investigators began to show that natural pregnancy after cancer was safe and did not affect overall survival rates (Ariel & Kempner, 1989; Danforth, 1991). In one of the earliest reports examining the reasons young women desire a natural pregnancy following a cancer diagnosis, Dow (1994) interviewed 16 breast cancer survivors about their decision to establish a natural pregnancy following cancer. Three central themes emerged that centered on (a) having children, which was often a long-standing desire that was interrupted by cancer; (b) desiring a sense of normalcy by reentering life and integrating their cancer experiences; and (c) reconnecting with others in their family and peer groups who were having or raising children (Dow, 1994). Little research followed Dow's report until 2004 when Partridge et al. surveyed 657 young women who survived breast cancer. In this report, 73% of the sample indicated they were concerned about fertility, and when asked whether they were either more concerned or less concerned about the possibility of becoming infertile with cancer treatment, 57% reported they were more concerned about their future fertility related to their cancer diagnosis and treatment. Similar to Dow's findings, many women who voiced their concern in the Partridge et al. study wanted children or more children. Furthermore, the Partridge et al. study included women (36%) who reported that they did not want future children or were unsure about future childbearing. These young women indicated they felt a future pregnancy could result in an increased risk of their breast cancer reoccurring. Other research completed by Avis, Crawford, and Manuel (2004) as well as by Connell, Patterson, and Newman (2006) would substantiate these early findings. It is noteworthy that some breast cancer survivors voiced their concern about establishing pregnancy and bringing a child into the world with knowledge that, as the child's mother, their life span could be limited due to their prior cancer, and thus, may potentially cause hardship to the child (Connell et al., 2006).

These early reports were foundational to understanding young women's reasons for fertility treatment decisions and played a key role in bringing awareness to the importance of motherhood among young women with cancer. As advances in the field of reproductive science took place, the increased awareness of the importance of motherhood and the increasing success rates, safety, and availability of both traditional fertility treatments (e.g., embryo freezing) and new fertility treatments (e.g., egg freezing) led to the groundbreaking recommendations in 2006 by the American Society of Clinical Oncology ([ASCO]; see Lee et al., 2006). Essentially, the ASCO recommendations stated that clinicians should engage in discussions about the possibility of fertility loss with patients of reproductive age and be prepared to address questions about fertility preservation options or refer appropriate and interested patients to experienced reproductive clinicians (Lee et al., 2006).

## SECOND WAVE OF RESEARCH TARGETS YOUNG WOMEN WITH CANCER

Following the ASCO recommendations, clinicians and scientists recognized the burgeoning need for research that would facilitate young women's informed decisions about fertility preservation following a cancer diagnosis (Lamar & DeCherney, 2009; Peate, Meiser, Hickey, & Friedlander, 2009; Quinn et al., 2010). To address this need, investigators were able to gain insight into young women's reasons about fertility preservation treatment for the first time, from women who had actually made a decision whether to undergo fertility preservation treatment following a cancer diagnosis. Klock, Zhang, and Kazer (2010) described their fertility clinic's initial experience with offering fertility preservation to young women with cancer. In this study that included women with several cancer types (e.g., ovarian, lymphoma, leukemia), 41 accepted treatment and 18 declined treatment. Among the women who accepted fertility preservation, seven had previous chemotherapy. Women who declined fertility preservation indicated they were in shock on learning of their cancer diagnoses and preferred to focus on cancer treatment. Other young women were emotionally overwhelmed, or, as reported in the early research findings (Partridge et al., 2004), were fearful of recurrence or exacerbating their cancer. However, the Klock et al. study presented an underlying reason for deciding not to undergo fertility preservation treatment: financial cost. This was an underlying reason that other investigators would later report (Mersereau et al., 2013).

### Effects of Clinical Counseling

Components of clinical counseling (Bastings et al., 2014; Goodman, Balthazar, Kim, & Mersereau, 2012; Hill et al., 2012; King et al., 2008; Mersereau et al., 2013) including processes about the exchange of information between clinicians and young women (Balthazar et al., 2012; Jukkala, Azuero, McNees, Bates, & Meneses, 2010; Thewes et al., 2005) can impact young women's reasons regarding whether to undergo fertility preservation treatment. For example, in a study from the United Kingdom where the reasons or factors that affected both men's and women's decisions about fertility preservation treatment were examined, Peddie et al. (2012) interviewed 6 men and 18 women who were diagnosed with cancer and 15 clinicians involved with cancer care. The investigators found that women's reasons in particular for declining fertility preservation were because of the way that information was provided to them by their clinicians, which often depicted an urgent need for cancer treatment. As an illustration, the investigators provided this quote from a female participant (age 35 years) who stated, "And then, the way they [clinicians] put it was, 'Well, you can freeze some but it is a big, long process and chances are that it won't work anyway, so we just need to get on with the [cancer] treatment'" (Peddie et al., 2012, p. 1052). In my research with colleagues about young women's decisions regarding the use of fertility preservation treatment following a cancer diagnosis, our findings support the work of Peddie et al. (Hershberger, Finnegan, Altfeld, Lake, & Hirshfeld-Cytron, 2013). As one young woman in our study stated about her interactions with clinicians regarding fertility preservation: "I think that [fertility] should have been addressed from the outset, and you know…it wouldn't have hurt for them [clinicians] to put in, you know…an information packet" (Hershberger et al., 2013, p. 265). Other investigators have found similar occurrences about lack of information, low rates for clinical referrals for fertility counseling, and clinician encouragement affecting young women's decisions regarding fertility preservation (Hill et al., 2012; Mersereau et al., 2013; Peate et al., 2011; Thewes et al., 2005).

## Effects of Sociodemographics and Other Factors

In part, to control for the lack of information and counseling about fertility preservation and as fertility counseling became the standard of care (see Lee et al., 2006; Practice Committees of the American Society for Reproductive Medicine and the Society for Assisted Reproductive Technology, 2013), investigators began to require counseling sessions as an eligibility criteria for study participation, which led to further knowledge about a variety of factors, albeit at times conflicting, about young women's underlying reasons for fertility preservation. Kim et al. (2012) examined patient databases from three fertility clinics in the United States in an effort to identify which breast cancer patients accept fertility preservation. The findings noted differences across the three clinics and indicated that, of the 185 patients who met the criteria for inclusion (e.g., age less than or equal to 42 years, diagnosis of breast cancer, participation in fertility preservation counseling), 58% ($n = 108$) accepted fertility preservation. However, further analysis of these data revealed that women had varying rates of accepting fertility preservation across the three clinics (i.e., 27.8%, 70.7%, 48.5%, respectively), leaving investigators to question possible differences within the fertility counseling sessions or other underlying reasons. However, the key underlying reasons identified in the sample of women who accepted fertility preservation were that they were typically older (i.e., 36.1 years), wealthier, of lower parity, had a lower mean body mass index, had a lower cancer stage, and were significantly less likely to have undergone neoadjuvant chemotherapy (typically prescribed for patients with advanced disease and begun soon after diagnosis) compared with women who declined fertility preservation (Kim et al., 2012). In another large multicenter study, investigators analyzed data from 70 fertility centers located in Germany, Switzerland, and Austria and found that, of the 1,280 patients counseled (15–40 years of age), women who accepted fertility preservation were typically childless (87%) and about 27 to 28 years of age (Lawrenz, Jauckus, Kupka, Strowitzki, & von Wolff, 2011). Although the age of the women in the Lawrenz et al. (2011) study is much lower than the 36.1 years reported by Kim et al. (2012), the low parity is consistent across these studies and adds to earlier findings (Dow, 1994; Partridge et al., 2004) that the desire for children or more children often drives young women's decisions. In recent research, my colleagues and I have also demonstrated the importance of a strong desire for motherhood or additional children as an important reason for young women's decisions (Hershberger, Sipsma, Finnegan, & Hirshfeld-Cytron, in review). However, Peate et al. (2011) surveyed 111 young women in Australia and found that having a strong desire for more children did not predict women's intentions to pursue fertility preservation. This idea was supported by Hill et al. (2012), who found that young women's decisions about fertility preservation were not affected by having a child. Another interesting finding by Peate et al. was that being in a committed relationship was also not a predictor of undergoing fertility preservation treatment. It is noteworthy that in the Lawrenz et al. study, the options for fertility preservation included the non-freezing methods of ovarian transposition and use of a gonadotropin-releasing hormone agonist. This latter option is often viewed as a protective versus a preservation method and evidence about its effectiveness is evolving (Trudgen & Ayensu-Coker, 2014).

In an informative study based in the United States that examined egg, embryo, and ovarian tissue freezing, investigators surveyed 52 young women about their fertility counseling sessions and the sociodemographic and cognitive factors that affected their decisions about fertility preservation (Kim et al., 2013). In this sample of young women who underwent fertility preservation counseling at one of the two clinics, 37% ($n = 19$) accepted fertility preservation (Kim et al., 2013). Regarding the reasons, women completed a web-based survey 5 to 10 months post-counseling and ranked the most influential reasons in their decision about fertility preservation. Options included "religious beliefs," "feeling overwhelmed," "increased chance of recurrence," and "my oncologist's opinion" (p. 101). Among women who opted for treatment, the most commonly reported factors were "desire for future children" (63%) and "partner's wishes" (11%; p. 99). For young women who decided not to undergo treatment, the top reasons selected were: "[lack of] desire for future children" (27%), "cost" (21%), and "the amount of time needed for treatment" (12%; p. 99). Lack of time for decision making had been reported a year earlier by Hill et al. (2012). Yet, Hill et al.'s findings did not support the notion that financial cost was a decisive reason for young women in Canada to decline treatment.

## Effects of Culture, Society, and Policies

Little in the scientific literature has addressed the effects of cultural, societal, and political influences on young women's reasons to undergo or not undergo fertility preservation treatment following a cancer diagnosis. Yet, underlying political, cultural, and societal factors often affect fertility decisions, especially for assisted reproductive treatments (Nachtigall, 2006). In related research, my colleagues and I have demonstrated the impact of underlying reasons such as financial cost on assisted reproductive technology, with preimplantation genetic diagnosis treatment decisions among couples at high genetic risk and who live in states within the United States where insurance incentives were available for assisted reproduction treatments. Furthermore, in a recent review examining culture and assisted reproduction, Inhorn and Birenbaum-Carmel (2008) describe the reciprocal effects of assisted reproduction on culture and culture on the sociopolitical forces that affect individual decision making about the use of assisted reproductive technologies. In Israel, for example, the provision of assisted reproductive technology treatments is almost completely state subsidized (Birenbaum-Carmeli, 2004; Kahn, 2000), while in Muslim countries, gamete (egg, sperm) donation and use of a gestational surrogate have received strong objections (Hudson, Culley, Rapport, Johnson, & Bharadwaj, 2009; Inhorn, 2006a, 2006b).

## CONCLUSION

Young women's reasons for deciding whether to undergo fertility preservation treatment are complex and preference based. Current research findings about sociodemographic and other underlying reasons should be contextualized within the sociopolitical systems in which the decision occurs. For example, financial cost was identified as a reason for opting not to undergo fertility preservation treatment in several studies conducted in the United States (Kim et al., 2013; Klock, Zhang, & Kazer, 2010; Mersereau et al., 2013), leaving many young women or their families faced with incurring large financial costs or not undergoing treatment. In other studies, such as one completed in Canada where 42% of the sample of young women reported having a drug plan that would cover the cost of the fertility medications, young women were no more likely than the other women in the study to pursue treatment (Hill et al., 2012). The underexplored cultural, societal, and political factors that affect the decisions of young women with cancer are an area that is ripe for future research.

### Recommendations

Despite the relative wide range of reasons that affect young women's decisions, clinicians and others who are actively assisting young women with cancer in their decision-making processes about whether to undergo fertility preservation can benefit from awareness of the information detailed in this review. Several studies indicated that some young women's reasons for deciding to undergo fertility preservation was because of their desire for children or more children, especially if the woman was older, of high socioeconomic status, and at a lower cancer stage, as well as had a partner who desired children. Clinicians, who play a key role in the decision process, may be able to provide young women with this information, which may be helpful to young women. Noteworthy is that some investigators have reported conflicting findings; therefore, not all women that have similar desires or traits will opt for fertility preservation. In preference-sensitive decisions such as deciding whether to undergo fertility preservation following a diagnosis of cancer, researchers and clinicians need to work closely to find ways that will optimize the exchange of information and the ability to help young women identify and, when necessary, formulate their personal decision about fertility preservation. Working together, young women will be able to make an informed, personally relevant decision about fertility preservation treatment that aligns with her own underlying reasons and personal preferences and values.

This review provides an analysis of literature beginning in the 1990s and moves to recently published literature about what is known regarding the reasons that drive young women's decisions about whether to undergo fertility preservation treatment. Clinicians, policy makers, scientists, and others interested in assisted reproductive technologies may want to compare and contrast this review with other populations where fertility preservation treatment is available or emerging into other health care treatment plans. For example, fertility preservation treatment is available to young men and children with cancer (Gardino & Emanuel, 2010). Fertility preservation treatment is also expanding to young women who are diagnosed with an autoimmune disorder (e.g., systemic lupus erythematosus, rheumatoid arthritis) and to those with conditions such as sickle cell disease where hematopoietic stem cell transplantation is a growing treatment option (Trudgen & Ayensu-Coker, 2014). A rapidly expanding area of fertility preservation is among young women who are opting to postpone pregnancy for social reasons (Stoop, Nekkebroeck, & Devroey, 2011). Findings from this review may be beneficial to others who care for, or care about, individuals with whom compromised or potential loss of fertility is a concern.

# REFERENCES

American Cancer Society. (2014). *Cancer treatment and survivorship facts & figures 2014–2015.* Atlanta, GA: Author.

Ariel, I. M., & Kempner, R. (1989). The prognosis of patients who become pregnant after mastectomy for breast cancer. *International Surgery, 74*(3), 185–187.

Avis, N. E., Crawford, S., & Manuel, J. (2004). Psychosocial problems among younger women with breast cancer. *Psycho-Oncology, 13*(5), 295–308. doi:10.1002/pon.744

Balthazar, U., Deal, A. M., Fritz, M. A., Kondapalli, L. A., Kim, J. Y., & Mersereau, J. E. (2012). The current fertility preservation consultation model: Are we adequately informing cancer patients of their options? *Human Reproduction, 27,* 2413–2419. doi:10.1093/humrep/des188

Bastings, L., Baysal, Ö., Beerendonk, C. C., IntHout, J., Traas, M. A., Verhaak, C. M., ... Nelen, W. L. (2014). Deciding about fertility preservation after specialist counselling. *Human Reproduction, 29,* 1721–1729. doi:10.1093/humrep/deu136

Birenbaum-Carmeli, D. (2004). "Cheaper than a newcomer": On the social production of IVF policy in Israel. *Sociology of Health and Illness, 26,* 897–924. doi:10.1111/j.0141–9889.2004.00422.x

Connell, S., Patterson, C., & Newman, B. (2006). A qualitative analysis of reproductive issues raised by young Australian women with breast cancer. *Health Care for Women International, 27,* 94–110. doi:10.1080/07399330500377580

Danforth, D. N., Jr. (1991). How subsequent pregnancy affects outcome in women with a prior breast cancer. *Oncology, 5*(11), 23–30, dis 30–31, 35.

De Vos, M., Smitz, J., & Woodruff, T. K. (2014). Fertility preservation in women with cancer. *Lancet, 384*(9950), 1302–1310. doi:10.1016/S0140–6736(14)60834–5

Dow, K. H. (1994). Having children after breast cancer. *Cancer Practice, 2*(6), 407–413.

Epstein, R. M., & Peters, E. (2009). Beyond information: Exploring patients' preferences. *JAMA, 302,* 195–197. doi:10.1001/jama.2009.984

Gardino, S. L., & Emanuel, L. L. (2010). Choosing life when facing death: Understanding fertility preservation decision-making for cancer patients. *Cancer Treatment and Research, 156,* 447–458. doi:10.1007/978–1-4419–6518-9 34

Goodman, L. R., Balthazar, U., Kim, J., & Mersereau, J. E. (2012). Trends of socioeconomic disparities in referral patterns for fertility preservation consultation. *Human Reproduction, 27,* 2076–2081. doi:10.1093/humrep/des133

Hamilton, B. E., Martin, J. A., Osterman, M. H. S., & Curtin, S. C. (2014). *Births: Preliminary data for 2013* (National Vital Statistics Reports Vol. 63, No. 2). Retrieved from http://www.cdc.gov/nchs/data/nvsr/nvsr63/nvsr63_02.pdf

Hershberger, P. E., Finnegan, L., Altfeld, S., Lake, S., & Hirshfeld-Cytron, J. (2013). Toward theoretical understanding of the fertility preservation decision-making process: Examining information processing among young women with cancer. *Research and Theory for Nursing Practice: An International Journal, 27,* 257–275. doi:10.1891/1541–6577.27.4.257

Hershberger, P. E., Finnegan, L., Pierce, P. F., & Scoccia, B. (2013). The decision-making process of young adult women with cancer who considered fertility cryopreservation. *Journal of Obstetric, Gynecologic, and Neonatal Nursing, 42,* 59–69. doi:10.1111/j.1552–6909.2012.01426.x

Hershberger, P. E., Sipsma, H., Finnegan, L., & Hirshfeld-Cytron, J. (In press). Understanding young women's reasons for accepting or declining fertility preservation treatment following a cancer diagnosis. *Journal of Obstetric, Gynecologic, & Neonatal Nursing.*

Hill, K. A., Nadler, T., Mandel, R., Burlein-Hall, S., Librach, C., Glass, K., & Warner, E. (2012). Experience of young women diagnosed with breast cancer who undergo fertility preservation consultation. *Clinical Breast Cancer, 12,* 127–132. doi:10.1016/j.clbc.2012.01.002

Hudson, N., Culley, L., Rapport, F., Johnson, M., & Bharadwaj, A. (2009). "Public" perceptions of gamete donation: A research review. *Public Understanding of Science, 18*(1), 61–77.

Inhorn, M. C. (2006a). "He won't be my son": Middle Eastern Muslim men's discourses of adoption and gamete donation. *Medical Anthropology Quarterly, 20*(1), 94–120.

Inhorn, M. C. (2006b). Making Muslim babies: IVF and gamete donation in Sunni versus Shi'a Islam. *Culture, Medicine, and Psychiatry, 30*(4), 427–450. doi:10.1007/s11013–006-9027-x

Inhorn, M. C., & Birenbaum-Carmeli, D. (2008). Assisted reproductive technologies and culture change. *Annual Review of Anthropology, 37,* 177–196. doi:10.1146/annurev.anthro.37.081407.085230

Jukkala, A. M., Azuero, A., McNees, P., Bates, G. W., & Meneses, K. (2010). Self-assessed knowledge of treatment and fertility preservation in young women with breast cancer. *Fertility and Sterility, 94,* 2396–2398. doi:10.1016/j.fertnstert.2010.03.043

Kahn, S. M. (2000). *Reproducing Jews: A cultural account of assisted conception in Israel.* Durham, NC: Duke University Press.

Kim, J., Deal, A. M., Balthazar, U., Kondapalli, L. A., Gracia, C., & Mersereau, J. E. (2013). Fertility preservation consultation for women with cancer: Are we helping patients make high-quality decisions? *Reproductive BioMedicine Online, 27,* 96–103. doi:10.1016/j.rbmo.2013.03.004

Kim, J., Oktay, K., Gracia, C., Lee, S., Morse, C., & Mersereau, J. E. (2012). Which patients pursue fertility preservation treatments? A multicenter analysis of the predictors of fertility preservation in women with breast cancer. *Fertility and Sterility, 97,* 671–676. doi:10.1016/j.fertnstert.2011.12.008

King, L., Quinn, G. P., Vadaparampil, S. T., Gwede, C. K., Miree, C. A., Wilson, C., ... Perrin, K. (2008). Oncology nurses' perceptions of barriers to discussion of fertility preservation with patients with cancer. *Clinical Journal of Oncology Nursing, 12,* 467–476. doi:10.1188/08.CJON.467–476

Klock, S. C., Zhang, J. X., & Kazer, R. R. (2010). Fertility preservation for female cancer patients: Early clinical experience. *Fertility and Sterility, 94,* 149–155. doi:10.1016/j.fertnstert.2009.03.028

Lamar, C. A., & DeCherney, A. H. (2009). Fertility preservation: State of the science and future research directions. *Fertility and Sterility, 91,* 316–319. doi:10.1016/j.fertnstert.2008.08.133

Lawrenz, B., Jauckus, J., Kupka, M. S., Strowitzki, T., & von Wolff, M. (2011). Fertility preservation in >1,000 patients: Patient's characteristics, spectrum, efficacy and risks of applied preservation techniques. *Archives of Gynecology and Obstetrics, 283,* 651–656. doi:10.1007/s00404–010-1772-y

Lee, S. J., Schover, L. R., Partridge, A. H., Patrizio, P., Wallace, W. H., Hagerty, K., ... Oktay, K. (2006). American Society of Clinical Oncology recommendations on fertility preservation in cancer patients. *Journal of Clinical Oncology, 24,* 2917–2931. doi:10.1200/JCO.2006.06.5888

Mersereau, J. E., Goodman, L. R., Deal, A. M., Gorman, J. R., Whitcomb, B. W., & Su, H. I. (2013). To preserve or not to preserve: How difficult is the decision about fertility preservation? *Cancer, 119,* 4044–4050. doi:10.1002/cncr.28317

Nachtigall, R. D. (2006). International disparities in access to infertility services. *Fertility and Sterility, 85,* 871–875. doi:10.1016/j.fertnstert.2005.08.066

Ory, S. J., Devroey, P., Banker, M., Brinsden, P., Buster, J., Fiadjoe, M.,…Sullivan, E. (2014). International Federation of Fertility Societies Surveillance 2013: Preface and conclusions. *Fertility and Sterility, 101*, 1582–1583. doi:10.1016/j.fertnstert.2014.03.045

Partridge, A. H., Gelber, S., Peppercorn, J., Sampson, E., Knudsen, K., Laufer, M.,…Winer, E. P. (2004). Web-based survey of fertility issues in young women with breast cancer. *Journal of Clinical Oncology, 22*, 4174–4183. doi:10.1200/JCO.2004.01.159

Peate, M., Meiser, B., Friedlander, M., Zorbas, H., Rovelli, S., Sansom-Daly, U.,…Hickey, M. (2011). It's now or never: Fertility-related knowledge, decision-making preferences, and treatment intentions in young women with breast cancer—An Australian fertility decision aid collaborative group study. *Journal of Clinical Oncology, 29*, 1670–1677. doi:10.1200/JCO.2010.31.2462

Peate, M., Meiser, B., Hickey, M., & Friedlander, M. (2009). The fertility-related concerns, needs and preferences of younger women with breast cancer: A systematic review. *Breast Cancer Research and Treatment, 116*, 215–223. doi:10.1007/s10549-009-0401-6

Peddie, V. L., Porter, M. A., Barbour, R., Culligan, D., MacDonald, G., King, D.,…Bhattacharya, S. (2012). Factors affecting decision making about fertility preservation after cancer diagnosis: A qualitative study. *BJOG: An International Journal of Obstetrics and Gynaecology, 119*, 1049–1057. doi:10.1111/j.1471-0528.2012.03368.x

Practice Committees of the American Society for Reproductive Medicine and the Society for Assisted Reproductive Technology. (2013). Mature oocyte cryopreservation: A guideline. *Fertility and Sterility, 99*, 37–43. doi:10.1016/j.fertnstert.2012.09.028

Quinn, G. P., Vadaparampil, S. T., Jacobsen, P. B., Knapp, C., Keefe, D. L., & Bell, G. E. (2010). Frozen hope: Fertility preservation for women with cancer. *Journal of Midwifery and Women's Health, 55*, 175–180. doi:10.1016/j.jmwh.2009.07.009

Stoop, D., Nekkebroeck, J., & Devroey, P. (2011). A survey on the intentions and attitudes towards oocyte cryopreservation for non-medical reasons among women of reproductive age. *Human Reproduction, 26*, 655–661. doi:10.1093/humrep/deq367

Thewes, B., Meiser, B., Taylor, A., Phillips, K. A., Pendlebury, S., Capp, A.,…Friedlander, M. L. (2005). Fertility- and menopause-related information needs of younger women with a diagnosis of early breast cancer. *Journal of Clinical Oncology, 23*, 5155–5165. doi:10.1200/JCO.2005.07.773

Trudgen, K., & Ayensu-Coker, L. (2014). Fertility preservation and reproductive health in the pediatric, adolescent, and young adult female cancer patient. *Current Opinion in Obstetrics and Gynecology, 26*, 372–380. doi:10.1097/GCO.0000000000000107

# CHAPTER 11

# ACCOMMODATING ASSISTED REPRODUCTIVE TECHNOLOGIES TO RABBINIC LAW

*Tsipy Ivry*

## CULTURALLY AND RELIGIOUSLY APPROPRIATE REPRODUCTIVE MEDICINE: WHOSE INITIATIVE? WHOSE RESPONSIBILITY?

The importance of taking "culture" into account in health care contexts gained institutional recognition in Israel when, on February 2011, the Israel Ministry of Health (IMOH) issued a white paper demanding that all health care providers make their services linguistically and culturally appropriate and accessible. Like American and European cultural competence enterprises, which served as its role models, the Israeli initiative places responsibility for culturally appropriate care with health care professionals, allocating a passive role to their patients.

The IMOH initiative conceptualizes clinical encounters as interactions between two mutually exclusive groups of people: culture-full patients and supposedly culture-less biomedical practitioners. Biomedical professionals are expected to become aware of the possible effects that cultural/religious factors might bear on their patients' health and styles of communication. Whether these factors are conceptualized as religious beliefs and/or taboos, cultural traits, local explanatory models, culturally specific idioms of distress, or even culture-bound syndromes, the purpose of practitioners' heightened awareness to them is, ideally, to negotiate treatment possibilities in patients' own terms; patients presumably lack scientific literacy. Moreover, underlying cultural competence initiatives involve a dyadic vision of patient–doctor clinical encounters operating in conjunction with an ethos of patient autonomy. Such a scheme tends to overlook the possible involvement of authority figures, other than biomedical practitioners, in the most practical details of medical treatment. This chapter is about a mode of reproductive health care provision mindful of observant Judaism that calls the aforementioned assumptions into question.

The rabbis, whose interventions into medical care are outlined here, say that they have acted on an initiative by a prominent rabbinic leader among Zionist religious communities—the late Rabbi Mordechai Eliyahu—rather than by a governmental initiative. Following the advent of assisted reproductive technologies (ARTs) in Israel during the late 1980s (more than 20 years before the Ministry of Health initiative was published) Rabbi Mordechai Eliyahu entrusted his disciple, Rabbi Menachem Burstein, with the mission of accommodating ARTs to rabbinic law and thus making them usable and accessible to religiously observant Jews (see PUAH Institute website [n.d.]). Over the past two decades, Rabbi Burstein and a growing group of rabbis that he trained have been negotiating with doctors and health care institutions, in the latter's own biomedical language, adaptations of infertility treatments to a range of requirements stemming from *halacha*—rabbinic law. Their efforts have been effective to the extent that currently one can trace an emergent mode of biomedical care provision that can be called kosher medicine with its own treatment protocols and modes of communication between rabbis, doctors, and patients (Ivry, 2010b). Since 2006, I have documented the social dynamics of providing and consuming "kosher" reproductive medicine through in-depth ethnographic interviews with rabbis, doctors, and infertility patients (Ivry, 2010b, 2013, 2015).[1] This chapter briefly outlines these findings as a way to advance discussion of the challenges, experienced by patients and care providers, that might arise when scientifically literate religious experts that are also well networked in biomedical circles get involved in the treatment process.[2]

The "hands-on" interventions of religious authority figures, I suggest, change the fabric of health care provision. Rabbis do not only introduce religious beliefs and/or restrictions into medical procedures but they also offer their authority on medical and ethical issues. Importantly, rabbis' readiness to provide an authoritative decree on difficult questions—such as whether to give up trying in vitro fertilization (IVF) and proceed to egg donation (a decision that echoes compromised kinship ties with the resultant offspring), or decisions with heavy moral implications such as post-diagnostic terminations of pregnancy—might signify meaningful relief for patients (Ivry, 2015). Health care professionals opt to provide care while exercising their professional commitment to nondirective consultation, which is further enforced under a constant heavy threat of lawsuits, both malpractice and wrongful birth cases (Ivry, 2010a). Patients, on the other hand, are often perplexed and sometimes overwhelmed by the expectation that they ultimately exercise autonomy by using medical information to decide on options of medical treatment, especially when these carry moral dilemmas. Thus, in the tension saturated and ethically turbulent field of reproductive medicine, patients (and their providers) might welcome the offer to shoulder burdens of decision making (see also Hershberger et al., 2012; Hershberger, Klock, & Barnes, 2007; Hershberger & Pierce, 2010).

Rabbis' willingness to accept responsibility over heavy moral decisions is one aspect of their intervention (Ivry, 2015). Scientifically literate rabbis also introduce hierarchies of authority and complex power relations into the patient–provider dyad to the extent that the classic division of labor between providers and religious authority figures is no longer at work.

Instead of the classic doctor–patient relations, we find triadic provider–patient–rabbi relations, which bear significant dynamics that can be both empowering and disempowering for fertility patients and the medical professionals that treat them (Ivry, 2010b). Within the complex social relations of kosher medical care, some care providers may feel that their professional integrity is being put to trial, particularly when questions of safety are negotiated vis-à-vis rabbinic requirements.

## FERTILITY AND MEDICINE ACCORDING TO THE HALACHA

PUAH (the Hebrew initials of fertility and medicine according to the halacha) is the not-for-profit institution that stands at the center of this exploration.[3] PUAH appeals to observant Jewish clients belonging to the full range of religious affiliations, estimated at 30% of the Israeli population. However, the 12 rabbis that currently comprise PUAH are all of religious Zionist orientation. The rabbis have no formal medical education but have learned to speak medical language and are tuned to all new developments in fertility medicine. They regularly attend professional conferences in various fields of reproductive medicine and maintain ongoing relations with medical doctors through face-to-face, phone, and e-mail conversations on medical issues on behalf of their patients. PUAH's rabbis establish a new kind of medico-religious expertise grounded in mastering two systems of authoritative knowledge: biomedicine and rabbinic law. PUAH's main goal, as they phrase it in their mission statements, is to assist religious couples who have problems conceiving in navigating the double labyrinth of fertility treatments in Israeli biomedical institutions (and abroad) and rabbinic law. To achieve this goal, PUAH provides information and services that opt to be consistent with both systems of authoritative knowledge and practice. They regularly furnish couples with information about doctors who are highly acclaimed in their fields and accustomed to working with religious clients; hence, they are well aware of their special restrictions and needs. This information is conveyed in couples' private consultations with PUAH's rabbis, as well as in round the clock telephone consultations.

Of the three monotheistic religions, Judaism through rabbinic law presents the longest list of concerns over technologically assisted reproduction. Unlike the Catholic Church that condemned ARTs outright for their potential to destroy reproductive cells (Roberts, 2006), rabbinic Judaism, like Sunni Islam, is much more concerned with the legitimacy of the children who result from ARTs (Clarke, 2009; Inhorn, 2006; Kahn, 2000). Like Sunni Muslim scholars, rabbis consider the kinship ties between the ARTs users and their resultant children, as well as lineage and national–religious affiliation. These concerns apply to donor technologies but also to any manipulation of patients' reproductive cells outside their bodies; rabbis are particularly apprehensive about unintentional mismatches of sperm, eggs, and embryos, producing "mamzer" children. (Hebrew *mamzer* is defined by rabbinic law as the child of a married woman and a man who is not her husband, or a person born as a result of incest. Mamzers are subject to severe restrictions by rabbinic law; they are forbidden to marry, to take one prominent example.) Furthermore, under rabbinic law, any medical procedure that involves widening the cervix and may cause bleeding could render a woman ritually impure, thereby prohibiting sexual relations between the partners until after her ritual bathing. As for masturbation, the common method for obtaining male sperm for diagnostic or fertility treatments (e.g., IVF), some deciders consider it as a violation of the prohibition against "spilling sperm in vain." There are many more examples.

Rabbis who have publicly identified with different religious sects and factions have voiced a range of opinions on technologically assisted reproductive options; sometimes these converge, sometimes they diverge considerably. A halachic opinion, however, is not a ruling that is handed down case by case. "Rabbinic law"—as it is often called in English, rather monolithically—is an extremely wide array of opinions and practical attitudes, which draw on the same pool of written sources to reach markedly different conclusions. PUAH's idea is to constitute an information center that can offer consultees the full range of rabbinic opinions juxtaposed to the full range of medical options (Ivry, 2010b). If the couple is affiliated with the Zionist religious stream, they can ask PUAH's rabbis to give them a ruling appropriate to their circumstances. If they belong to another faction or sect of observant Judaism, PUAH can provide their rabbi with the full range of precedent rulings and medical information to assist him to rule for them.

Maybe their highlight service is halachic "supervision" (*hashgacha*), provided by a an ultra-orthodox woman trained by PUAH who traces the couple's semen and ovum from the time they are extracted from their bodies throughout the fertilization process at the IVF laboratory until they are retransplanted as an embryo in the woman's womb. Finally, halachic supervisors also ensure that the extra embryos are frozen for future treatment in a separate sealed tank called PUANIT, reserved especially for PUAH's couples. The aim of supervision is to prevent unintentional mismatching of ovum, semen, and embryos that may produce mamzer children. PUAH's rabbis see biomedicine as *the* solution to infertility, but they are on guard about medical practitioners. That PUAH managed to secure entrance into the sacred spaces of the fertility lab is an achievement owing to their unique position within the field of reproductive medicine. Fertility is never a closed issue for many religiously devout Jewish couples, sometimes even when a couple has six children. Embodying their rabbinico–medical expertise, PUAH's rabbis are situated as the authoritative agents who have access and influence over a broad potential clientele.

## RELIGIOUSLY OBSERVANT FERTILITY PATIENTS BETWEEN THEIR RABBIS AND THEIR DOCTORS

The generous state subsidization of fertility treatments in Israel (until the couple has two children) produces an exceptionally overloaded biomedical realm of assisted conception (Birenbaum-Carmeli, 2004). In such context, PUAH may offer a refuge by their very mediation.

Women who embarked on treatment with a practitioner whom they met through PUAH suffered less friction with the biomedical system: first, because PUAH gave its blessing, they were less suspicious of the doctor; second, because the physician was very much aware of having gained a patient due to PUAH, he or she was ready for the negotiations with PUAH's rabbis. Such women were often full of praise to PUAH for "saving us all the torments, by directly referring us to the right place," and for the combination of medical expertise and divine providence that PUAH brings.

However, in the context of the very same effective relations between physicians and PUAH, women may also be "skipped" while the health care provider and the rabbi negotiate the medical procedures. Significantly, some of the women reported relief when a rabbi assumed responsibility over the interaction with medical care providers as well as over medical decision making pertaining to interventions practiced on her body. Such instances illuminate the confusion and the burden of decision making experienced by patients in the context of nondirective medical consultation as well as the potentially liberating power of patriarchal authority.

However, when PUAH steps into an already established provider–patient relationship the consequences for the patients depend on the readiness of both providers and rabbis to cooperate. Antagonistic relations between PUAH's rabbis and medical professionals have the distinct potential of putting women under heavy pressures in an already tense situation. A key example is the diagnostic testing of sperm. Medical procedures usually require that male factors including sperm be evaluated for infertility in conjunction with female factors. However, some rabbinical opinions require that several IVF cycles be attempted before the male factor is tested because the test might entail "extraction of sperm in vain" (*hotsa'at zera levatala*). In other cases, the couples are required to undergo a postcoital test (PCT). In this procedure, the man ejaculates the sperm during sexual intercourse with his wife into a halachically kosher condom, perforated and without spermicidals, that is then brought to the clinic for diagnostic testing. Because most of the practitioners I spoke to considered PCT unreliable, the suggestion that the diagnosis and treatment be based on the PCT results might introduce tension into clinical practice decisions.[4] One informant, a successful lawyer, told me how she tearfully begged PUAH's rabbis to give her and her husband halachic permission to undergo sperm testing because their doctor refused to proceed with the treatment without it. She told me: "I felt that it was impossible that the halacha would interfere with biomedicine. It seemed illogical to me."

Nevertheless, although she found herself squashed between the rabbi and the doctor (being reproached by both), this informant also disclosed that "It was clear to me that I would do nothing against what they said, otherwise I would not have gone to persuade them."

## MEDICAL PRACTITIONERS ON TRIAL

Some of the medical practitioners I spoke with admitted that they cooperate with rabbis despite various frictions. One informant, a famous fertility expert, explicated the economic constraints involved, saying: "we have no other choice—we want this population (the religious patients) and there is a lot of competition out there." Other practitioners, however, insist on the meaningful merits of rabbi-health care provider collaboration. For religiously devout patients, they claim, rabbinic involvement "makes a huge difference" contributing to the religious patients' peace of mind.

In informal conversations, however, some doctors complain about transgressions of medical confidentiality when patients' medical documents become available to their rabbis (a common occurrence in kosher medical care), as well as about transgressions into what they see as their professional domain, when rabbis offer alternative courses of medical treatment. Their critiques of rabbis' referrals to other physicians reveal the providers' constant awareness of the ways in which rabbinic involvement influences the rating of their medical services. Finally, a number of fertility experts talked about challenges that rabbinic interventions pose for their professional integrity.

Physicians' illustrations of their exercise of medical integrity, as discussed in the following, reveal instances in which rabbis attempted to solve halachic problems by proposing medical procedures. From the perspective of some practitioners, rabbinic considerations lack adequate attention to the health consequences of medical procedures for women. One head of a gynecology and obstetrics department in a public hospital described a disagreement between a PUAH rabbi and himself over the latter's request to treat a 46-year-old woman with IVF. The PUAH rabbi forwarded a demand by the woman's religious authority figure (an ultraorthodox rabbi) who insisted that she first undergo one cycle of IVF before asking his halachic permission for egg donation. The medical expert refused, citing the age threshold for IVF designated in IMOH guidelines and proposed egg donation. He explained angrily that he refused to endanger a woman for a procedure that "certainly won't work" and proceeded with a list of risks beginning with hyperstimulation and culminating in the possibility that the woman may lose her womb. PUAH's rabbi sent the woman to a private clinic to undergo IVF.

Kosher medicine flourishes in public institutions. Rabbis may turn to private medicine after they have exhausted the potential of public medicine as well as put pressure on practitioners working in public institutions. However, beyond the institutional dimensions of kosher medicine in Israel, the earlier story reveals that rabbinic interventions can not only give rise to new procedures and practices to make medicine kosher but also instigate medicalization of rabbinic law. In this process, medical interventions are not merely "allowed" under specific conditions—they become imperative (preconditions) to observing God's commandments.

While some rabbinic demands, such as treating women older than 45 years with IVF to solve halachic problems, are perceived by doctors as exaggerated, other demands have become normalized in medical practice. A prominent example is the hormonal treatment of "halachic infertility." A woman with this condition is a healthy and physiologically fertile woman whose menstrual cycles are relatively short, so she cannot take the ritual bath early enough to resume sexual relations in time to conceive. The source of this infertility problem is the length of abstinence prescribed by contemporary halacha (Haimov-Kochman, Rosenak, Orvieto, & Hurwitz, 2010; Ivry, 2013; Yairi-Oron, Rabinson, & Orvieto, 2006). It is hard to find rabbinic authorities willing to allow shortening of the period of abstinence. Instead, rabbis refer women with short cycles to doctors to prescribe hormonal treatments to delay ovulation. In 2006, a religious OB/GYN started speaking out publicly against the prescription of hormones to healthy women, offering instead a reform in rabbinic ruling (Rosenak, 2011). Few doctors joined his struggle. Rabbinic involvement may alleviate the burden of moral decision making on certain issues for certain patients, but may create ethical problems on other issues for certain health care providers.

## CONCLUSION

### Religiously Mindful Fertility Treatments and Their Discontents

Kosher medicine reminds anybody who is interested in providing religiously sensitive health care that religion may bring not only "beliefs" and restrictions into the clinic, but also networks of power and authority that might change the course of treatment. The configurations that the relational dynamics among care providers, patients, and religious experts may take depend on a myriad of factors. Of course, religious perceptions of the beginning of life and its meaning are important. However, of no less importance are the size of the religious clientele within the general population and the social and political positioning of religious scholars within the general population and especially among health care providers and policy makers. Furthermore, the scientific literacy of religious experts seems a crucial factor in their ability to negotiate treatment courses with medical practitioners. PUAH's involvement introduces both possibilities of relief and additional tensions into fertility treatments. The popularity of PUAH reminds us that patients might not necessarily share with their doctors the ethos of patient autonomy and might not necessarily welcome nondirective counseling; quite on the contrary, it seems that especially in reproductively challenging situations, some patients long for unequivocal authority, even when this quest puts them between the "devil and the deep blue sea." Furthermore, PUAH's success reminds us that taking religion into consideration in the clinic might sometimes demand that providers compromise their professional and even ethical standards of medical care. Whether such compromises contribute to the health and well-being of religiously devout fertility patients is a question for further research and discussion.

## NOTES

1. Since 2006, I have collected 85 in-depth ethnographic interviews along with many informal conversations, and participated in study days and annual conferences organized by PUAH featuring lectures by rabbis and doctors on issues surrounding fertility medicine.
2. For an exploration of the challenges that kosher medicine presents for PUAH's rabbis who must navigate the complex structure of rabbinic authority, see Ivry (2015).
3. Susan Kahn (2000) mentions PUAH in her groundbreaking book *Reproducing Jews*, but focuses on rabbinical debates on matters of assisted conception without tending to the actual relations between the rabbis and medical care providers.
4. For a discussion of the prognostic power of PCT, see Glazener, Ford, and Hull (2000).

## REFERENCES

Birenbaum-Carmeli, D. (2004). "Cheaper than a newcomer": On the social production of IVF policy in Israel. *Sociology of Health & Illness, 26*(7), 897–924.

Clarke, M. (2009). *Islam and new kinship: Reproductive technology and the shariah in Lebanon.* New York, NY and Oxford, UK: Berghahn Books.

Glazener, C. M. A., Ford, W. C. L., & Hull, M. G. R. (2000). The prognostic power of the postcoital test for natural conception depends on duration of infertility. *Human Reproduction, 15*(9), 1953–1957. doi:10.1093/humrep/15.9.1953

Haimov-Kochman, R., Rosenak, D., Orvieto, R., & Hurwitz, A. (2010). Infertility counseling for Orthodox Jewish couples. *Fertility and Sterility, 93*(6), 1816–1819.

Hershberger, P., Klock, S. C., & Barnes, R. B. (2007). Disclosure decisions among pregnant women who received donor oocytes: A phenomenological study. *Fertility and Sterility, 87*(2), 288–296.

Hershberger, P. E., & Pierce, P. F. (2010). Conceptualizing couples' decision making in PGD: Emerging cognitive, emotional, and moral dimensions. *Patient Education and Counseling, 81*(1), 53–62.

Hershberger, P. E., Gallo, A. M., Kavanaugh, K., Olshansky, E., Schwartz, A., & Tur-Kaspa, I. (2012). The decision-making process of genetically at-risk couples considering preimplantation genetic diagnosis: Initial findings from a grounded theory study. *Social Science & Medicine (1982)*, *74*(10), 1536–1543.

Inhorn, M. C. (2006). Making Muslim babies: IVF and gamete donation in Sunni versus Shi'a Islam. *Culture, Medicine and Psychiatry*, *30*(4), 427–450.

Ivry, T. (2010a). *Embodying culture: Pregnancy in Japan and Israel*. New Brunswick, NJ: Rutgers University Press.

Ivry, T. (2010b). Kosher medicine and medicalized halacha: An exploration of triadic relations among Israeli rabbis, doctors, and infertility patients. *American Ethnologist*, *37*, 662–680. doi:10.1111/j.1548-1425.2010.01277.x

Ivry, T. (2013). Halachic infertility: Rabbis, doctors and the struggle over professional boundaries. *Medical Anthropology: Cross-Cultural Studies in Health and Illness*, *32*(3), 208–226. doi:10.1080/01459740.2012.674992.

Ivry, T. (2015). Les dilemmes du diagnostic prénatal cacher et la montée d'un nouveau leadership rabbinique [The predicaments of koshering prenatal diagnosis and the rise of a new rabbinic leadership]. *Ethnologie Française*, *45*, 281–292. doi:10.3917/ethn.152.0281

Kahn, S. M. (2000). *Reproducing Jews: A cultural account of assisted conception in Israel*. Durham, NC: Duke University Press.

PUAH Institute (n.d.). PUAH Institute [website]. Retrieved from http://www.puahonline.org; http://www.puah.org.il/Default.aspx

Roberts, E. F. S. (2006). God's laboratory: Religious rationalities and modernity in Ecuadorian in vitro fertilization. *Culture, Medicine and Psychiatry*, *30*(4), 507–536. doi:10.1007/s11013-006-9037-8

Rosenak, D. (2011). *To restore the splendor: The real meaning of severity in applying Jewish marital traditions*. Tel Aviv, Israel: Miskal.

Yairi-Oron, Y., Rabinson, J., & Orvieto, R. (2006). A simplified approach to religious infertility. *Fertility and Sterility*, *86*(6), 1771–1772. doi:10.1016/j.fertnstert.2006.05.050

# CHAPTER 12

# "IF SOME IS GOOD, MORE MUST BE BETTER": DIVERGING GOALS BETWEEN PATIENT AND PROVIDER ABOUT MULTIFETAL PREGNANCIES IN ART

*Alexandra Cooper, Kathryn E. Flynn, and Elizabeth A. Duthie*

"If some is good, more must be better." This colloquialism captures a common feeling that can pervade many aspects of our lives, childbearing certainly among them. If a singleton pregnancy is a cause for joy, news of a twin pregnancy must be twice as joyful. Certainly, it is easy to understand how prospective parents, particularly parents who have struggled to conceive, might rejoice at learning that they have two babies on the way, and with twins increasingly common, almost everyone can think of a pair of happy, healthy twins, and the wonderful relationship that they have with one another and with others in their family.

Yet, twin and higher order pregnancies are risky. Since the development of contemporary infertility treatments, most have been iatrogenic, and the field of reproductive endocrinology has devoted considerable efforts to examining how it contributes to multifetal pregnancies and how its contribution to this phenomenon can be reduced. Indeed, the American Society for Reproductive Medicine (ASRM) defines the goal of infertility treatment as being "for each patient to have *one* healthy baby at a time" (emphasis added; Practice Committee of the American Society for Reproductive Medicine, 2012, p. 825).

Yet, despite some progress over the past decade, this goal remains elusive. Infertility treatment remains a significant cause of twin- and higher order multifetal pregnancies and births; in 2012, 6% of multifetal births in the United States were the result of in vitro fertilization (IVF) treatment—a proportion that sounds modest, until one considers that fewer than 1% of pregnancies result from IVF. Indeed, as many as half of the babies that are born as a result of infertility treatment in the United States may be the result of a multiple gestation (Centers for Disease Control and Prevention, American Society for Reproductive Medicine, & Society for Assisted Reproductive Technology, 2014; Martin, Hamilton, Osterman, Curtin, & Mathews, 2013).

In fact, the precise number of multifetal pregnancies that result from most infertility treatment is uncertain, because the outcome of many courses of treatment is unknown—there is no system in place in the United States to record or track the outcome of all such cycles—relatively "older" and less invasive approaches to treatment such as ovarian stimulation and intrauterine insemination (IUI) do not require any tracking or reporting. However, any treatment that involves handling of oocytes and sperm *does* require that its outcome be reported, so data about IVF treatment (and variants, such as gamete intrafallopian transfer [GIFT] and zygote intrafallopian transfer [ZIFT], which reduce or eliminate the amount of time an egg and/or embryo remains outside the woman's body, but nonetheless involve surgical retrieval of oocytes) do provide detailed information about the number of multifetal pregnancies that result from this approach to treatment.

However, because IVF involves transferring a select number of embryos to the uterus after conception as compared with other, less invasive treatments, IVF is more closely managed and monitored; therefore, it offers more control over the likelihood of multiple gestation. As a result, both ovulation induction and ovulation enhancement through controlled ovarian stimulation using injectable gonadotropins are more, not less, likely to lead to twin (particularly), triplet, or higher order pregnancies than IVF (Corchia et al., 1996; Derom, Derom, Vlietinck, Maes, & Van den Berghe, 1993; Evans et al., 1995; Jones, 2007; Levene, Wild, & Steer, 1992; Wilcox, Kiely, Melvin, & Martin, 1996). We can therefore assume that in examining the rates of multiples that result from IVF, we are more likely to underestimate, rather than overestimate, the total rate of multifetal pregnancies that result from infertility treatment overall.

Since 1996, the Centers for Disease Control and Prevention (CDC) has collected data on all IVF procedures performed in fertility clinics in the United States. Examining the most recent data available from the CDC at the time of writing, in 2012, there were 157,662 IVF cycles in the United States intended for immediate treatment (as opposed to egg/embryo banking). From these, 35,840 pregnancies resulted, of which approximately one in three (29%) was of twins or higher order multiples (65% were singleton pregnancies, while 7% ended before the number of fetuses involved could be determined). In contrast, among pregnancies achieved without medical assistance, slightly more than 3% are multifetal (and the vast majority of those, twin), so the proportion of multifetal pregnancies that result from IVF treatment represents approximately a tenfold increase over the proportion of multifetal pregnancies that occur in conceptions that do not involve medical intervention (Centers for Disease Control and Prevention, American Society for Reproductive Medicine, & Society for Assisted Reproductive Technology, 2014).[1]

Multiple gestation is, of course, associated with greater risks for infants and their mothers, including higher rates of miscarriage, prematurity, low birth weight, infant death, and infant disability—some of which may resolve with treatment, whereas others will persist throughout the life course. Maternal complications include increased risk of anemia, gestational diabetes, pregnancy-induced hypertension, placenta previa, placental abruption, and preeclampsia. Additionally, twin and higher order pregnancies are also far more likely than singleton pregnancies to be delivered by cesarean section, which carries additional risk and cost related to major surgery.

Given the extensive medical risks associated with multiple gestation, it is a source of both surprise and concern that medical treatment is the cause of so many such pregnancies. To understand why iatrogenic multifetal pregnancies are so common, it is essential to consider how the processes involved in reproduction, and the way they are manipulated by those who would assist infertile patients in navigating them—and understood by those patients themselves—shape the decision-making process of both care providers and patients. It is also important to have a basic knowledge of the history and regulation of infertility treatment in the United States. It is to these issues that we now turn.

## REPRODUCTIVE PROCESSES AND INFERTILITY TREATMENTS

Human reproduction (like reproduction generally) is a process replete with attrition, one with many stages at which things can go wrong and where, once they have failed, one must begin again "from scratch." Taking a woman's menstrual cycle as the relevant unit of analysis, for any fertile cycle, a woman's ovaries must ripen an egg and release it through ovulation so that it can be fertilized. If this process fails, and the egg does not ripen, or ovulation does not occur, the cycle loses its utility for achieving pregnancy.

Once ovulation occurs, the egg can be fertilized, if it is exposed to viable semen in the fallopian tube. But the woman may not experience intercourse during her fertile window, the semen may not be of adequate quality,[2] or other problems (such as a blocked fallopian tube on the side where the ovary that ripened the egg lies) may prevent conception. If the solitary egg likely released in an unmedicated cycle does unite with a sperm and conception occurs, the resulting zygote must, in turn, undergo mitosis, dividing from one cell into two, and those resulting cells must themselves then divide repeatedly, that is, the incipient embryo must develop. Early in its development it must also implant into the uterine wall and begin the processes that will lead to the development of a healthy placenta that will sustain it during gestation.

Any number of these steps may fail. An egg may not ripen; a ripened egg may not be released through ovulation; an ovulated egg may not come into contact with adequately numerous, motile, or healthy sperm or may not be fertilized; a fertilized egg may not cleave; a developing embryo may not implant; or its implantation may not succeed. Even an embryo that has implanted successfully may not be genetically normal and it may, therefore, not survive to be born; such genetic abnormalities are common. Examining the many stages in the process where failure can occur can make it seem startling that humans manage to reproduce at all. And the appeal of a strategy that is used in many treatments for infertility in order to overcome these obstacles—overproduction of eggs and embryos—becomes clear.

It is important to recognize that a key element common to many infertility treatments *is* intentional, medically induced overproduction. Ovarian stimulation ripens *many* eggs, not the one that is typical of the unmedicated cycle; having many eggs available increases the likelihood that one or more of them will successfully traverse the numerous hurdles that lie ahead of it, if it is to lead to pregnancy. Ovulation may be hormonally stimulated as well, to ensure its occurrence (or control its timing). Whether surgically retrieved (as for IVF) or left in the body to allow fertilization to occur in the fallopian tubes (as with IUI), the multiple eggs that ripen and release *all* have a chance to be fertilized; through IVF, if fertilization is in doubt (due to male factor diagnoses or prior experience), intracytoplasmic sperm injection (ICSI) may be employed, with an embryologist selecting a single sperm to inject directly into *every* available egg.[3] Yet even with medical intervention, any woman's ovaries can be coaxed into ripening only so many eggs in any given cycle (exactly how many will vary by woman and is shaped by factors such as her age). Of these eggs, it is likely that not all will fertilize, and not all that fertilize will cleave and survive. That is, at each stage of the process, attrition will winnow the resources available to the goal of creating a pregnancy.

Nonetheless, in many instances, the couple may have more than one embryo as a result of a stimulated cycle. And the availability of *multiple* healthy embryos available to implant in the uterus (either after transfer in an IVF cycle, or in vivo in the case of controlled ovarian stimulation with or without IUI) increases the likelihood of a clinically detectable pregnancy—but again, many embryos that appear to be able to cleave, implant, and thrive will not do so for reasons not completely understood.

Thus, even with this overproduction of key elements of successful reproduction, notably eggs and embryos, and the potential manipulation of other critical steps such as ovulation and fertilization, most infertility treatments fail. Nearly four decades after IVF was first successfully implemented—a treatment far more effective, on average, than other less expensive and less invasive alternatives—it is still true that, in any given cycle, across almost all types of treatment (the one exception being donor-egg IVF), more women will fail to get pregnant than will succeed.

Of course, couples (and individuals) do not undergo infertility treatment because they want to achieve a pregnancy. They undergo infertility treatment because they want to have a baby—to give birth to a healthy infant. Yet a pregnancy is not a guarantee of bearing a child. It is necessary, but not sufficient. Infertility treatment helps patients achieve a critical step, but even among those for whom it works, for whom conception and implantation succeed, it does not ensure that a baby will result. Indeed, in 2012, nearly one in five pregnancies achieved using assisted reproductive technologies (ART) did not result in a live birth (Centers for Disease Control and Prevention, American Society for Reproductive Medicine, & Society for Assisted Reproductive Technology, 2014).

This discrepancy between the immediate goal of treatment—pregnancy—and the underlying motivation of patients—a baby—creates a tension. That tension is that the overproduction (of eggs and, subsequently, embryos) on which infertility treatment relies is an important component of its effectiveness—of achieving pregnancy. But ironically, overproduction at the point of successful implantation, that is, the inception of multifetal pregnancies, is contraindicated in terms of patients' ultimate goal of having a baby.

The reason for this is simple. Multifetal pregnancies are less likely to end in live birth than are singleton pregnancies. Examining the 2012 data for fresh non-donor cycles shows us that a woman who (using ART) became pregnant with a singleton through IVF had a 92% chance of a live birth, whereas women who became pregnant with twins had an 81% chance of a live birth. And a woman who became pregnant with triplets or a still higher order pregnancy had only a 41% chance of a live birth (Centers for Disease Control and Prevention, American Society for Reproductive Medicine, & Society for Assisted Reproductive Technology, 2014).[4]

This reality creates a difficult quandary for practitioners and their patients. On the one hand, it is entirely clear that the best way to ensure that a pregnancy endures to become what is colloquially described as a "take-home baby" is to ensure that that pregnancy is of a singleton. This is true when focusing (only) on infant survival, and extends also to child and maternal health. Yet on the other hand, babies are not born unless pregnancy is achieved, and achieving pregnancy is, in fact, best accomplished by giving multiple embryos the opportunity to implant.

Looking again at the 2012 data, among women younger than 35 years who set aside extra embryos for future use, which is the group most likely to become pregnant from treatment, those who opted for single-embryo transfer (SET) had a 50% likelihood of becoming pregnant in any given cycle. Those in this group who transferred two embryos achieved a pregnancy rate of 57%, of which *more than half* (57%) were *singleton* pregnancies, and 41% were twins (1% were triplet or higher pregnancies due to post-transfer embryo division; for the same reason, 2% of pregnancies resulting from SET were twin pregnancies). Women who transferred three embryos had a 47% pregnancy rate: with 58% of those being singleton, 35% twin, and 7% triplet or higher. Even among women who transferred four or more embryos (45% of whom realized pregnancy), a majority (52%) was singletons and 48% were twins (Centers for Disease Control and Prevention, American Society for Reproductive Medicine, & Society for Assisted Reproductive Technology, 2014).

There are confounding factors that affect these proportions. Women who have never had a pregnancy, particularly women who have undergone repeated failed treatment cycles, are more likely to be advised and ultimately to choose to have multiple embryos transferred. And women whose embryos appear to be poorer quality are, similarly, more likely to have more transferred than are women with what appear to be good, healthy embryos. These confounding factors alone may explain why women having more than two embryos transferred are actually slightly less likely to realize any type of pregnancy, single or multifetal, than are women having one or two embryos transferred. Yet the reality is that transferring two embryos increases the chance of pregnancy, relative to transferring one (and, of course, given the confounding factors mentioned, that for any given woman—even though this does not appear in the aggregate data—that transferring more embryos may improve the likelihood of achieving a pregnancy relative to transferring fewer).

In fact, at the point of deciding between transferring one or two embryos, transferring two increases the likelihood of having a take-home baby, though only slightly. All else equal, the 2012 data indicate a 49% likelihood that a woman who has two embryos transferred will take home a live baby, as compared with a 46% likelihood for a woman (younger than 35 years with more embryos available than are transferred) who has just one embryo transferred. Yet, it is equally clear that, in general, transferring multiple embryos, even just two embryos, drives the multifetal pregnancy rate up to a dramatically high level. Moreover, the evidence suggests that even the *transfer* of two embryos has detrimental effects on a resulting singleton pregnancy when one occurs, including an increased risk of preterm birth (Pinborg et al., 2013) and low birth weight (Almog et al., 2010; Grady, Alavi, Vale, Khandwala, & McDonald, 2012).

With this information as background, the high prevalence of multifetal pregnancies that result from ART seems unsurprising. Moreover, imagining the typical

infertile patient seeking treatment as one focused (correctly) on achieving pregnancy as a critical step toward the end goal, there is perhaps little surprise that multiple gestation pregnancies are as common as they are. Yet, beyond the probabilities
involved in achieving pregnancy and a live birth, there are other aspects of policy
and practice that drive this phenomenon. Many believe that the ways in which the
United States regulates infertility clinics may further augment the willingness of
many patients and practitioners to accept a risk of multifetal pregnancies.

## REGULATING CARE: IVF AND THE FERTILITY CLINIC
## SUCCESS RATE AND CERTIFICATION ACT

The first baby conceived through IVF in the United States was born in 1981, 3 years
after the procedure was first successfully pioneered in the United Kingdom. IVF's
availability increased throughout the 1980s, and as this happened, practitioners and
consumers expressed concern about patients' (and prospective patients') ability to
access accurate information about clinics' practices and success rates—a concern
made all the more pressing by the reality that, as of 1992, half of all U.S. IVF programs had achieved *no* pregnancies (137 Cong. Rec. E961, 1992).

Patients cannot make informed decisions regarding whether available therapies offer them a reasonable chance of conceiving a child, nor about whether any
given clinic offers a good chance of success if they cannot access accurate data about
success rates. Responding to concerns about the quality of treatment available
and about patient access to information about treatments' effectiveness, in 1992,
Congress passed the Fertility Clinic Success Rate and Certification Act (FCSRCA;
Public Law 102–493, 42 U.S.C. 263a-1(a)), mandating that all clinics performing ART
provide data annually for all ART procedures performed to the CDC in a standardized manner. The FCSRCA defines ART as including procedures that involve handling of oocytes and sperm in establishing pregnancy, but not those that engage only
in artificial insemination (i.e., IUI) or the use of fertility drugs, including injectable
gonadotropins. The CDC, in turn, is required to prepare and publish clinic-specific
success rates and certification of embryo laboratories annually. Initially published
in paper format, today these annual reports can be easily accessed via the Internet
in a user-friendly structure that provides detailed clinic level as well as aggregate
statistics.

The FCSRCA, as described by Congressman Ron Wyden, who sponsored the
act, requires that clinics report and that the government publish "their *pregnancy*
success rates" (emphasis added). The FCSRCA is intended to empower consumers
"with good, sound information about patient outcomes," thereby allowing them
to "reward the best fertility clinics." As he told his congressional colleagues, "The
legislation we are considering today will establish a meaningful set of consumer
protections to help these couples get what they want most—a *child*" (emphasis
added; 137 Cong. Rec. E961, 1992). Thus, we see again in the Congressional Record
a tension between what is commonly used as the measure of treatment success—
pregnancy—and what infertility patients in fact seek—a child. Neither the FCSRCA
itself nor the dialogue leading up to its passage explicitly acknowledge or address
this tension. As IVF was a relatively little-used treatment at that time, having only

initiated 37,955 cycles in 1992 with a low success rate (only 7,355 deliveries resulted from those 37,955 pregnancies, about 19%), the tension may not have been widely recognized (Assisted Reproductive Technology in the United States and Canada: 1992 Results Generated From the American Fertility Society/Society for Assisted Reproductive Technology Registry, 1994). Perhaps because of this shortcoming, the reporting system this law put in place is believed to have contributed to—and perhaps continues to contribute to—the problem of iatrogenic multifetal pregnancies.[5]

As described previously, patients may have good reasons to focus on achieving pregnancy rather than having a live birth, even though both are essential to achieving their goals. Patients may focus on pregnancy as an essential and hard-to-realize step without considering how the type of pregnancy achieved affects the likelihood of bearing a healthy infant. The FCSRCA's focus on pregnancy rates may have exacerbated this tendency among both practitioners and patients. From the beginning of its IVF data collection efforts, the CDC has gathered data not only on pregnancy rates but also on live birth rates, singleton birth rates, and average number of embryos transferred per cycle. Yet, as recently as 2012 (when the report for 2010 outcomes was made available), the CDC has presented implantation and pregnancy rates as the first outcomes listed for cycles, by clinic, and only in 2013 (for its report on 2011 outcomes) did it shift to reporting live-birth rates before presenting the data on pregnancy rates. The Society for Assisted Reproductive Technology (SART), which also provides the CDC data online in a readily searchable format, still lists information about pregnancy rates before it provides information on live-birth rates. The CDC seeks to offer patients some guidance about how to read clinic data, for example, stating that:

> Success rates for the birth of a single live infant (a singleton live birth)
> are emphasized in the table because they are an important measure
> of success. Multiple-infant births are associated with increased risk of
> adverse outcomes for mothers and infants, including higher rates of
> caesarean section, prematurity, low birth weight, and infant disability
> or death. (Centers for Disease Control and Prevention, American
> Society for Reproductive Medicine, & Society for Assisted Reproductive
> Technology, 2013, p. 17)

SART, however, does not provide advice on its website about how to interpret a clinic's success rates for pregnancy or live birth, nor does it address what shortcomings such data may have or what risks patients may want to be aware of as they evaluate clinical outcomes.

In short, certainly historically and even, to some extent, today, the data provided to prospective patients may encourage them to focus on pregnancy rates rather than live-birth rates. Clinics, in turn, may have an incentive to focus on maximizing their patients' pregnancy rate. Of course, the clinical tools of reproductive endocrinology already focus on achieving pregnancy; once an infertility patient has a confirmed clinical pregnancy, she will see her care managed by an obstetrician, not a reproductive endocrinologist. This is not to suggest that reproductive endocrinology as a field is insensitive to or unconcerned about pregnancy health, but rather the contrary. But a practitioner in this specialty has far more regular contact with patients seeking to achieve pregnancy than with patients seeking to navigate it. It may be natural, then, that consumers use information about clinics' pregnancy success rates to "reward the best fertility clinics" with a focus on achieving pregnancy, which was the initial insight of Representative Wyden. This focus has the potential to endanger the health of the very pregnancy it brings about if viewed too single-mindedly.

Leaders in the field of reproductive endocrinology are aware of this possibility and have established guidelines to reduce the occurrence of multifetal pregnancy, which has been characterized as "the principal problem associated with assisted reproductive technology" (Rebar & DeCherney, 2004). We turn next to an examination of the development and revision of these guidelines and a consideration of their effects.

## ART PRACTICE AND GUIDELINES TO MANAGE THE LIKELIHOOD OF MULTIFETAL PREGNANCY

As described previously, ART procedures rely on the overproduction of eggs and embryos to compensate for the high likelihood that any given egg or embryo will not develop successfully to become a healthy pregnancy and lead to a live birth. In the context of IVF, the development of embryo cryopreservation, which makes it possible to preserve the viable embryos for subsequent attempts at conception, has been crucial to facilitating decisions to limit the number of embryos transferred in any given treatment cycle. Techniques for successful cryopreservation of human embryos developed not long after IVF itself was introduced. The first pregnancy to result from a cryopreserved embryo occurred in 1983, though that pregnancy subsequently terminated in miscarriage (Trounson & Mohr, 1983). The first live birth to result from transfer of a cryopreserved embryo occurred in 1984 (Zeilmaker, Alberda, van Gent, Rijkmans, & Drogendijk, 1984). By 1992, there were 5,814 treatment cycles initiated with embryos that had previously been cryopreserved; 14% of those cycles resulted in live births (Assisted Reproductive Technology in the United States and Canada: 1992 Results Generated From the American Fertility Society/Society for Assisted Reproductive Technology Registry, 1994). The possibility of cryopreservation and subsequent use of embryos for treatment opened the door to systematic, careful decision making about how many embryos should be transferred in a "fresh" cycle, and how many frozen for subsequent use. With this technology in place, the ASRM turned its attention to providing guidance on this important issue.

The ASRM first released guidelines for limiting the numbers of embryos transferred in January 1998, and again in 1999 (Practice Committee of American Society for Reproductive Medicine & Practice Committee of Society for Assisted Reproductive Technology, 1998, 1999). By 2000, for patients who had conceived through ART during the three preceding years, 19% of deliveries among women 40 years of age or older and 42% of deliveries among women 39 years of age or younger were of twins or higher order multiples; the average number of embryos transferred per cycle was 3.5, with little variation across age group (Reynolds, Schieve, Martin, Jeng, & Macaluso, 2003). This may have been in part because older women using ART to conceive are likely to have fewer embryos available to transfer than are younger women. The early guidelines recommended limiting to two the number of embryos transferred in women younger than 35 years of age with good-quality embryos and additional embryos available for cryopreservation—those with the most favorable prognosis. Among women younger than 35 years with a less favorable prognosis, the guidelines recommended transferring no more than three embryos; for women aged 35 to 40 years, four embryos; and for women 40 years or older or with a history of failed ART cycles, five embryos.

Some combination of the ASRM guidelines as well as the science and clinical experience that led to their development seems to have had an impact on practice. Even before the first set of guidelines was issued, the average number of embryos transferred per cycle began decreasing in 1997, a decline that accelerated in 1998 and 1999. The impact of this change can be seen in a corresponding decline in the rate of high-order multiple pregnancies, which declined over the same time period, with its steepest decline from 10.6% of all ART pregnancies to 8.4% of all ART pregnancies (a 21% decrease) between 1998 and 1999, shortly after the publication of that first set of guidelines. However, the percentage of twin pregnancies did not change significantly during this interval (Jain, Missmer, & Hornstein, 2004).

ASRM has continued to refine its guidelines, and published updates in 2004, 2006, 2008, 2009, and 2013; without exception, its goal has been to reduce the rate of multifetal pregnancies. Results have been mixed. The success at reducing higher order multiples has been dramatic, with the rate dropping by 92% from when it was first tracked. In 1997, the rate was an enormous 11.4%; by 2012, that rate dropped to 0.8%. This is, of course, still a huge number of triplet pregnancies as compared with unassisted conceptions, but it is a stark improvement. In contrast, the rate of twin pregnancies has remained stubbornly high, indeed, depending on what year one chooses as the baseline. The incidence of twins appears to have even slightly increased. In 1997, the rate of twins was 27%, whereas in 2012 it was 29%. Although this increase in proportions is modest in size, it is highly statistically significant and not simply a "blip" in the data. Moreover, the raw numbers are far more dramatic, as the number of ART cycles has increased over the same time period, such that nearly three times as many ART-conceived twins are being born in 2012 compared with 1997.[6]

Examining current guidelines suggests reasons for this situation. First, even in its most recent guidelines, in only one case does ASRM clearly recommend transferring only one embryo: for a patient younger than 35 years with a good prognosis and a blastocyst available to transfer, that is, a young woman who has had at least one embryo survive 5 days to reach blastocyst stage. For patients 35 years or younger with a good prognosis and only day 3 (or younger) embryos available, ASRM recommends transferring one or two embryos.[7] For patients younger than 35 years with less favorable prognoses, patients older than 35 years but younger than 38 years with favorable prognoses, or even those 38 to 40 years but with favorable prognoses and blastocysts available, it again recommends two embryos; for patients in still older categories, without blastocysts available, or with poor prognoses, it recommends transferring anywhere from three to five embryos.

Examining actual practice shows that a large majority of transfers still involve two (or more) embryos. Per cycle in 2012, the average number of embryos transferred was 2.2; only among women younger than 35 years did the average fall below 2, and then only to 1.9. Among women with more than one embryo available to transfer, only 15% of those younger than 35 years, 10% of those between 35 and 37 years, and 2% of those 38 years or older opted to transfer just one (Centers for Disease Control and Prevention, American Society for Reproductive Medicine, & Society for Assisted Reproductive Technology, 2014).

In short, although the rate of triplet (or higher order) pregnancies has been brought down dramatically, nothing has changed with regard to the rate of twin gestations that result from infertility treatment over the past two decades. Moreover, the problems associated with iatrogenic twin pregnancies have increased, simply because more women are using medical treatment to conceive. There are more ART pregnancies, and thus, more twin pregnancies resulting from ART. The reason the rate of twin pregnancies has not declined is simple. Treatment itself, and thus pregnancy rates, has improved as a result of improved and refined techniques, and embryo transfer practice continues to present numerous opportunities for twins to implant. And although embryo transfer guidelines have been revised downward, they are not strictly enforced. Even if there could be more enforcement of these recommendations, they continue to provide plentiful opportunities for the development of twin pregnancies.

## PATIENT DECISION MAKING

Moreover, although clinic guidelines, practitioner ethics, and medical advice may all provide significant constraints, patients themselves are central to decision making when it comes to questions involving their care, including questions such as how many embryos to transfer. As patients consider the options available to them, they are far less concerned about the risks multifetal pregnancies involve than are care providers. Indeed, many patients express an explicit desire to bring two (or more) babies into their family through a single course of treatment. Patients see several advantages to multifetal pregnancies. Many view them as a tool that can produce cost savings, and not without reason. The costs associated with such pregnancies notwithstanding, patients pay a far higher proportion of treatment costs out-of-pocket to achieve the pregnancy, whereas most will have insurance coverage to defray the significant costs associated with high-risk pregnancy and neonatal care outcomes. Beyond financial cost, patients find treatment stressful, and hope to succeed in getting pregnant and ultimately bringing home a baby (or, again, babies), without needing to undergo multiple cycles of treatment. They may value the possibility of having a baby, or babies, without regard to that child's health status. They may embrace the risk of having a child with a significant disability over the risk of never having a child (Scotland, McNamee, Peddie, & Bhattacharya, 2007). They also overestimate the extent to which transferring an additional embryo increases their chances of becoming pregnant (Newton, McBride, Feyles, Tekpetey, & Power, 2007).

To examine how couples considering infertility treatment understand their options and make decisions about the tradeoffs that such treatment can involve, the authors of this chapter (and others) conducted a mixed-method study following 37 couples over the year during which they first sought an evaluation from a reproductive specialist (RS) and subsequently underwent diagnosis and (potentially) treatment. Among the topics we examined were respondents' attitudes toward the possibility of multiple gestation. Describing what they see as the positive and negative aspects of such outcomes sheds valuable light on patients' perspectives on this issue.

The couples who participated in this project were recruited from a specialty clinic for reproductive medicine at a large, midwestern academic medical center. Couples were recruited from May to November 2013 through letters from the physician (either a reproductive endocrinologist or an urologist) with whom they had scheduled an initial consultation. The letters described the research study and were sent to patients who met the following preliminary inclusion criteria: (a) living within 30 miles of the clinic; (b) having a partner who had not yet been contacted about the study; and (c) the scheduled initial consultation was at least 1 week away ($N = 339$). Ninety patients (26.5%) contacted the research team in response to the letter. Of these, 27 patients chose not to participate and 22 patients did not meet the additional inclusion criteria, including their partner was willing to participate, they had not previously had a child using ART, they spoke English comfortably, and they were willing and able to meet in person to be interviewed prior to their first appointment with the RS.

Forty-one couples enrolled in the study. After the first interview, one couple withdrew from the study for an unknown reason; two couples were removed because of difficulties communicating in English, and one couple was removed because of difficulties with scheduling. Of the remaining 37 participating couples, 35 of them consisted of a man and a woman, and two couples were same-sex female couples.

Couples met with trained interviewers six times over the 12 months after scheduling the initial consultation: (a) about 1 week prior to the first appointment with the RS; (b) about 1 week after the first appointment; (c) about 2 months after the first appointment if no testing was done, or if testing was done, then about 1 week after receiving test results; (d) about 4 months after the first appointment; (e) about 8 months after the first appointment; and (f) about 12 months after the first appointment. All data collection was done individually, that is, each member of each couple was interviewed and completed self-administered questionnaires separately from his or her partner. Participants were paired with one of two trained interviewers and remained paired with the same interviewer across all six data collection points. When couples became pregnant or completed an adoption (and so were no longer making fertility-related decisions) they completed surveys but not interviews at the 2-, 4-, and 8-month time points. Participants provided written informed consent; the study was approved by the institutional review board at Froedtert and the Medical College of Wisconsin.

Participants were explicitly asked about multiple-gestation pregnancies in interviews 1 and 3 (pre-consult and posttest results) and also had the opportunity to introduce the topic themselves at any point due to the semi-structured nature of the interviews. All interviews were recorded and subsequently transcribed. They were coded to identify and categorize all mentions of the possibility of such a pregnancy where this outcome was described in positive or negative terms (or both, as many did), or identified a multifetal pregnancy as something the respondent either desired or hoped to avoid. Between interview questions about multiple gestation and participant-initiated discussions, the topic was broached in ways that addressed these categories in 205 interviews (of 412 total interviews) and was discussed in at least one interview by 34 (of 39) female participants and 31 (of 35) male participants.

Examining positive and negative mentions of the prospect of twins (or, in some cases, an explicit mention of the prospect of higher order multiples, almost without exception triplets), respondents spoke clearly about both advantages and disadvantages to becoming pregnant with or parenting multiples. A number expressed a general sense that having twins would be "fun" or "cool," or "a blessing" (mentioned by 16 respondents), would complete the desired family or move the respondent closer to achieving the desired family (32 respondents), and/or would reduce the need for further infertility treatment. Several respondents also expressed a sense that transferring a higher number of embryos (for IVF) or having more eggs available for fertilization (for IUI) would increase the likelihood of achieving pregnancy (10 respondents). Other advantages respondents linked to multiple gestation included excitement associated with parenting two children of the same age at one time, the bonds felt between twins, and cost savings by reducing or eliminating a need for further infertility treatments. Patients who identified risks or expressed concern spoke in some cases about health risks to the mother and/or babies (13 respondents), but many more (36 respondents) focused on hassles and costs that they identified as part of the postpartum period—costs associated with any infant and not related, for example, to increased care needs associated with preterm birth. In this context, they mentioned items such as loss of sleep; the cost of items needed in larger quantities such as car seats, diapers, and childcare services; or the desire to be able to devote individual attention to each of their children (in turn) as they raise them. We turn next to comments profiling the types of perspectives respondents offered on each of these issues.

As noted, 16 of 74 respondents expressed—either directly or indirectly—a desire for twins (or in some cases higher order multiples). One 32-year-old woman expressed her enthusiasm for the possibility of a multifetal pregnancy in the direct and explicit "more is better" language that introduced this chapter by saying simply, "then I will get more babies." Similarly, a 29-year-old female respondent commented that twins would "definitely [be] a blessing. I think it would be a very cool experience. I would then say that that would be having your cake and eating it, too."

In the same vein, a 24-year-old man expressed a desire for multiples that he shared with his wife, together with the sense that having multiples would complete his family. He also referred to the presence of several sets of twins in his extended family—suggesting his perception of the normalcy of twins as an outcome, saying,

> We'd be more than happy to have multiple [babies] at once so we could just [be] one and done. Have as many kids as we can and then not have to worry about it, so I'm sure we'd be happy to. My mom is a twin. We have a couple other twins in the family, and they love it, so I'm sure we'd be happy if that were the case.

A 27-year-old woman described not thinking of herself and her husband as having an increased chance of multiples because they were exploring less-invasive treatment strategies, but being enthusiastic about the idea of twins:

> I think because IVF isn't really something that we think we're going to be faced with it right now, there have just been kind of fun conversations not real serious one but for us, it would be kind of like awesome to get the twins because it would just make everything easier.

This idea of twins as being easier is clearly linked for many respondents to another point that many expressed explicitly—the desire to grow their families quickly. This was true for respondents who wanted only two children, but also for those who wanted larger families. The 41-year-old man cited previously who references twins in his family tells the interviewer: "We know that we would like to have at least three children, four would be best. [My wife] and I have both talked about it and so if we could have twins and be able to get that number up then that would be a very positive thing."

Similarly, a 28-year-old woman commented that,

> Two would be awesome because I feel like we're getting a later start with the kid thing than we wanted to in life, so I kind of feel like, great, we can play some catch up and get two going right away and get caught back up and then have another one later.

A number of respondents linked this desire for completing their families to avoiding a need for additional infertility treatment down the road. The same 29-year-old woman who characterized twins as "having your cake and eating it too" (previously) continued, saying,

> You get two right off the bat and not have to worry about, you know, wanting—okay, we had one! What an awesome experience. Now I want another one! Here we go again! Another struggle! So two off the bat would be pretty much a wonderful thing.

Her husband, aged 35 years, contrasted the treatment option the couple had identified as within its budget with IVF (which they were not planning to pursue) using similar language, saying,

> Insemination is closer to the price point we can afford. It's like a grand per time and it's not guaranteed but neither is in vitro and that's like ten to eleven grand and it's not necessarily guaranteed but there's a higher chance. The thing I like about [IVF] is the possibility of twins. It would make it a little bit easier, that we wouldn't have to go through this whole process again in another 2 or 3 years.

Similarly, without explicitly referring to avoiding additional treatment, a 25-year-old female respondent nonetheless brought the cost of treatment into the picture by saying, "I think maybe it'd be almost like a bonus. Maybe then we'd be done, two for the price of one, three for the price of one."

A 33-year-old man was less explicit about what he saw as the advantages of twins, but nonetheless presented them as a "solution" to the stress he and his wife were facing, saying, "I think if we had twins, we could stop worrying about everything. It would be wonderful to stop worrying about everything."

In short, many respondents desire twin (or even higher order multiple) pregnancies, and are excited at the possibility of welcoming multiple babies into their family, increasing their family size, and, potentially, saving money on treatment. Yet respondents' reactions to the prospect of multiple gestation were not uniformly positive. Many respondents identified both positive and negative aspects to such pregnancies, such as a 32-year-old woman who noted the advantages to bringing two children into the family at once while also expressing concern about the postpartum challenges involved in raising twins:

> It's good and bad. If it happens, oh that would be great. If it's a boy and a girl that would be awesome. We'll be done. We'll be complete. I don't think we want any more kids. He just wants one, at least one healthy and that's it. But if it's twins then we've talked about it, but we'll definitely—we're thinking about relocating back to [where our parents live]. I think with the pregnancy of one child I think we still have an option to kind of move [elsewhere], but with two it's going to be hard. We might have to consider just staying here with help and everything on both sides of the family.

Another respondent, a 25-year-old man, raised similar concerns, commenting on the cost of multiples (though particularly on the prospect of triplets), saying,

> I think it would be hard for us financially to have especially triplets—to do that right away. I know that my family—our families would help and support us in any way they can so we're not—cost I don't think—it would be hard for start of things—like strollers and things like that— but we're not big spenders on clothes and things so it's—there are definite ways that we could be able to afford it. I'd probably have to get another job in the summer outside of teaching and that's—whatever it takes to provide for my family.

In a later interview, he attributed the concerns about the financial difficulties involved in raising multiples to his wife, saying "My wife hopes for one at a time, please. That [having twins] is a financial burden." But he then continued to describe his willingness to embrace the possibility of twins, contrasting that possibility as one he preferred to childlessness, "But if it's either having twins or having no kids, bring them on."

Indeed, asked about whether they desired to have or to avoid a multifetal pregnancy, some respondents spoke of a discrepancy between their wishes and their partner's. Describing what multiples would entail, one woman commented,

I see four times as much work, frustration, overwhelmed, what am
I to do with two babies at once? And he sees it as I only have to get
pregnant once and go through labor once. That's how he sees it because
he knows I want two children, so he's like well, just get it over.

Some respondents did incorporate discussion of the health risks associated
with multifetal pregnancies, particularly higher order multiples. One 42-year-
old woman made reference to the possibility of cryopreserving embryos for later
attempts at pregnancy. Commenting about how many embryos to transfer in an IVF
cycle, she said,

I think the health risks [of transferring more than two] are just too great.
I know the health risks are great. They're greater for the kids. I would
rather have one healthy child instead of having three very small, sick
little babies. I really would. And I get that that can happen in utero, that
you can have twins, I get that. But I don't need to be implanted with
three. I would rather save that embryo for a different shot...And I told
my husband cause he's like, "Triplets?" And I looked at him and I was
like, "You're nuts!" He kind of said it funny and I was like, "We need
to be very clear. I don't want three kids. I don't want to be selfish about
this. I just want a healthy child. I'll take one."

Yet in this same interview, this respondent commented that she felt "totally
fine" about having twins, going on to say, "[My husband and I] are both very much
okay with that. I'm not holding out great hope for that because [of what I've been
able to gather about the success rates for women my age treated at this clinic]."
Indeed, a number of respondents distinguished between twin pregnancies,
which many see as fairly ordinary, with triplet pregnancies. Considering how many
embryos to transfer in an anticipated IVF cycle, a 49-year-old male respondent said,

So how do you strike a balance between giving yourself the most bang
for your buck so to speak and I suppose guarding against being wildly
successful?...That is probably something we'll want to think about as
we approach this because how do you strike a balance between really
wanting one, two, or boy on the outside three? Ah. That's a lot to ask. It
would be a blessing no doubt, but I suppose we would aim for two.

A 45-year-old woman considering this same issue—the number of embryos to
transfer—expressed similar ideas, going on to identify herself as a good candidate
for a twin pregnancy because of her body type. She said,

I don't know because we've always been open to having twins, and
I have no problem with that, so I'd—if it's medically okay, and it's
approved and there's no problem with it, I would say yes. Because
the chances of having one [baby] if you've got two [embryos] is better,
you know, the odds. I just don't—I don't like the idea of doing—
probably doing—more than the max because I'm not interested in the

potential multiple like triplets or more. Just because you have a higher opportunity for something to go wrong, or premature births and I don't want to set my potential children up for a difficult future as a result. But you know, being a tall and bigger woman, I think I can handle twins just fine. They could probably grow to be pretty big babies, as long as everything else is alright.

Some respondents did identify what they perceived as more significant negatives with multiples. A 33-year-old man, speaking of the possibility of high-order multiples and his and his wife's decision to pursue adoption rather than treatment, identified the possibility of needing selective reduction as the deciding factor, saying,

I think what put us over the edge toward the adoption was [my wife] wouldn't have to take shots, there would be no possibility of having multiple babies. They had said sometimes if there's too many that they will only keep one or two. And with our faith we wouldn't want to get rid of any babies. If we were going to have six, we'd want to have all six of them.

And within the context of comparing treatment options, a 28-year-old female respondent said,

Then, I wouldn't be opposed to having twins, but then that can also be a more challenging pregnancy and greater chances of having premies or low-weight babies, which cause issues, and so with IUI and no drugs, there's less of a chance of having twins, so that's an advantage as well, I think personally.

Another 28-year-old female respondent drew on memories of her family history to label *any* multiple-gestation pregnancy as "scary," telling the interviewer:

My aunt carried three sets of multiples and only one came to term because the others didn't. I know how sick she was and how scary it was for her and my mom had me young so I'm actually pretty close in age to my aunts. They're 10 years or less older than me. So, I was old enough to understand what was going on and how scary it was. Two aunts on bed rest at the same time and nobody to help them because everybody's on bed rest.

A 38-year-old male respondent identified a similar awareness, again based on the experience of someone in his wife's family, saying

Well, you know, we're worried about risks of multiples. And we know her cousin has multiples, twins, and she's on bed rest. There seems like complicated pregnancies with multiples and then you always have to worry about the babies too because maybe they're low birth weight or stuff like that. It just doesn't seem like it's as healthy as a pregnancy compared to having just one.

In short, some patients are aware of multiple-gestation pregnancies as high risk. Yet that fact notwithstanding, overall most respondents appeared more positive than negative at the prospect of becoming pregnant with or parenting multiples. Indeed, almost half of the negatives respondents mentioned in connection with parenting multiples involved postpartum concerns. This reality puts practitioners in a difficult position, and it is to this that we now turn.

## Infertility Treatment, Multiple Gestation, and the Practitioner's Role

The patient considering or pursuing infertility treatment is in a difficult position. The female patient for whom most treatments are provided, regardless of the source of the infertility, is seeking medical assistance to achieve what is for many people a basic and much desired part of the life course. Treatment can be expensive and its cost is often prohibitive because it is often not covered by insurance. Also, patients typically present as one member of a couple seeking to have a child together, and may have a different perspective than their partner about what to prioritize as they seek to grow their families (and realize other, perhaps conflicting, goals) and how to balance the different costs and benefits that different courses of treatment entail. Moreover, by the time they seek treatment, couples have typically been trying to conceive for a year or more, may have experienced pregnancy loss, and are often facing a narrowing window of time available to have children, particularly children with a genetic link to their mother.

In this context, many patients perceive the possibility of having multiple children at once as a positive outcome. Having struggled to conceive, they may be excited by the prospect of twins, enticed by the apparent cost savings and efficiency of getting two for one, and/or motivated by a desire to avoid a need for further treatment at a later date in order to bring another child into their family. They pursue their goals in a context where much of what practitioners do is focused on achieving pregnancy, rather than maximizing pregnancy health. This often means that the tools of treatment themselves dramatically increase the likelihood of multifetal pregnancies. Existing guidelines, regulation, and regulatory history may in some ways foster an environment that welcomes multiple gestation and that has certainly failed to curtail its propensity to create twin pregnancies, even as it has grappled with and largely succeeded at bringing down the rate of iatrogenic higher order multiples.

Practitioners must be aware of these forces as they are needed as a source of guidance for patients, many of whom are surprisingly ill-informed of the risks associated with multiple gestation. Patients more often focus not on such important problems as pregnancy loss, low birth weight, and preterm birth, but rather, if they have concerns at all, on the cost of childcare and car seats once the babies are born.

The truth is that multifetal pregnancies have long-lasting effects. They are much more likely than singleton gestations to end in miscarriage or stillbirth, outcomes no one wants to face. This is in a context where many patients come to treatment having already navigated losses and often numerous losses. Even when they are successful and result in live birth, such pregnancies also bring with them a significant likelihood of lifelong effects for the babies whose lives begin in such pregnancies. These effects may be large or small; twins are much more common today than they were in earlier eras because of infertility treatments. Most individuals can think of twins who live happy, healthy, productive lives. The contrast to this is the fact that even a baby born from a singleton pregnancy resulting from an IVF cycle involving the transfer of two embryos is less healthy, on average, than a singleton who results from a SET (Grady et al., 2012; Poikkeus & Tiitinen, 2008). It is also the case that as infertility treatments have improved, transferring an additional embryo has a relatively low (though positive) impact on the pregnancy rate.

## CONCLUSION

Every patient seeking treatment for infertility is unique, and patients must have the opportunity to make decisions about the risks they are willing to assume, both for themselves and for their prospective children. Yet, at the same time, it is critical that patients receive accurate, evidence-based information to make informed choices. Providers are charged with providing information about the risks associated with multifetal pregnancies as well as the relatively low value of adding embryos (in the case of IVF) or ripened eggs (in the case of IUI) to improve the pregnancy and live-birth rate. The provision of this key information is an important service that infertility patients need, and yet is not currently being delivered effectively. The practitioner who makes this information available offers a needed service to a vulnerable population: patients making decisions in a high-stress, time-sensitive context. Not only does this impact patients but also their prospective children who have no voice of their own and who must rely on their aspiring parents, and those parents' care providers, to provide for their future well-being.

## NOTES

1. Worldwide, the iatrogenic multifetal pregnancy rate is somewhat lower, estimated at close to 24% for IVF cycles (Mansour et al., 2014). Many nations regulate IVF more stringently than does the United States, including by requiring SET in patients who are good candidates for achieving a pregnancy. Many also fund health care (including infertility treatments) in ways that reduce patients' out-of-pocket costs, reducing the extent to which financial concerns may encourage patients to seek to maximize their likelihood of pregnancy in any given cycle. However, throughout this chapter, our focus is on the United States.

2. Of course, the semen provided by the male partner offers perhaps the most dramatic example of the attrition that pervades the reproductive process; a typical healthy ejaculation contains a hundred million or more sperm, at most one of which will, by fertilizing an egg, pass its genes along to the next generation. Yet, although only one sperm will fertilize the egg, millions more must be present in the ejaculate if conception is to occur without medical assistance.

3. Although ICSI does not guarantee fertilization, it does increase the chances of it occurring in cases where issues such as low sperm count, poor morphology, or poor motility otherwise reduce the availability of sperm.

4.   These numbers may be slightly misleading, as they are calculated based on the assumption that something that started as a twin or triplet pregnancy remained a twin or a triplet pregnancy. It is possible that triplet or higher order pregnancies were reduced, and ended with the live birth of a singleton or twins. But working on the assumption that most pregnancies that started as multifetal remained multifetal, these proportions are accurate. Indeed, they likely *understate* the extent of loss for multifetal pregnancies, because 7% of ART pregnancies in 2012 failed before the number of fetuses that had implanted could be established, and we know that multifetal pregnancies are more likely than singleton pregnancies to end in miscarriage.

5.   It is difficult to know what effect the passage of the FCSRCA had on ART practice, which, in general, was increasing as adoption of this new tool for treatment spread. In 1992 and 1993, the number of clinics in the United States increased, as did the number of treatment cycles. In 1994, the number of clinics declined though the overall number of cycles increased. By 1995, both the number of clinics and the number of cycles were again on the rise. Overall treatment success increased across all years, but by very modest amounts—only a small percent each year.

6.   All data are derived from the CDC Fertility Clinic Success Rates Report for the relevant years; all cited sources can be accessed online through this link: http://www.cdc.gov/art/reports/index.html.

7.   This is in stark contrast to current practice in many other nations, which are much more likely than the United States to endorse SET and where such endorsement is often implemented not as a recommendation, but as a requirement for a subset of patients. The impact of SET is disputed (and certainly is in part a function of the subpopulation of infertile women in which it is applied); a number of studies find success rates similar to dual-embryo transfer, particularly if SET is coupled with a follow-up transfer of a cryopreserved embryo if pregnancy is not realized for the fresh transfer cycle (Béraud et al., 2013; Fauque et al., 2010; Gremeau et al., 2012; Pandian, Marjoribanks, Ozturk, Serour, & Bhattacharya, 2013). However, some studies find that it diminishes pregnancy rates (Scotland et al., 2012; Vélez, Connolly, Kadoch, Phillips, & Bissonnette, 2014).

# REFERENCES

Almog, B., Levin, I., Wagman, I., Kapustiansky, R., Lessing, J. B., Amit, A., & Azem, F. (2010). Adverse obstetric outcome for the vanishing twin syndrome. *Reproductive Biomedicine Online, 20*, 256–260. doi:10.1016/j.rbmo.2009.11.015

Assisted Reproductive Technology in the United States and Canada: 1992 Results Generated From the American Fertility Society/Society for Assisted Reproductive Technology Registry. (1994). *Fertility and Sterility, 62*, 1121–1128.

Béraud, E., Brugnon, F., Gremeau, A.-S., Dejou, L., Pons, H., Janny, L.,...Pouly, J.-L. (2013). Reduction of multiple pregnancies in ART with large SET procedures over the period 2001–2010. *Gynécologie Obstétrique & Fertilité, 41*, 20–26. doi:10.1016/j.gyobfe.2012.09.025

Centers for Disease Control and Prevention, American Society for Reproductive Medicine, & Society for Assisted Reproductive Technology. (2013). *2011 Assisted reproductive technology fertility clinic success rates report.* Retrieved from http://www.cdc.gov/art/pdf/2011-report/fertility-clinic/art_2011_clinic_report-full.pdf

Centers for Disease Control and Prevention, American Society for Reproductive Medicine, & Society for Assisted Reproductive Technology. (2014). *2012 Assisted reproductive technology fertility clinic success rates report.* Retrieved from http://www.cdc.gov/art/pdf/2012-report/art-2012-fertility-clinic-report.pdf

Corchia, C., Mastroiacovo, P., Lanni, R., Mannazzu, R., Currò, V., & Fabris, C. (1996). What proportion of multiple births are due to ovulation induction? A register-based study in Italy. *American Journal of Public Health, 86*, 851–854. doi:10.2105/AJPH.86.6.851

Derom, C., Derom, R., Vlietinck, R., Maes, H., & Van den Berghe, H. (1993). Iatrogenic multiple pregnancies in East Flanders, Belgium. *Fertility and Sterility, 60,* 493–496.

Evans, M. I., Littmann, L., St. Louis, L., LeBlanc, L., Addis, J., Johnson, M. P., & Moghissi, K. S. (1995). Evolving patterns of iatrogenic multifetal pregnancy generation: Implications for aggressiveness of infertility treatments. *American Journal of Obstetrics and Gynecology, 172,* 1750–1753. doi:10.1016/0002-9378(95)91407-2

Fauque, P., Jouannet, P., Davy, C., Guibert, J., Viallon, V., Epelboin, S.,...Patrat, C. (2010). Cumulative results including obstetrical and neonatal outcome of fresh and frozen-thawed cycles in elective single versus double fresh embryo transfers. *Fertility and Sterility, 94,* 927–935. doi:10.1016/j.fertnstert.2009.03.105

Fertility Clinic Success Rate and Certification Act of 1991, 137 Cong. Rec. E961 (daily ed. April 3, 1992) (statement of Rep. Wyden).

Grady, R., Alavi, N., Vale, R., Khandwala, M., & McDonald, S. D. (2012). Elective single embryo transfer and perinatal outcomes: A systematic review and meta-analysis. *Fertility and Sterility, 97,* 324–331. doi:10.1016/j.fertnstert.2011.11.033

Gremeau, A.-S., Brugnon, F., Bouraoui, Z., Pekrishvili, R., Janny, L., & Pouly, J.-L. (2012). Outcome and feasibility of elective single embryo transfer (eSET) policy for the first and second IVF/ICSI attempts. *European Journal of Obstetrics & Gynecology and Reproductive Biology, 160,* 45–50. doi:10.1016/j.ejogrb.2011.09.032

Jain, T., Missmer, S. A., & Hornstein, M. D. (2004). Trends in embryo-transfer practice and in outcomes of the use of assisted reproductive technology in the United States. *The New England Journal of Medicine, 350,* 1639–1645. doi:10.1056/NEJMsa032073

Jones, H. W., Jr. (2007). Iatrogenic multiple births. *Fertility and Sterility, 87,* 453–455. doi:10.1016/j.fertnstert.2006.11.079

Levene, M. I., Wild, J., & Steer, P. (1992). Higher multiple births and the modern management of infertility in Britain. *British Journal of Obstetrics and Gynaecology, 99,* 607–613. doi:10.1111/j.1471-0528.1992.tb13831.x

Mansour, R., Ishihara, O., Adamson, G. D., Dyer, S., de Mouzon, J., Nygren, K. G.,...Zegers-Hochschild, F. (2014). International Committee for Monitoring Assisted Reproductive Technologies world report: Assisted Reproductive Technology 2006. *Human Reproduction, 29,* 1536–1551. doi:10.1093/humrep/deu084

Martin, J. A., Hamilton, B. E., Osterman, M. J., Curtin, S. C., & Mathews, T. J. (2013). *Births: Final data for 2012* (National Vital Statistics Reports Vol. 62, No. 9). Retrieved from http://www.cdc.gov/nchs/data/nvsr/nvsr62/nvsr62_09.pdf

Newton, C. R., McBride, J., Feyles, V., Tekpetey, F., & Power, S. (2007). Factors affecting patients' attitudes toward single- and multiple-embryo transfer. *Fertility and Sterility, 87,* 269–278. doi:10.1016/j.fertnstert.2006.06.043

Pandian, Z., Marjoribanks, J., Ozturk, O., Serour, G., & Bhattacharya, S. (2013). Number of embryos for transfer following in vitro fertilisation or intra-cytoplasmic sperm injection. *Cochrane Database of Systematic Reviews, 7*(CD003416). doi:10.1002/14651858.CD003416.pub4

Pinborg, A., Wennerholm, U. B., Romundstad, L. B., Loft, A., Aittomaki, K., Söderström-Anttila, V.,...Bergh, C. (2013). Why do singletons conceived after assisted reproduction technology have adverse perinatal outcome? Systematic review and meta-analysis. *Human Reproduction Update, 19,* 87–104. doi:10.1093/humupd/dms044

Poikkeus, P., & Tiitinen, A. (2008). Does single embryo transfer improve the obstetric and neonatal outcome of singleton pregnancy? *Acta obstetricia et gynecologica Scandinavica, 87,* 888–892. doi:10.1080/00016340802307787

Practice Committee of American Society for Reproductive Medicine & Practice Committee of Society for Assisted Reproductive Technology. (1998). *Guidelines on numbers of embryos transferred.* Birmingham, AL: American Society for Reproductive Medicine.

Practice Committee of American Society for Reproductive Medicine & Practice Committee of Society for Assisted Reproductive Technology. (1999). *Guidelines on numbers of embryos transferred.* Birmingham, AL: American Society for Reproductive Medicine.

Practice Committee of the American Society for Reproductive Medicine. (2012). Multiple gestation associated with infertility therapy: An American Society for Reproductive Medicine Practice Committee opinion. *Fertility and Sterility, 97*, 825–834. doi:10.1016/j .fertnstert.2011.11.048

Rebar, R. W., & DeCherney, A. H. (2004). Assisted reproductive technology in the United States. *The New England Journal of Medicine, 350*, 1603–1604. doi:10.1056/NEJMp048046

Reynolds, M. A., Schieve, L. A., Martin, J. A., Jeng, G., & Macaluso, M. (2003). Trends in multiple births conceived using assisted reproductive technology, United States, 1997–2000. *Pediatrics, 111*(Suppl. 1), 1159–1162.

Scotland, G. S., McLernon, D., Kurinczuk, J. J., McNamee, P., Harrild, K., Lyall, H.,...Bhattacharya, S. (2012). Minimising twins in in vitro fertilisation: A modelling study assessing the costs, consequences and cost-utility of elective single versus double embryo transfer over a 20-year time horizon. *British Journal of Obstetrics and Gynaecology, 118*, 1073–1083. doi:10.1111/j.1471–0528.2011.02966.x

Scotland, G. S., McNamee, P., Peddie, V. L., & Bhattacharya, S. (2007). Safety versus success in elective single embryo transfer: Women's preferences for outcomes of in vitro fertilisation. *British Journal of Obstetrics and Gynaecology, 114*, 977–983. doi:10.1111/j.1471–0528.2007.01396.x

Trounson, A., & Mohr, L. (1983). Human pregnancy following cryopreservation, thawing and transfer of an eight-cell embryo. *Nature, 305*, 707–709. doi:10.1038/305707a0

Vélez, M. P., Connolly, M. P., Kadoch, I.-J., Phillips, S., & Bissonnette, F. (2014). Universal coverage of IVF pays off. *Human Reproduction, 29*(6), 1313–1319. doi:10.1093/humrep/ deu067

Wilcox, L. S., Kiely, J. L., Melvin, C. L., & Martin, M. C. (1996). Assisted reproductive technologies: Estimates of their contribution to multiple births and newborn hospital days in the United States. *Fertility and Sterility, 65*, 361–366.

Zeilmaker, G. H., Alberda, A. T., van Gent, I., Rijkmans C. M., & Drogendijk, A. C. (1984). Two pregnancies following transfer of intact frozen-thawed embryos. *Fertility and Sterility, 42*, 293–296.

# CHAPTER 13

# *Exemplar:* MEDICALLY HIGH-RISK CONDITIONS NECESSITATING UTILIZATION OF A GESTATIONAL CARRIER

## Eleanor L. Stevenson

For three decades, surrogates and gestational carriers have been part of assisted reproductive technology (ART) treatment options for situations in which the intended mother is physically unable to gestate a fetus (Utian, Sheean, Goldfarb, & Kiwi, 1985). Traditionally, a surrogate is one who provides her oocytes as well as carries the pregnancy (Anchan & Ginsburg, 2012; Utian et al., 1989), whereas a gestational carrier is a woman who carries a nonbiological child for another intended parent, and therefore only has a gestational, not genetic, relationship to the child (Anchan & Ginsburg, 2012; Marrs, Ringler, Stein, Vargyas, & Stone, 1993). The oocytes either come from the intended mother or another third-party donor. There is a continued rise in the need and use of gestational carriers (Burrell & Edozien, 2014). Gestational carriers are not legal in all countries, and even within countries there are differing regulations based on regions. For example, within the United States, some states do not allow the legal use of gestational carriers; therefore, intended parents who live in these states will contract with gestational carriers outside of their home state.

Gestational carriers should be used when a woman has a true medical condition that precludes her from carrying a pregnancy or would result in significant risk, harm, or death to either the woman or the fetus. Additionally, gestational carriers can be used when there is a biological inability to conceive or carry a child, as is the case for single and homosexual men (Practice Committee of the American Society for Reproductive Medicine & Practice Committee of the Society for Assisted Reproductive Technology, 2015). A specific case exemplar about the use of a gestational carrier is presented, and then considerations that are essential for both the intended parents and gestational carrier are discussed.

## CASE STUDY

E.M. is a 38-year-old woman who presents to her local fertility clinic in the United States desiring a pregnancy. She reports being married to K.D. for 2 years. They are seeking services for assistance because of E.M.'s complex medical history. She reports autosomal dominant polycystic kidney, which was diagnosed in child-hood, and despite medical management, led to the necessity of a known-donor kidney transplant at the age of 36 years. Although many women who receive solid-organ transplants can carry a pregnancy, they are not without risk. Risks for the woman and her pregnancy include potential negative effect of the pregnancy on long-term allograft function, graft rejection, hypertension, gestational diabetes, anemia, and infections such as urinary tract infections. The maternal transplant recipient is also at increased risk of infection as a result of the use of immunosup-pressive medications (McKay & Josephson, 2008). The fetus may have potentially negative effects of in utero exposure to medications during organogenesis and development. There is no option other than to expose the fetus to immunosup-pressive agents, because all immunosuppressive medications pass through the maternal–fetal circulation (McKay & Josephson, 2006). Because of some postop-erative complications and her age, it was advised that E.M. not carry a pregnancy herself. Complicating her path to parenthood, due to her transplant status, E.M. and K.D. knew they would be ineligible for adoption, thus limiting their options for family building.

On consultation with the fertility specialist, use of a gestational carrier was discussed with E.M and K.D. The decision to use a gestational carrier is chal-lenging for potential parents. It is recommended that those considering using a gestational carrier be offered psychosocial education and counseling to help with the decision-making process. Included in the counseling should be psycho-logical testing in accordance with American Psychological Association (2010) Ethical Standards, with appropriate follow-up as necessary. The areas that must be explored during the counseling include the potential impact of the relation-ship between the intended parent and carrier and plans about disclosing iden-tity and future contact between the gestational carrier, intended parents, and baby (Practice Committee of the American Society for Reproductive Medicine & Practice Committee of the Society for Assisted Reproductive Technology, 2015). Evidence suggests there are no negative relationships when there is contact between the family and gestational carrier and no increase in regret. Most gesta-tional carriers report being satisfied in their relationship with the intended par-ent (Imrie & Jadva, 2014).

In addition to counseling, the intended parents will be provided extensive screening and testing, as well as a complete medical evaluation, to ensure that they are healthy to proceed with the treatment cycle. Intended parents will have genetic screening, and in some countries such as the United States, prospec-tive genetic parents with any identified risk factors based on screening ques-tions are considered ineligible according to guidelines issued by the Food and Drug Administration; embryos created can still be transferred into a gestational carrier as long as the tissue is labeled to indicate any possible increased risks. Although not a requirement, the best practice would be to inform the gestational carrier of the screening results (Practice Committee of the American Society for Reproductive Medicine & Practice Committee of the Society for Assisted Reproductive Technology, 2015).

Both physical and psychological evaluations of E.M. and K.D. were per-formed and it was determined that they were eligible to utilize a gestational carrier with the use of their own gametes. Using the resources within their center, the couple was able to identify an appropriate gestational carrier for the pregnancy. As important, gestational carriers as well as their partners are also recommended to receive psychosocial evaluation and counseling, which would include a clinical interview and possibly psychological testing. Although research indicates the children of surrogate mothers do not experience any negative consequences as a result of their mother's decision to be a gestational carrier (Jadva & Imrie, 2014), it is critical that the evaluation should consider the impact of the pregnancy on family and community dynamics. An ideal carrier would be between the ages of 21 and 45 years; should have had at least one, term, uncomplicated pregnancy but not more than five previous deliveries or three deliveries via cesarean section; and be in a stable family environment with adequate support. All potential gestational carriers should be evaluated and cleared for a pregnancy and have risk factors evaluated (Practice Committee of the American Society for Reproductive Medicine & Practice Committee of the Society for Assisted Reproductive Technology, 2015).

Gestational carriers and their partners have significant needs when they consider entering into a relationship with intended parents. One of the most important needs is that they have full informed consent about the risks associated with both the ART process and medication used to achieve a pregnancy as well as potential complications of a resulting pregnancy, including health sequelae and the possibility of prolonged bed rest, hospitalization, and a possible surgical birth. Gestational carriers must have their own independent legal representation to support them throughout the entire process, especially in situations when the intended parents reside in areas that do not allow the legal use of gestational carriers. Women who become gestational carriers need to understand the extent of screening and testing of the fetus during pregnancy, and contingency plans for management of specific complications (e.g., abnormal genetic testing of the fetus, birth defects, etc.) should be discussed and agreed on before beginning treatment. Lifestyle and other habits, such as travel, exercise, and diet, also need to be discussed between the gestational carrier and intended parents. Finally, compensation paid to the gestational carrier should be agreed on in writing in the legal contract before any treatment begins, if allowed (Practice Committee of the American Society for Reproductive Medicine & Practice Committee of the Society for Assisted Reproductive Technology, 2015). For example, compensation to gestational carriers is legal in the United States and can be as high as US$30,000, though the total cost to the intended parent is much higher, nearing US$100,000 (Herron, n.d.). Countries such as Canada do not allow gestational carriers to received monetary reimbursement.

Once the gestational carrier was identified and all necessary screening was conducted, the intended mother's cycle was coordinated with the gestational carrier such that the carrier would be ready to have embryos transferred into her uterus, created from the stimulation cycle of the intended mother. This process is highly coordinated to ensure that the gestational carrier is ready to receive the embryo created by E.M. and K.D., because they desired a fresh embryo cycle. Because the gestational carrier lived several hundred miles away from E.M. and K.D., they were only able to participate in prenatal visits that included ultrasonography, but were able to be participatory in the birth process. All of the details about the birth had been previously arranged, and while the gestational carrier's partner was also present, E.M. and K.D. were able to be present at the birth of their baby, and participatory in the newborn care prior to being discharged with them to their home.

The use of gestational carriers is challenging. In many countries, the practice is not legal. In others, it is very cost prohibitive, for example, in the United States the out-of-pocket cost to intended parents can near US$100,000 (Herron, n.d.), depending on whether donor gametes are needed and if the intended parents have private insurance to cover the in vitro fertilization (IVF) procedures. For many people for whom adoption is either not available or desirable, the use of a gestational carrier provides an option toward parenthood. The clinical team supporting both the intended parents and carrier must work collaboratively to ensure that all parties are having their needs met to ensure a positive outcome.

## Sample Discussion Questions

1. What are the primary concerns of E.M. and K.D. regarding the use of a gestational carrier?
2. Are there any issues in the process that E.M. and K.D. have overlooked?
3. What other concerns from the point of view of the gestational carrier are there?

## REFERENCES

American Psychological Association. (2010). *Ethical principles of psychologists and code of conduct.* Retrieved from http://www.apa.org/ethics/code/index.aspx

Anchan, R. M., & Ginsburg, E. S. (2012). Gestational carrier pregnancy. In D. S. Basow (Ed.), *UpToDate.* Retrieved from www.uptodate.com/home

Burrell, C., & Edozien, L. C. (2014). Surrogacy in modern obstetric practice. *Seminars in Fetal & Neonatal Medicine, 19,* 272–278. doi:10.1016/j.siny.2014.08.004

Herron, J. (n.d.). *The cost of adoption vs. surrogacy.* Retrieved from http://www.bankrate.com/finance/smart-spending/costs-adoption-vs-surrogacy.aspx

Imrie, S., & Jadva, V. (2014). The long-term experiences of surrogates: Relationships and contact with surrogacy families in genetic and gestational surrogacy arrangements. *Reproductive Biomedical Online, 29,* 424–435. doi:10.1016/j.rbmo.2014.06.004

Jadva, V., & Imrie, S. (2014). Children of surrogate mothers: Psychological well-being, family relationships and experiences of surrogacy. *Human Reproduction, 29,* 90–96. doi:10.1093/humrep/det410

Marrs, R. P., Ringler, G. E., Stein, A. L., Vargyas, J. M., & Stone, B. A. (1993). The use of surrogate gestational carriers for assisted reproductive technologies. *American Journal of Obstetrics & Gynecology, 168,* 1858–1863. doi:10.1016/0002-9378(93)90702-K

McKay, D. B., & Josephson, M. A. (2006). Pregnancy in recipients of solid organs—Effects on mother and child. *New England Journal of Medicine, 354,* 1281–1293. doi:10.1056/NEJMra050431

McKay, D. B., & Josephson, M. A. (2008). Pregnancy after kidney transplantation. *Clinical Journal of the American Society of Nephrology, 3*(Suppl. 2), S117–S125. doi:10.2215/CJN.02980707

Practice Committee of the American Society for Reproductive Medicine & Practice Committee of the Society for Assisted Reproductive Technology. (2015). Recommendations for practices utilizing gestational carriers: A committee opinion. *Fertility and Sterility, 103,* e1–e8. doi:10.1016/j.fertnstert.2014.10.049

Utian, W. H., Goldfarb, J. M., Kiwi, R., Sheean, L. A., Auld, H., & Lisbona H. (1989). Preliminary experience with in vitro fertilization-surrogate gestational pregnancy. *Fertility and Sterility, 52,* 633–638.

Utian, W. H., Sheean, L., Goldfarb, J. M., & Kiwi, R. (1985). Successful pregnancy after in vitro fertilization and embryo transfer from an infertile woman to a surrogate. *New England Journal of Medicine, 313,* 1351–1352. doi:10.1056/NEJM198511213132112

# PART III

# POLICY: EXPLORING ACCESS AND CHALLENGES IN ART

"The right to health is a fundamental part of our human rights and of our understanding of a life in dignity" (Office of the United Nations High Commissioner for Human Rights & World Health Organization, 2008, p. 1). Individuals and couples with fertility challenges who need assisted reproductive technology (ART) not only face medical challenges, but very often have to navigate a complex and inconsistent system in order to receive high-quality care.

In this part, many considerations related to access to fertility care are discussed. Collura and Stevenson examine the challenges facing access to care in the United States. Stevenson and Kanehl present data from many European and other developed countries from the perspective of legal access to specific ARTs and qualifications for publicly funded care. The authors also discuss some reasons why many people are going to other countries to receive the care that is needed. Dhont and Ombelet approach fertility care in developing countries with two chapters: one that presents the challenge of utilization in these countries and the other about emergent lower cost options in these settings. Scholten and Mol challenge the current approach of timing of care for couples with fertility challenges as a way to equitably use the current services available, and Everett, Apatira, and McCabe consider how those in a same-sex relationship have challenges in receiving the same level of fertility care as those in opposite-sex relationships.

## REFERENCE

Office of the United Nations High Commissioner for Human Rights & World Health Organization. (2008). *The right to health. Fact sheet no. 31.* Retrieved from http://www.ohchr.org/Documents/Publications/Factsheet31.pdf

# CHAPTER 14

# CHALLENGES TO INFERTILITY ADVOCACY IN THE UNITED STATES: DEFINING INFERTILITY AND BARRIERS TO ACCESS TO CARE

*Barbara Collura and Eleanor L. Stevenson*

Determining the incidence of infertility in the United States should be fairly straightforward, as identifying the burden of other diseases such as diabetes, cancer, and even gout has been described (American Cancer Society, n.d.; Christine et al., 2015; Macovei & Brujbu, 2015). But identifying the incidence of infertility, which seems like a straightforward number to determine, is actually much more difficult to quantify. This chapter discusses the incidence of infertility and utilization of services, as well as barriers to access in the United States from the perspective of RESOLVE: The National Infertility Association, a nonprofit patient advocacy organization whose mission is to improve the lives of people living with the disease of infertility. Every day, the media, policy makers, government agencies, insurers, and regulators in the United States look to RESOLVE to provide data on infertility (RESOLVE, n.d. a).

In order for the information that comes from RESOLVE to be viewed as credible, it must reflect accurate statistics that come from reliable sources. There are key reasons for this: The first is that we, as a community, must be able to challenge our government to do better for people with infertility. The second is that when working with legislators, media, and the general public in order to advance the cause of infertility, statistical jargon must be boiled down into digestible sound bites that are easy to communicate and remember. Finally, it is imperative to have a universally accepted definition of infertility, which currently does not exist (Chandra, Copen, & Hervey, 2013; European Society of Human Reproduction and Embryology, n.d.; Practice Committee of the American Society for Reproductive Medicine, 2013; Zegers-Hochschild et al., 2009). If the statistics and the definitions are not consistent among our government agencies and the nonprofits within the community, it becomes increasingly difficult to best represent the interests of an individual with this disease.

# INCIDENCE OF INFERTILITY AND UTILIZATION OF SERVICES

## Source of the Data

Organizations such as RESOLVE must ensure that the source of the data used is credible and verifiable. Ideally, the source is a government entity or other reputable source that has been compiling data using approved and reliable procedures consistently over time. For example, the National Survey of Family Growth (NSFG) was created in 1973 and gathers information on family life, marriage and divorce, pregnancy, infertility, use of contraception, and men's and women's health. These data have been collected seven times since its creation (Centers for Disease Control and Prevention [CDC], n.d.). The survey results are used by the U.S. Department of Health and Human Services and others to plan health services and health education programs and to serve as a statistical dataset for research that examines families, fertility, and health. The NSFG is administered by the National Center for Health Statistics, which became part of the CDC in the 1980s. To the best of our knowledge, these are the only data collected in the United States that capture the number of people living with infertility. Key leaders at RESOLVE, along with many other leaders in professional groups, including the CDC, jointly decided many years ago to use the data from the NSFG in our communications as it is the most credible data source available. Although the NSFG has its limitations and the data can be complicated to understand, these are considered the most accurate when working toward doing advocacy goals for those with infertility.

## Definition of Infertility

In order to give the statistics meaning and be able to effectively communicate findings to the public, the statistics used must match the definition of infertility. The challenge becomes determining the exact definition of infertility. Surprisingly, there is no universally agreed-upon definition.

The American Society for Reproductive Medicine (ASRM) defines infertility as "the result of a disease (an interruption, cessation, or disorder of body functions, systems, or organs) of the male or female reproductive tract which prevents the conception of a child or the ability to carry a pregnancy to delivery" (American Society for Reproductive Medicine, n.d., p. 1). ASRM further suggests that earlier evaluation is warranted after 6 months of failure to achieve a successful pregnancy in women older than 35 years, yet does not include recurrent pregnancy loss (two or more miscarriages or stillbirths) in their definition of infertility.

The World Health Organization and the International Committee for Monitoring Assisted Reproductive Technology define infertility as "a disease of the reproductive system defined by the failure to achieve a clinical pregnancy after 12 months or more of regular unprotected sexual intercourse" (Zegers-Hochschild et al., 2009, p. 1522). When reporting data about infertility, the NSFG breaks out the data based on two different definitions. The first group is infertility, which they define as:

> When neither the respondent [to the Survey] nor her current husband or cohabiting partner is surgically sterile, a woman is defined as

infertile at time of interview if, during the previous 12 months or longer, she and her husband or partner were continuously married or cohabiting, were sexually active each month, had not used contraception, and had not become pregnant. (Chandra et al., 2013, p. 2)

They use a second category called fecundity or impaired fecundity, which "describes the physical ability (or with impaired, the inability) of a woman to have a child and not simply to conceive a pregnancy. This measure is defined for all women, regardless of their relationship status" (Chandra et al., 2013, pp. 2–3). The key differences between "infertility" and "impaired fecundity" are that one (infertility) is based on married or cohabitating women and is limited to problems getting pregnant, and the other (impaired fecundity) is for all women and includes the inability to carry a pregnancy to a live birth. Additionally, the NSFG does include one measure of male infertility and it shows that 12% of men aged 25 to 44 years experience some form of infertility.

Given these two definitions, organizations such as RESOLVE have chosen to use the statistics associated with impaired fecundity, as that definition is more in line with what the general public views as "infertility"—a woman who cannot get pregnant or who cannot carry a pregnancy to term. This is the most inclusive definition and the one those working on behalf of RESOLVE feel is the most accurate about the experience of those in the United States.

## Incidence of Infertility

Based on this definition, the incidence of infertility in the United States is one in eight couples, or 12%. It is important to note that the most recent data from the NSFG were analyzed and published in 2013, but are based on data collected from 2006 to 2010. Before this, the last dataset available was from 2002, so more recent figures are definitely needed. At this pace, the data on infertility are analyzed on a very inconsistent schedule.

A commonly reported number of the incidence of infertility is one in six couples. This number came from a study conducted by researchers at the National Institutes of Health (NIH) from 2012 to 2013, and became used by the media in their reporting about infertility; therefore, it received a significant amount of public attention. For this study, they relied on the same data from the NSFG (though they used the older 2002 data) and employed a different statistical method called "current duration approach." In this method, the approach is to look at the answers to the question, "How long have you been trying to get pregnant?" They felt that the NSFG definition of infertility, which only included married women, was too narrow, and the changing sociodemographic data (number of unmarried women, delayed childbearing, etc.) impacted the magnitude and scope of infertility, which older datasets may not have taken into consideration. When they applied the current duration approach methodology, the prevalence of infertility went way up—from 7.0% from the NSFG data to 15.5% or one in six couples (Thoma et al., 2013). As the authors noted, this study was the "first application of the current duration design for estimating infertility" in U.S. women. It is not the method investigators/statisticians from the CDC are using to determine the number of infertile individuals at this time, but it may gain authority in the future.

## Call to Action

Because of the confusing and conflicting approach to defining and gauging the incidence of infertility in the United States, some effort has been made to help arrive at a consensus. Several years ago, RESOLVE participated in a meeting at the CDC to discuss the need for an "Action Plan" on infertility, resulting from advocacy by RESOLVE to Congress for the prioritization to create this "National Action Plan" by the CDC (2014). The Action Plan was drafted and was released on July 16, 2014; it calls for the need for a clear definition of infertility and better data on the prevalence of infertility in the United States. The National Public Health Action Plan for the Detection, Prevention, and Management of Infertility discusses infertility as a public health issue, and in each section, outlines the challenges—and opportunities—for the entire community to come together to advance the cause of infertility. The limitations of this plan, however, are the action steps that follow. What is necessary is that this plan needs to be set in action and the thoughtful plans that are drafted need to be implemented.

## Utilization of Services

The NSFG also looks at how many people use infertility services. This report examines the types of services that a woman or man accessed in her or his lifetime, including medical advice, testing, medications, and in vitro fertilization (IVF). The data based on the 2006 to 2010 survey showed that 12% of women will have had infertility services in their lifetime, which is one in eight (7.4 million) women. Only 38% of all nulliparous women with infertility problems ever used infertility services, a significant drop from 56% in 1982. Furthermore, those most likely to use the services were older, nulliparous, non-Hispanic White women with higher levels of education and household income (Chandra, Copen, & Stephen, 2014), which is not representative of all individuals who are in need of these services.

## BARRIERS TO ACCESS

Once an individual or couple is diagnosed with infertility, or is unable to conceive a child after 12 months of unprotected intercourse, they soon discover that where they live, who they work for, and how much disposable income they have determine the extent of medical care they can actually receive for their infertility and what family building options are available to them (Drazba, Kelley, & Hershberger, 2014). Although the most commonly used fertility services are advice, testing, and medical treatment to prevent miscarriage and the use of ovulation drugs, many contributory factors will determine what the infertile individual or couple have available to them and if they seek out additional necessary services.

### Infertility Is Not Covered by Insurance

To date, there has been little in the way of a coordinated national effort for collaboration between the medical community and the patient advocacy community on working toward ART coverage by our nation's health insurance providers. There have been some efforts and positive results for infertility coverage recently, but the challenge to see larger successes requires time to develop positive working relationships with insurers. Some of the challenges for insurers in the decisions to provide coverage include the lack of basic data and consensus around issues such as the standard of care for infertility and its corresponding allowable insurance reimbursements; the total burden of infertility in the United States; current and defendable actuarial data on the cost of coverage for infertility treatments, such as clomiphene citrate, controlled ovarian stimulation, intrauterine inseminations, and IVF; and birth outcomes and risks of various treatments. Advocates' message to insurers for health insurance coverage for the disease of infertility has not been strong, partly hindered by old and incomplete data. To help bridge the information gap and provide additional resources that advocates can use when working with insurers, two documents are available publicly that outline the need for insurance coverage for infertility treatments: The Hastings Center/Yale School of Medicine report, commissioned by the March of Dimes, which was released in April 2014, and the CDC's National Public Health Action Plan for the Detection, Prevention, and Management of Infertility, which was released in July 2014 (Centers for Disease Control and Prevention, 2014; Johnston, Gusmano, & Patrizio, 2014). Despite these efforts, there is still more work necessary to ensure that infertility is treated as a disease and coverage is comprehensive but cost-effective for employers to offer to their employees.

## The Status of the State Mandates

In the absence of health insurers covering infertility as a disease, the community has sought other ways to achieve coverage over the years. State mandates, specifically those in eight states that have a mandate to cover IVF (Arkansas, Connecticut, Hawaii, Illinois, Maryland, Massachusetts, New Jersey, and Rhode Island), have allowed thousands of people to access care and many of them to have children (RESOLVE, n.d. b). However, many of these mandates are out of date with current medical practice. Additionally, all mandates provide exclusion of self-insured plans. Exclusions in some of the mandates, specifically Arkansas, Hawaii, and Maryland, make it difficult for many people to even receive coverage. Advocates have supported recent attempts to update and improve the mandates in Hawaii and Maryland, though have not had any success. The challenge in working with the different states to consider updating their infertility insurance mandate bills is related to broader issues including state-specific budget/financial crises and the passage and roll-out of the Affordable Care Act (ACA), which left state lawmakers unsure about costs in this new structure. These two larger issues diverted attention from the key issues surrounding insurance coverage. An example of state lawmakers not wanting to fully consider the issues of infertility care in the unclear setting of the ACA was that a widely supported bill in California in 2013 to mandate insurance coverage for fertility preservation for cancer patients was vetoed by a Democratic governor, citing uncertainty about the ACA and its implementation. Finally, due to provisions in the ACA, states and advocacy groups have been hesitant to update the current mandates or add new ones as the federal government stated that any changes to any state mandate (or new ones added) after December 31, 2011, would impose a host of financial issues for the states.

## Complacency in States With Mandates

The patient and provider communities in the states with mandates that do cover IVF have not worked together to ensure that elected officials and insurance commissions, including governors, state legislators, and regulators, know the positive impact of the existing policy. The infertility community has become complacent and has taken the current mandates for granted. Some of the mandates have been in place for many years and newly elected state officials may not even know or appreciate the positive impact the mandate has had on their state and its residents. The strength and organization of the community helps ensure that attempts to weaken or remove the mandate will not happen. This effort allows legislators and regulators to have a clear understanding that an existing policy has a vocal constituency that cares about keeping it in place. More effort is needed to protect the existing mandates.

## Personhood and Other Anti-Family State Bills

Since 2008, representatives from RESOLVE and ASRM have been extremely active (and successful) in opposing state bills that would limit or outlaw access to IVF. Many of these bills may seem small in nature, but undermine the ability to allow both science to continue to expand and develop as well as provide innovative solutions to some of the most complex infertility challenges. These bills have included provisions such as embryo tracking, outlawing donor compensation, outlawing gestational carrier surrogacy, regulating donor and IVF consent, and the most significant—Personhood. Personhood defines a fertilized egg as a person. Groups including RESOLVE strongly believe that all of these proposed laws would alter the standard of care so profoundly that access to IVF and other ART in a state may be reduced or altogether eliminated. Although the Personhood movement (see www .personhoodusa.com) has not yet been realized, those who support the movement continue to attempt the passage of bills and ballot initiatives. For example, in 2014, Colorado and North Dakota had Personhood ballot initiatives on their state ballots in November, which did ultimately both fail passage. To date, 26 states have had a Personhood bill or ballot initiative introduced since 2008, yet the infertility community is not organized fully to properly fight these challenges to access to care, and more effort is required to handle these and future initiatives.

## The Affordable Care Act

The ACA, widely deemed as a policy initiative passed to improve access to medical care across the United States, may in fact have a significantly negative effect on infertility coverage. This act may end existing infertility state mandates, dramatically *reducing* access to infertility medical care. Although there is a great deal of uncertainty at this point, what is known is this: The Department of Health and

Human Services has waived certain provisions in the ACA law for calendar years 2014, 2015, and 2016 that would negatively impact the mandates. Those working toward expanded infertility coverage still need clarity on the following: whether the Department of Health and Human Services will extend that waiver past 2016; if they will release a rule that in essence makes the bad provision in the law go away; if the waiver is not extended, what is the impact on the state mandates; will the consolidation of the online exchanges affect the possible creation of a standard Essential Health Benefits (EHB) plan that may exclude procedures such as IVF; and, if a standard EHB plan is created and IVF is excluded, what is the impact on employer plans, which are not under the EHB rules, but may voluntarily adopt the "standard" EHB plan. There are so many unknowns surrounding this issue, but the worst-case scenario is a profoundly negative outcome for individuals and couples who need IVF in states with existing mandates.

## Restrictive Federal Benefits

There is significant opportunity to increase access to infertility treatments within the federal government. Currently, the Department of Defense insurance plan for active duty military, TRICARE, specifically excludes coverage for IVF. Active duty military can pay out of pocket at a handful of Military Treatment Facilities (MTF) that offer IVF for a reduced price, but obstacles, such as deployments, taking time off to seek treatment, the waiting lists, and the cost, make this option out of reach for most in the military. Veterans do not fare much better: if they have a service-related injury that caused their infertility, the Veterans Administration is banned from offering IVF, and it will require congressional action to reverse that ban. There has been, however, some potential positive change in this area. The Women Veterans and Families Health Services Act of 2015 was introduced in February 2015 in the Senate by Senator Patty Murray, a revised version of the legislation Senator Murray has introduced in previous sessions of Congress. This legislation is a result of collaboration with and support of organizations such as ASRM and, if passed, would allow the Department of Veterans Affairs and the Department of Defense to provide reproductive services (including IVF) to service members, veterans, and their families who have suffered catastrophic wounds during war that prevent them from starting families without medical assistance. Additionally, it would expand the current fertility services offered to service members and their families by the Department of Defense, and end the ban on IVF services at the Veterans Administration (American Society for Reproductive Medicine, 2015).

As for the civilian workforce, the Office of Personnel Management does not include infertility in their standard benefit plans for federal employees. A few plans offered by the feds include some coverage for IVF, but with high deductibles and exclusions, it is not coverage that is helpful to the masses. The missing piece has been a coordinated effort from the infertility community to correct these inequities so that the military and our federal government serve as examples of the coverage that should be available to everyone. What are needed are data, a coordinated strategy, and the means by which to focus on these efforts to achieve positive outcomes and gain coverage for our federal workforce, our military, and our veterans.

## Federal Research Restrictions

Since 1995, the Department of Health and Human Services and the NIH are prevented from funding any research on human embryos. This restriction is attached to the NIH funding appropriations (a bill rider) each year by Congress. It was first attached as an amendment, called the Dickey–Wicker Amendment, in 1995 and has been included in NIH funding authorizations ever since. This means that our ability to advance the field of research in the United States, where federal protections and oversight mechanisms are in place, is nonexistent. This limits advances in the field or allows investigators in other countries to advance the field, leaving valuable research contributions outside the United States. Ultimately, the effectiveness of treatment is hampered by restrictive federal research funding.

## CONCLUSION

There are many challenges in advocating for the needs and rights of individuals and couples who are dealing with fertility challenges. Working collectively, patients, clinicians, policy leaders, and others can support RESOLVE's mission to provide advocacy for those living with the disease of infertility. In order to do this work effectively, it is essential to have a clear message, particularly when working with governmental agencies to bring about a change: the definition of infertility needs to be clear as it helps one to understand the true scope of the problem. The current inconsistency of defining infertility by leading professional organizations makes it difficult to adequately voice needs for particular populations: Therefore, providing an accurate picture of the incidence of impaired fecundity and infertility is difficult, taking away meaning from the message about the need to increase attention to this problem.

Because some of the biggest barriers for quality care for those with fertility challenges include inadequate insurance coverage and the status of the state mandates, particularly with the introduction of the ACA, advocacy groups such as RESOLVE must support the work on a state and national level with a goal of expanded coverage and access for all people, regardless of their economic situation. The ever-evolving and complex political landscape necessitates that organizations such as RESOLVE stay current and active to be able to advocate and help the continued development of the science that supports fertility care, and ultimately be the voice for those who are directly and indirectly affected by this disease.

## REFERENCES

American Cancer Society. (n.d.). *What causes cancer?* Retrieved from http://www.cancer.org/cancer/cancercauses/index

American Society for Reproductive Medicine. (n.d.). *Infertility.* Retrieved from https://www.asrm.org/topics/detail.aspx?id=36

American Society for Reproductive Medicine. (2015, February 11). ASRM endorses The Women Veterans and Families Health Services Act of 2015. *ASRM Bulletin, 17*(6). Retrieved from http://www.asrm.org/ASRM_Endorses_The_Women_Veterans_and_Families_Health_Services_Act_of_2015

Centers for Disease Control and Prevention. (n.d.). *National survey of family growth*. Retrieved from http://www.cdc.gov/nchs/nsfg.htm

Centers for Disease Control and Prevention. (2014). *National public health action plan for the detection, prevention, and management of infertility*. Atlanta, GA: Author.

Chandra, A., Copen, C. E., & Hervey, S. E. (2013). *Infertility and impaired fecundity in the United States, 1982–2010: Data from the National Survey of Family Growth* (National Health Statistics Reports No. 67). Retrieved from http://www.cdc.gov/nchs/data/nhsr/nhsr067.pdf

Chandra, A., Copen, C. E., & Stephen, E. H. (2014). *Infertility service use in the United States: Data from the National Survey of Family Growth, 1982–2010* (National Health Statistics Reports No. 73). Retrieved from http://www.cdc.gov/nchs/data/nhsr/nhsr073.pdf

Christine, P. J., Auchincloss, A. H., Bertoni, A. G., Carnethon, M. R., Sánchez, B. N., Moore, K.,....Diez Roux, A.V. (2015). Longitudinal associations between neighborhood physical and social environments and incident type 2 diabetes mellitus: The multi-ethnic study of atherosclerosis (MESA). *JAMA Internal Medicine, 175,* 1311–1320. doi:10.1001/jamainternmed.2015.2691

Drazba, K. T., Kelley, M. A., & Hershberger, P. E. (2014). A qualitative inquiry of the financial concerns of couples opting to use preimplantation genetic diagnosis to prevent the transmission of known genetic disorders. *Journal of Genetic Counseling, 23,* 202–211. doi:10.1007/s10897–013-9638–7

European Society of Human Reproduction and Embryology. (n.d.). *Assisted reproductive technology (ART)—Glossary*. Retrieved from http://www.eshre.eu/Guidelines-and-Legal/ART-glossary.aspx

Johnston, J., Gusmano, M. K., & Patrizio, P. (2014). Preterm births, multiples, and fertility treatment: Recommendations for changes to policy and clinical practices. *Fertility and Sterility, 102,* 36–39. doi:10.1016/j.fertnstert.2014.03.019

Macovei, L. A., & Brujbu, I. C. (2015). Clinical and epidemiological aspects of gout, a dysmetabolic disabling disorder. *Revista Medico-chirurgicala a Societatii de Medici si Naturalisti din Iasi, 119,* 62–68.

Practice Committee of the American Society for Reproductive Medicine. (2013). Definitions of infertility and recurrent pregnancy loss: A committee opinion. *Fertility and Sterility, 99,* 63. doi:10.1016/j.fertnstert.2012.09.023

RESOLVE. (n.d. a). *About us*. Retrieved from http://www.resolve.org/about/

RESOLVE. (n.d. b). *Insurance coverage*. Retrieved from http://www.resolve.org/family-building-options/insurance_coverage/

Thoma, M. E., McLain, A. C., Louis, J. F., King, R. B., Trumble, A. C., Sundaram, R., & Buck Louis, G. M. (2013). Prevalence of infertility in the United States as estimated by the current duration approach and a traditional constructed approach. *Fertility and Sterility, 99,* 1324–1331. doi:10.1016/j.fertnstert.2012.11.037

Zegers-Hochschild, F., Adamson, G. D., de Mouzon, J., Ishihara, O., Mansour, R., Nygren, K.,...Vanderpoel, S. (2009). International Committee for Monitoring Assisted Reproductive Technology (ICMART) and the World Health Organization (WHO) revised glossary of ART terminology, 2009. *Fertility and Sterility, 92,* 1520–1524. doi:10.1016/j.fertnstert.2009.09.009

# CHAPTER 15

# UTILIZATION OF ART SERVICES IN DEVELOPED COUNTRIES AND IMPACT ON CROSS-BORDER REPRODUCTIVE CARE

*Eleanor L. Stevenson and Jamie Kanehl*

Infertility is a worldwide problem that affects about 9% of the population, with one in six couples experiencing infertility problems (European Society of Human Reproduction and Embryology, 2014). This translates to 48.5 million infertile couples worldwide, and rates for women between the ages of 20 and 44 years have remained relatively stable in the past 20 years (Mascarenhas, Flaxman, Boerma, Vanderpoel, & Stevens, 2012). Reproductive health is a priority topic across the globe, yet resources and access for infertility are less consistently available for multifactorial reasons. Although technology continues to advance, European and other developed countries use various treatment options to different extents, in part based on public versus private funding, and availability of certain treatments based on governmental regulations, among others. These differences between countries have a direct impact on individuals and couples who are affected by infertility and their ability to access services within their country. This chapter discusses the current utilization of assisted reproductive technology (ART) services, presents country-specific data about public funding for these services, and considers how different factors, including money and government regulation, are driving patients out of their own country to seek care elsewhere.

Many countries use ART services at increasing rates. However, the regulations for eligibility and public financing for ART vary, leading to utilization discrepancies between countries. According to the most recent data in 2011, Europe is the leader in ART cycles at approximately 55% of all reported cycles (European Society of Human Reproduction and Embryology, 2014). The United States and Japan are the most active countries, followed by France, Germany, Australia, Spain, and Italy. Other countries such as Ireland, which currently does not offer government-funded ART, have very low rates of ART cycles. One estimate is that 1,500 in vitro fertilization (IVF) cycles per million habitants are required to meet each country's treatment needs, yet currently only a third of the countries are meeting this need (Brigham, Cadier, & Chevreul, 2013). When a country does not meet the needs of the citizens for reasons including government funding, individuals and couples either seek services outside their own country or do not receive the care they need.

# FUNDING FOR ART

## Eligibility and Restrictions for Publicly Funded ART

In many developed countries, there is some level of government funding for ART. Each country in which these benefits exist sets its own parameters for who qualifies for the benefit. One driving factor in the utilization of ART services in countries that publicly fund treatment is the eligibility for those seeking care (Table 15.1). Because age, particularly of the female partner, is strongly associated with success of ART (Lee et al., 2015), most countries that offer public financing impose specific age requirements. Some countries, such as Belgium, Denmark, France, Greece, and The Netherlands, cite specific age limits for the female partner. Germany and Austria impose both a female and male limit in which the female must be below the age of 40 years and the male partner younger than 50 years. Others, such as Spain, Sweden, and Italy, set a "soft guideline" for the woman to be "childbearing age," although they do not specify an exact age limit (Shenfield et al., 2010). Japan,

**TABLE 15.1 Coverage for ART (Publicly Funded)**

| | COVERAGE LEVEL | MAXIMUM CYCLES COVERED | AGE LIMIT | ONLY MEDICAL INDICATIONS |
|---|---|---|---|---|
| Australia | Partial | — | — | Yes |
| Austria | Partial | 4 | Female < 40, Male < 50 | Yes |
| Belgium | Full | 6 | < 40 | Yes |
| Denmark | Partial | 3 | < 40 | No |
| Finland | Partial | Varies | No | No |
| France | Full | 4 | < 43 | Yes |
| Germany | Partial | 3 | Female < 40, Male < 50 | Yes |
| Greece | Partial | Varies | < 50 | Yes |
| Italy | Partial | Varies | Childbearing age | Yes |
| Japan | Partial | 10, two per year for 5 years | None | Yes |
| Portugal | Partial | Varies | None | Yes |
| Spain | Partial | 3 | Childbearing age | Yes |
| Sweden | Full | Varies | Childbearing age | Yes |
| The Netherlands | Full | 3 | < 45 | Yes |
| United Kingdom | Partial | Varies | < 40 | Yes |

*Source:* Publicly funded restrictions for coverage for ART are from Brigham et al. (2013), Study Group of Reproductive Technology and Healthcare (2013), and Svitnev (2012).

Finland, and Portugal do not have age limits for public funding of ART. Japan, however, is currently undergoing proposed revisions to change the regulation to include an age restriction requiring the woman to be younger than 43 years (Study Group of Reproductive Technology and Healthcare, 2013).

Other social restrictions must also be met for those seeking public services for ART regardless of publicly funded care. France, Germany, Italy, Austria, and Portugal require those using ART to be in a heterosexual relationship with specific diagnosed medical indications for ART treatment. Sweden also specifies that there be a specific medical indication for ART treatment and also excludes single women, but provides homosexual couples with access to treatment. Eight of these countries do not specify a medical indication for ART treatment eligibility; however, seven require there be a medical indication for ART services provided (Table 15.2) (Brigham et al., 2013).

Even when eligibility restrictions are met by individuals and couples with infertility in countries that provide public financing, there are additional parameters about the use of services. The number of cycles of ART treatment financially covered also varies by the country (Table 15.2). The majority of the countries that

TABLE 15.2 Restrictions for Eligibility for ART

|  | ONLY COUPLES | AGE LIMIT | ONLY HETEROSEXUALS | ONLY MEDICAL INDICATIONS |
|---|---|---|---|---|
| Australia | No | None | No | No |
| Austria | Yes | None | Yes | Yes |
| Belgium | No | Yes < 45 | No | No |
| Denmark | No | Yes < 45 | No | No |
| Finland | No | None | No | No |
| France | Yes | Yes, child-bearing age | Yes | Yes |
| Germany | Yes | None | Yes | Yes |
| Greece | No | Yes < 50 | No | No |
| Italy | Yes | Yes, child-bearing age | Yes | Yes |
| Portugal | Yes | None | Yes | Yes |
| Russia | No | None | No | No |
| Spain | No | None | No | No |
| Sweden | Yes | Yes, child-bearing age | No | Yes |
| The Netherlands | No | Yes < 45 | No | Yes |
| United Kingdom | No | None | No | No |

Source: Restrictions for eligibility for each country are from Brigham et al. (2013), Study Group of Reproductive Technology and Healthcare (2013), and Svitnev (2012).

offer public financing cover at least three cycles of ART. Belgium and Japan cover the most number of cycles at six and ten, respectively. More specifically, Japan funds two cycles per year up to 5 years. This is another regulation under review for Japan in which the 2016 proposal suggests a maximum of six cycles with unlimited cycles per year (Study Group of Reproductive Technology and Healthcare, 2013). There is also discrepancy between coverage levels of different countries for each cycle. France, Belgium, The Netherlands, and Sweden offer full public financial coverage for ART, whereas countries such as Germany, Australia, and Japan offer approximately 50% coverage.

It is important to note that in many instances, individuals and couples who do not meet these criteria often have the option of paying for treatment themselves through private providers. For many, however, the cost can be prohibitive, as it often is in the United States. Because of the privatization of health care in the United States, laws about coverage for private insurance coverage for infertility services fall to the state level. Currently, 15 of 50 states mandate coverage, leaving a significant number of people without coverage, thus paying for services out-of-pocket (RESOLVE, n.d.). Another factor that must also be considered is the availability of and restrictions on certain ART procedures such as preimplantation genetic diagnosis (PGD). The availability of these services is regulated by each individual government, regardless of whether there is public funding or not. This issue is discussed in greater detail later in this chapter.

One of the consequences of restrictions on publicly funded ART is increasing waitlists for services. An example of this is in the United Kingdom. Although the United Kingdom offers various ART services, even if individuals or couples meet eligibility requirements, there may be waiting times for services. This is particularly true for gamete donation, both male and female, which has experienced a decline in the availability of donors, thus increasing waiting lists (Blyth, 2002; Gudipati et al., 2013). Availability of donor sperm from in-country donors has dropped over the years and the waiting time has increased to 18 months in 2010, which has led many couples to import donor sperm from international banks (Gudipati et al., 2013). This drop is partially attributed to aspects of the law that allow for identity disclosure of donors of sperm (Hudson & Culley, 2011; Hudson et al., 2011). In an effort to expedite treatment and reduce waiting lists for those who have the inability to pay for services with their own funds for IVF, oocyte sharing was introduced in which a woman is offered free or reduced-cost ART in return for "donating" oocytes for the treatment of another woman in need of a donor oocyte (Blyth, 2002).

## ART Access and Cross-Border Reproductive Care

Often there are many obstacles for individuals and couples to receive comprehensive, timely care for their fertility challenges. Countries such as the United States and Ireland offer no government funding; therefore, ART services are sought through private clinics only. This can have significant implications for whether individuals and couples can afford the necessary treatment. Additionally, a high demand for ART in public clinics and reduced availability of donor gametes can lead to long waitlists, which leads to the inevitable underutilization of ART overall. Governmental restrictions on the specific types of services that are available to residents further challenge full utilization, regardless of public or private funding.

Cross-border reproductive care (CBRC), formerly called "medical tourism," is the growing phenomenon that applies to persons who are seeking infertility treatment in another country outside of their own (Pennings et al., 2008). In Europe and other developed countries, the reasons why people seek reproductive treatments outside their national boundaries are quite diverse, in part because regulations differ so much among countries. The many reasons that contribute to this phenomenon include legal restrictions such as age limits, requiring marriage, or forbidding same-sex couples from receiving treatment. Issues with availability for treatment such as long waitlists and high monetary costs are other reasons to seek CBRC, as well as religious constraints and quality/safety issues. The specific rates of CBRC are unknown but estimated to be substantially high (Shenfield et al., 2010). Motivations for CBRC have psychosocial implications because of the potential profound long-term impact for those involved in the process.

The top four "outgoing" countries that persons left to seek CBRC were Italy (31.8%), Germany (14.4%), The Netherlands (12.1%), and France (8.7%), very often due to their highly restrictive regulations including age, marital status, and medical indication. The "incoming" countries most used in providing care included Belgium (29.7%), Czech Republic (20.5%), Switzerland (16.3%), Spain (15.7%), Denmark (12.5%), and Slovenia (5.4%) (Shenfield et al., 2010). Social restrictions are one of the drivers for those in "outgoing" countries. Sweden, for example, requires marriage but does not discriminate against homosexual couples. Therefore, Sweden has a large number of single women seeking outgoing treatment. Sometimes, long waitlists for public services drive this activity, as is the case of those in the United Kingdom (Shenfield et al., 2010).

In some cases, money is the driving cost for seeking care outside of a couples' country. In the case of the United States, this is well documented. The U.S. fertility medical trade has been referred to as the "baby business," largely in part to its unregulated, for-profit structure (Spar, 2006, p. 49). Because of the high demand for services and the associated high profits, there is little incentive to reduce their prices (Spar, 2006), so many couples seek care internationally where costs out-of-pocket are significantly reduced.

Even when money for services is not a concern, many countries place certain practice restrictions on what type of ART services are available, based very often on religious and ethical constructs. Shenfield et al. (2010) cite that the main reason for increases in the utilization of CBRC is for the purpose of law evasion. For example, a particular ART technique is illegal or a specific group of individuals are excluded from treatment due to social characteristics in certain countries. This study found that 54.8% of patients in Europe traveling to other countries for ART traveled for legal reasons. This translates to at least 8,000 cycles across Europe annually (Shenfield et al., 2010).

Many patients do not have PGD available to them, a procedure performed in conjunction with IVF that helps many individuals avoid passing on a genetic condition to their offspring. There are major differences in Europe regarding the regulation of PGD, which is banned in Austria and Switzerland, whereas severe limitations affect practice in Germany, Ireland, and Italy (Shenfield et al., 2010).

IVF was previously forbidden by national law in Italy to treat fertile patients with known genetic conditions, but was reversed in 2010, allowing noninfertile couples access to PGD to help prevent the transmission of certain diseases, such as cystic fibrosis, to their offspring (Benagiano & Gianaroli, 2010). Since that time, the number of couples who received PGD within their IVF cycle has increased; thus, fewer couples are forced to make the choice to go outside of their country for care (Gianaroli et al., 2014).

Another legal restriction that drives CBRC is a ban on gamete donation in certain countries. For example, egg donation is currently prohibited in Germany under the Embryo Protection Act (1990), which mandates that practitioners who violate this Act are subject to possible imprisonment or fine should they transfer a donated gamete or attempt to fertilize an egg cell artificially for any purpose other than pregnancy for the intended woman from her egg (Bergmann, 2011). Similarly, Austria currently has a ban on gamete donation with IVF that has been challenged within the legal system and upheld (Gianaroli et al., 2014). In Australia and New Zealand, patients who need gamete donation have to seek those services elsewhere for reasons beyond legal constraints. In addition to some treatments being legally prohibited, there is a limited availability of gamete donors in some states, and some patients have difficulty in meeting treatment eligibility criteria (Rodino, Goedeke, & Nowoweiski, 2014). Single and lesbian women in need of donor sperm are legally prohibited, and therefore, seek these services most often in Belgium, which is a popular destination country for ART owing to its ease of access, liberal laws about ART usage, and quality care (Van Hoof, Pennings, & De Sutter, 2015). Japanese couples are increasingly traveling to the United States and Asian countries such as India or Thailand for third-party reproduction, as this option is not available in Japan (Study Group of Reproductive Technology and Healthcare, 2013).

When individuals and couples make use of CBRC to avoid legal restrictions, in most cases they will not be prevented from seeking care outside their country or punished when they return to complete their pregnancies. However, some countries are taking steps of prohibiting their citizens from going beyond borders to seek out certain ART services. One example of this involves gamete donation. As of March 2010, Turkey became the first country to legislate against the cross-border travel of its citizens seeking third-party reproductive assistance. Although the use of donor eggs, donor sperm, and surrogacy has been illegal in Turkey since 1987, men and women were free to access these treatments in other jurisdictions. In some cases, such travel for CBRC was even facilitated between IVF clinics in Turkey and in other countries (Gürtin, 2011). Additionally, several states in Australia have either enacted or are considering restrictions to prohibit international commercial surrogacy (Van Hoof & Pennings, 2011).

## Patient Consideration Surrounding CBRC

Reproductive treatment, in general, is a stressful and complex process (Boivin et al., 2012). Although research indicates that those who do ultimately seek out fertility services outside of their own country of residence have a positive experience (Rodino et al., 2014), the treatment process is further complicated when those seeking care across borders also have to deal with practical issues related to treatment abroad. For example, gamete donation often has counseling mandates for recipients, but for those seeking this treatment via CBRC, couples may not have their needs met. In one study, less than half the sample (47.5%) had accessed some form of counseling (Rodino et al., 2014). There is a need for individuals and couples to be able to explore the importance of donor information and disclosure, the personal impact of legislation, and ongoing support needs after CBRC treatment, which currently are not being met.

Data about cross-border treatment indicate the significant emotional, financial, and logistical impact of deciding to seek treatment abroad has on individuals and couples, though much of this work has focused on the females, as she often incurs the majority of care and carries the resulting pregnancy (Shenfield et al., 2010). In addition to the discomfort derived from the need to travel from home, miss employment obligations, and stay abroad for 10 to 15 days, concerns arise on the safety and the quality of the treatments as well as on the financial implications (Pennings et al., 2009).

Currently, there is a gap regarding how to best care for individuals and couples seeking cross-border care. In no area is this more obvious than in how men utilize these services. Research is needed to better understand the experience and role of men seeking care across borders as patients, partners, or donors, as there is essentially no research in this area. There is one exception; that of work done examining Middle Eastern male expatriates who go to Lebanon with their wives in order to seek culturally and religiously familiar treatment (Inhorn, 2012). Males are often missed from research, and thus, have unmet care needs.

Increasingly, the Internet is becoming essential for couples who seek out care. From this resource, much of the care needs that otherwise would be meet by seeking care at their local infertility center are being satisfied virtually. Research indicates that online sources are used significantly by patients seeking information about cross-border care (Kahlor & Mackert, 2009). Patients looking for treatment options abroad are especially inclined to search for information online (Speier, 2011) and most patients considering and whom actually seek out treatment across borders use the data for all types of information, including for clinical selection (Blyth, 2010; Van Hoof, Provoost, & Pennings, 2013).

## CONCLUSION

The growing phenomenon of cross-border cultural care represents a challenge with infertility services worldwide. Restrictive laws, lack of public financing, high costs of treatment, and long waitlists all contribute to patients seeking legal, more affordable, and better medical care in other countries. The utilization of ART has not met the growth in technology for infertility treatment and poses a threat to the effective and comprehensive care of individuals and couples dealing with fertility challenges. As the science that advances ART care continues to move forward, governments will continue to evaluate the aspects of care available to their citizens. It is imperative for those caring for patients to be fully informed of the key issues and health policies that drive the desire to seek care outside of patients' countries.

# REFERENCES

Benagiano, G., & Gianaroli, L. (2010). The Italian constitutional court modifies Italian legislation on assisted reproductive technology. *Reproductive Biomedical Online, 20*, 398–402. doi:10.1016/j.rbmo.2009.11.025

Bergmann, S. (2011). Reproductive agency and projects: Germans searching for egg donation in Spain and the Czech Republic. *Reproductive BioMedicine Online, 23*, 600–608. doi:10.1016/j.rbmo.2011.06.014

Blyth, E. (2002). Subsidized IVF: The development of "egg sharing" in the UK. *Human Reproduction, 17*, 3254–3259. doi:10.1093/humrep/17.12.3254

Blyth, E. (2010). Fertility patients' experiences of cross-border reproductive care. *Fertility and Sterility, 94*, e11–e15. doi:10.1016/j.fertnstert.2010.01.046

Boivin, J., Domar, A. D., Shapiro, D. B., Wischmann, T. H., Fauser, B. C. J. M., & Verhaak, C. (2012). Tackling burden in ART: An integrated approach for medical staff. *Human Reproduction, 27*, 941–950. doi:10.1093/humrep/der467

Brigham, K. B., Cadier, B., & Chevreul, K. (2013). The diversity of regulation and public financing of IVF in Europe and its impact on utilization. *Human Reproduction, 28*, 666–675. doi:10.1093/humrep/des418

European Society of Human Reproduction and Embryology. (2014). *ART fact sheet (July 2014)*. Retrieved from http://www.eshre.eu/guidelines-and-legal/art-fact-sheet.aspx

Gianaroli, G., Crivello, A. M., Stanghellini, I., Ferraretti, A. P., Tabanelli, C., & Magli, M. C. (2014). Reiterative changes in the Italian regulation on IVF: The effect on PGD patients' reproductive decisions. *Reproductive BioMedicine Online, 28*, 125–132. doi: 10.1016/j .rbmo.2013.08.014

Gudipati, M., Pearce, K., Prakash, A., Redhead, G., Hemingway, V., McEleny, K., & Stewart, J. (2013). The sperm donor programme over 11 years at Newcastle Fertility Centre. *Human Fertility, 16*, 258–265. doi:10.3109/14647273.2013.815370

Gürtin, Z. B. (2011). Banning reproductive travel: Turkey's ART legislation and third-party assisted reproduction. *Reproductive BioMedicine Online, 23*, 555–564. doi:10.1016/j .rbmo.2011.08.004

Hudson, N., & Culley, L. (2011). Assisted reproductive travel: UK patient trajectories. *Reproductive Biomedicine Online, 23*, 573–581. doi:10.1016/j.rbmo.2011.07.004

Hudson, N., Culley, L., Blyth, E., Norton, W., Rapport, F., & Pacey, A. (2011). Cross-border reproductive care: A review of the literature. *Reproductive Biomedicine Online, 22*, 673–685. doi:10.1016/j.rbmo.2011.03.010

Inhorn, M. C. (2012). *The new Arab man: Emergent masculinities, technologies and Islam in the Middle East*. Princeton, NJ: Princeton University Press.

Kahlor, L., & Mackert, M. (2009). Perceptions of infertility information and support sources among female patients who access the Internet. *Fertility and Sterility, 91*, 83–90. doi:10.1016/j.fertnstert.2007.11.005

Lee, H.-L., McCulloh, D. H., Hodes-Wertz, B., Adler, A., McCaffrey, C., & Grifo, J. A. (2015). In vitro fertilization with preimplantation genetic screening improves implantation and live birth in women age 40 through 43. *Journal of Assisted Reproduction and Genetics, 32*, 435–444. doi:10.1007/s10815–014-0417-7

Mascarenhas, M. N., Flaxman, S. R., Boerma, T., Vanderpoel, S., & Stevens, G. A. (2012). National, regional, and global trends in infertility prevalence since 1990: A systematic analysis of 277 health surveys. *PLoS Medicine, 9*(12), e1001356. doi:10.1371/journal.pmed.1001356

Pennings, G., Autin, C., Decleer, W., Delbaere, A., Delbeke, L., Delvigne, A., ... Vandekerckhove, F. (2009). Cross-border reproductive care in Belgium. *Human Reproduction, 24*, 3108–3118. doi:10.1093/humrep/dep300

Pennings, G., de Wert, G., Shenfield, F., Cohen, J., Tarlatzis, B., & Devroey, P. (2008). ESHRE Task Force on Ethics and Law 15: Cross-border reproductive care. *Human Reproduction, 23*, 2182–2184. doi:10.1093/humrep/den184

RESOLVE. (n.d.). *Insurance coverage in your state.* Retrieved from http://www.resolve.org/family-building-options/insurance_coverage/state-coverage.html

Rodino, I. S., Goedeke, S., & Nowoweiski, S. (2014). Motivations and experiences of patients seeking cross-border reproductive care: The Australian and New Zealand context. *Fertility and Sterility, 102,* 1422–1431. doi.org/10.1016/j.fertnstert.2014.07.1252

Shenfield, F., de Mouzon, J., Pennings, G., Ferraretti, A. P., Nyboe Andersen, A., de Wert, G., & Goossens, V. (2010). Cross border reproductive care in six European Countries. *Human Reproduction, 25,* 1361–1368. doi:10.1093/humrep/deq057

Spar, D. L. (2006). *The baby business: How money, science, and politics drive the commerce of conception.* Boston, MA: Harvard Business School Press.

Speier, A. R. (2011). Brokers, consumers and the Internet: How North American consumers navigate their infertility journeys. *Reproductive Biomedical Online, 23,* 592–599. doi:10.1016/j.rbmo.2011.07.005

Study Group of Reproductive Technology and Healthcare. (2013). *Assisted reproductive technology in Japan.* Retrieved from http://saisentan.w3.kanazawa-u.ac.jp/image/ART%20in%20Japan_20130626.pdf

Svitnev, K. (2012). New Russian legislation on assisted reproduction. *Journal of Clinical Research & Bioethics, 1*(3), doi:10.4172/scientificreports.207

Van Hoof, W., & Pennings, G. (2011). Extraterritoriality for cross-border reproductive care: Should states act against citizens travelling abroad for illegal infertility treatment? *Reproductive BioMedicine Online, 23,* 546–554. doi:10.1016/j.rbmo.2011.07.015

Van Hoof, W., Pennings, G., & De Sutter, P. (2015). Cross-border reproductive care for law evasion: A qualitative study into the experiences and moral perspectives of French women who go to Belgium for treatment with donor sperm. *Social Science & Medicine, 124,* 391–397. doi:10.1016/j.socscimed.2014.09.018

Van Hoof, W., Provoost, V., & Pennings, G. (2013). Reflections of Dutch patients on IVF treatment in Belgium: A qualitative analysis of Internet forums. *Human Reproduction, 28,* 1013–1022. doi:10.1093/humrep/des461

# CHAPTER 16

# UTILIZATION OF FERTILITY CARE IN DEVELOPING COUNTRIES: CHALLENGES IN FAMILY BUILDING AROUND THE GLOBE

## Nathalie Dhont and Willem Ombelet

The majority of infertile couples are living in developing countries (DCs) where infertility is probably one of the most neglected public health problems. Although the ability to reproduce is a core aspect of reproductive health, infertility care is totally absent from reproductive health programs in these countries. Only a few private centers are attempting to fill the gap, offering assisted reproductive technology (ART) at costs prohibitive for most of the inhabitants of low-income countries. In this chapter, we explore the challenging aspects of infertility and the barriers to infertility access in DCs. In the second part, we suggest a roadmap toward meeting some of these challenges.

## INFERTILITY IN DCs: THE FACTS

### Some Definitions

#### What Are DCs?

DCs are defined according to their gross national income (GNI) per capita per year. According to the World Bank (2015), countries with a GNI of US$11,905 and less are defined as developing. Most of these countries belong to Africa, Asia, and Central and South America. South and East Asia (SEA) and sub-Saharan Africa (SSA) are the least developed regions.

#### Primary and Secondary Infertility

Infertility can mean different things for different authors. This renders analysis and interpretation of data difficult and explains partly some of the divergent results in infertility prevalence studies. In the clinical definition of infertility, conception is the endpoint. A couple is suffering from infertility when there is no conception after 12 months of regular and unprotected sexual intercourse (Habbema et al., 2004).

It is directly based on the self-reports of patients. Demographers use (indirect) data from health surveys to estimate infertility prevalence. They define infertility as the inability of noncontracepting sexually active women to have a live birth during a certain period of time, usually 5 to 7 years, as measured using the demographic infertility measure, developed by the World Health Organization (WHO). In their definition, the endpoint is live births (as these are registered in surveys). A longer period of exposure is used as the surveys do not capture whether the couples are actually trying for pregnancy (Habbema et al., 2004).

Clinicians use primary infertility for couples without any conception and secondary for couples with at least one previous conception. According to this definition, many women with secondary infertility do not have children. Some researchers, however, use secondary infertility for women with at least one child (Mascarenhas, Flaxman, Boerma, Vanderpoel, & Stevens, 2012).

## Magnitude of the Problem of Infertility

The true prevalence of infertility in resource-poor countries is not known as there are very few clinical data on self-reported infertility and we rely mostly on estimates based on demographic surveys. Boivin, Bunting, Collins, and Nygren (2007) calculated the prevalence of clinical (12 months definition) infertility based on 25 population surveys. In the less-developed nations, between 5% and 25.7% of the surveyed couples had suffered from infertility in their lifetime. The current infertility rate in DCs ranged from 5% to 15% (median 9%) and was similar to the rates in the developed countries. Another study performed in collaboration with the WHO looked at the trend of infertility prevalence since 1990 through analysis of 277 demographic and reproductive health surveys (Mascarenhas et al., 2012). They used the demographic infertility measure based on a 5-year exposure period. In 2010, 12.4% of women experienced infertility, with levels up to 24% in many of the less-developed regions. Of the 48.5 million infertile couples, 10 million and 14.4 million are living in SSA and South Asia, respectively. In these regions, infertility decreased slightly in the 20-year period, although the absolute number of infertile couples increased due to population growth.

In an older analysis based on the Demographic Health Surveys of 27 African nations, considerable variation was seen in the infertility rates between nations across the continent (Ericksen & Brunette, 1996). The researchers found that sociocultural and behavioral factors, such as early age at first sexual intercourse and urban residence, were strongly associated with infertility prevalence; these factors put women at risk for sexually transmitted infections (STIs) and reproductive tract infections.

## Causes of Infertility

The major causes of infertility in developed countries include ovulatory dysfunction (15%–20%); tuboperitoneal pathology, which is mainly caused by infections (14%–35%); male factors (25%–35%); and uterine pathology (5%; Fritz, 2005). Another major cause of infertility is the age-related decline in female fertility.

Available data indicate that the contributory causes of infertility in DCs are very different from those of developed countries. Between 1979 and 1984, the WHO investigated infertile couples worldwide and found that in SSA tubal factor infertility is threefold higher compared with Western countries. They estimated that infertility is caused by infections in more than 85% of women compared with 33% worldwide (Cates, Farley, & Rowe, 1985). Approximately, 70% of pelvic infections are caused by STIs whereas the other 30% are attributable to pregnancy-related sepsis (Ericksen & Brunette, 1996). Similarly, many cases of male factor infertility are caused by previous infections of the male genitourinary tract (Kuku & Osegbe, 1989). Both conditions can often be effectively treated with ART, but it is important to note that these conditions are preventable, thus decreasing the need for specialized reproductive care services.

This explains why especially secondary infertility rates are high in DCs. Many initially fertile women acquire infertility during their sexually active years. The past pregnancies in these infertile women were often complicated by (unsafe) abortions or delivery complications rendering them infertile and/or ending in neonatal death, as do becoming infected with STIs during these reproductive years, both before marriage and under circumstances in which partners bring these infections back into the marriage (Dhont, Luchters, et al., 2011).

## Culture and Religion

### Consequences of Infertility

The consequences of involuntary childlessness are much more dramatic in DCs and can create more wide-ranging societal problems compared with Western societies, particularly for women. Motherhood is one of the most important ways for women to enhance their status within the family and the community, and a marriage without children is considered a failure. Women are usually blamed for infertility and can be isolated and assaulted by their families and ostracized by the local community. This may result in physical and psychological violence and polygamy (Dhont, van de Wijgert, Coene, Gasarabwe, & Temmerman, 2011; Dyer, Abrahams, Hoffman, & van der Spuy, 2002; van Balen & Bos, 2010). Because many families in DCs completely depend on children for economic survival, childlessness has to be regarded as a social and public health issue and not only as an individual medical problem (Gerrits, 1997; Nahar et al., 2000).

### Health-Seeking Behavior

The cultural importance of childbearing and the negative implications of infertility also affect the way infertile women and men use infertility services. Several authors point to the secrecy surrounding their health-seeking behavior: visits to the fertility clinic, the diagnosis, the use of a particular form of treatment (such as the use of donor material), and/or the birth of a child resulting from ARTs may all be hidden from the partner, family, and/or community at large. Moreover, study findings from Mali show that men are often unwilling to go to a clinic as they have already fathered a child in another relationship or because they fear being diagnosed as the one who is causing the problem; or they would rather opt for social solutions (taking a second wife or fostering a child) than taking the uncertain route of expensive treatments (Hörbst, 2012).

Traditional beliefs that poisoning and witchcraft have caused the infertility play an important role in the perceptions of infertile patients. Research in Chad, Gambia, and Bangladesh has shown that infertile patients consult both the traditional healers and the formal medical sector for their problem (Dhont et al., 2010; Leonard, 2002; Nahar et al., 2000; Sundby, 1997).

In Sudan, in vitro fertilization (IVF) is only offered in combination with intracytoplasmic sperm injection (ICSI). This might indicate that in case of female factor infertility, men will try to seek a child with another woman and no treatment will be sought, a tendency that has also been observed by Hörbst (2012) in Mali (Khalifa & Ahmed, 2012). The secrecy that may surround the use of infertility treatments and the unwillingness of men to be involved in these treatments may lead to undesirable ethical dilemmas in clinical and counseling practices (Gerrits, 2012).

## HIV and Infertility

HIV infection is affecting a large number of couples in DCs, especially in SSA. Several studies have shown that HIV and infertility are linked in various ways. HIV/AIDS can affect fertility desires; and outcomes and fertility/infertility can affect the risk of HIV/AIDS. The two also share common determinants: sexual exposure, contraceptive practices, and reproductive tract infections. Efforts to plan infertility care in many DCs will need to take on board the issue of HIV infection.

In 2013, there were 35 million (33.2–37.2 million) people living with HIV, of which 70% reside in SSA (United Nations UNAIDS, 2014). Further information about HIV/AIDS can be found within the United Nations UNAIDS website (www.unaids.org).

HIV is three times more prevalent in infertile couples when compared with fertile controls in the same population in countries such as Rwanda and Tanzania (Dhont, Muvunyi, et al., 2011; Favot et al., 1997). The relationship between HIV and fertility is probably bidirectional and highly complex (Zaba & Gregson, 1998). HIV is primarily a STI and shares with infertility the same determinant of high-risk sexual behavior. There is some limited evidence that HIV worsens the tubal damage caused by pelvic inflammatory disease (Kamenga et al., 1995). Whether HIV can directly cause tubal damage or infertility is not known.

Reversely, marital instability and polygamy secondary to infertility may in turn increase the spread of HIV infection (Ross et al., 1999).

More research is needed to understand the interplay between HIV and infertility. Basically, we would like to know how much of the infertility is directly or indirectly caused by HIV infection and how much HIV infections are attributable to infertility.

## Current Access to Infertility Care

There are no good data on the access of infertility care in DCs. The latest world report on ART provides international information on availability, effectiveness, and perinatal outcomes of ART treatment cycles performed during 2007, as well as describing ART practices in 55 countries worldwide (Ishihara et al., 2015). Most of these countries belong to the developed world. Not a single country from SSA was surveyed; a few countries from Latin America and only India from Southeast Asia represented the DCs. The availability of ART exhibited a wide range, from six cycles per million inhabitants in Guatemala to 4,140 per million inhabitants in Israel (Ishihara et al., 2015). Interestingly, the WHO analysis in 1999 found that IVF availability and utilization are better correlated with a country's infant mortality rate than with the gross domestic product or overall health spending (Collins, 2002). Likely reasons for this correlation is that infant mortality may best reflect the overall quality of a nation's health system and countries with high infant mortalities place a lower priority on IVF availability because there are other health priorities (Nachtigall, 2006).

We know from some literature reports that fertility care in SSA and SEA is delivered mainly through private centers of which we have no official reports (Gerrits, 2012). The reported cost of an IVF cycle in these private centers in SSA and SEA varies between 600 and 6,000 euro and is in most cases only an option for the upper class. It has been documented that some patients seek and pay for treatment despite the fact that they cannot afford it, thereby incurring crippling financial burdens. Recently, the economic implications of infertility and its treatment were reviewed by Dyer and Patel (2012). They concluded that infertility treatment is associated with a significant risk of catastrophic expenditure, even for basic or ineffective interventions.

## INFERTILITY CARE IN DCs: HOW TO PROCEED

### To Advocate the Right to Have Access to Fertility Care

#### A Controversial Issue

National health care policies in most developed countries recognize infertility care as a medical need and make provisions to cover infertility treatment; however, the same does not apply for DCs (Nachtigall, 2006). The provision of infertility treatment in DCs is controversial and a major mind shift is needed to convince policy makers and governments to invest in treatment. It is true for many DCs that the policy makers are influenced by the views of the donor agencies. It is, therefore, important to change the conceptualization of prioritizing public health problems by the donors and government policy makers, which principally is guided only by epidemiological data. Strong advocacy is needed to promote the point that epidemiological data do not capture the impact of this burden on the well-being of infertile people (Nahar, 2012). The most common arguments used against the application of infertility treatment are overpopulation, prioritization of limited resources, and prevention rather than cure (Pennings, 2012).

#### Prevention

There is no doubt that prevention is better than cure. Because many of the infertility problems in DCs are induced by STIs, a preventable condition, promoting safer sexual behavior and better obstetric care will decrease infertility rates. However, even with huge efforts, prevention will only decrease the infertility rate to some extent and this will not help the millions of infertile couples currently living in the world.

## Overpopulation

The argument of overpopulation suggests that in countries where overpopulation poses a demographic problem, infertility management should not be supported by the government. However, denying infertile couples access to infertility care is not a fair population restriction policy and it would go against the declaration of the international conference on population and development in Cairo 1994 stating: "population is not about numbers, but about people. Implicit in this rights-based approach is the idea that every person counts" (United Nations Population Fund, 1994). This approach is also reflected in the WHO (n.d.) definition: "reproductive health, therefore, implies that people are able to have a responsible, satisfying and safe sex life and *that they have the capability to reproduce* and the freedom to decide if, when and how often to do."

In other words, we cannot deny a couple access to infertility care because their neighbors have too many children. Population growth can be restricted much more effectively by other means that do not infringe people's rights such as educating women, providing contraception, safe abortions, and so on (Pennings, 2012).

## Limited Resources

According to the "limited resources" argument, it is hard to justify expensive fertility treatment in settings with few resources and more important challenges to deal with. Can expensive techniques be justified in countries where poverty is still an important issue and where health care systems still struggle with the huge problem of infectious diseases such as malaria, tuberculosis, and HIV? In most DCs, the reduction of maternal mortality and the promotion of contraception are considered to be the reproductive health priorities (Aboulghar, 2005). Limited resources are a fact but there are many reasons to allocate at least part of the (reproductive) health budget to infertility care. First, most couples consider childbearing as one of the most important goals in their life and for them it is probably reproductive health issue number one. Second, preventing and treating infertility might decrease HIV and other STIs, as explained previously. Third, by integrating infertility care in other reproductive health services, these services could be strengthened in many ways, as is discussed in Chapter 17.

## Infertility Care as Part of Reproductive Health Care

### Integrated Reproductive Health Services

All reproductive health issues such as STIs, HIV, family planning, postabortion care, and antenatal and delivery care are connected to each other and infertility is not an exception. In the past, most of these services have been delivered in a vertical manner without much linkage. Many authors have pleaded to better integrate these different reproductive health services. One of the main arguments in support of the integration is that it will improve women's health by encouraging greater use of services because the same woman needs all of these services at different moments in her life (Berer, 2003). Women with STIs/HIV, unsafe abortions, and complicated deliveries will often go on to suffer from infertility. Women who need family planning today might need fertility care tomorrow. Women who conceived with reproductive technologies will need proper pregnancy and delivery care.

## As Part of Family Planning

Offering infertility care hand in hand with contraception might make the family planning services more acceptable for the people. A recent report by the WHO about infertility in developing nations states:

> In a world that needs vigorous control of population growth, concerns about infertility may seem odd, but the adoption of a small family norm makes the issue of involuntary infertility more pressing. If couples are urged to postpone or widely space pregnancies, it is imperative that they should be helped to achieve pregnancy when they so decide, in the more limited time they will have available. (WHO, 2010, p. 881)

## As Part of HIV Care

The link between HIV and infertility represents an opportunity and indeed an obligation to put public infertility services in place. Treating infertility in HIV-negative couples will prevent them from looking for children in multiple relationships, and therefore, will reduce the risk of becoming HIV infected. Providing infertility services to couples with at least one partner infected can prevent HIV transmission to the uninfected partner, transmission from mother to child, and transmission to other sexual partners. Some authors even argue that HIV/AIDS-related funds could be used to put such services in place, as the funds available for infertility are scarce (Dyer, 2008). An important prerequisite for addressing the reproductive needs of HIV-positive couples is to acknowledge that some will desire children and that this desire is, in principle, legitimate. At present, their fertility needs are not addressed and patients do not receive the advice and input they require. Treatment with antiretroviral therapy has prolonged the potential of survival for HIV-infected patients and has decreased the risk of mother to child transmission. Therefore, the arguments for excluding HIV-infected infertile couples from infertility treatment need to be reviewed. In fact, it can even be argued that all couples with HIV should be offered infertility investigations and this should happen preconceptionally, not after 12 to 24 months of trying. On the other hand, it is evident that HIV testing should be an integrated part of the exploration of all infertile couples. HIV counseling and testing in infertility clinics may identify many new HIV infections and increase opportunities for HIV care and treatment. When putting infertility services in place in DCs, integration of these services within the existing reproductive health services needs careful consideration. Infertility care cannot be successful without proper antenatal, delivery, and childcare and, when needed, HIV treatment.

## How to Avoid Risk

Risks of implementing ART in DCs include the inability to deal with complications following infertility treatment. Ovarian hyperstimulation syndrome, multiple pregnancies, premature babies, and ectopic pregnancies are not uncommon after ART. These complications should be avoided at all cost and the facilities and knowledge of the staff should be adequate to handle these problems. The presence of an accreditation body to regulate issues such as the quality and safety of care, laboratory procedures, training requirements, and pregnancy rates is an important tool but absent in many countries where IVF is only offered in private clinics. The lack of ART regulation implies that the full responsibility for these aspects of care rests on the shoulders of the professionals running the private clinics. In most countries where ARTs have been introduced, their use has preceded their regulation and legislation. Worldwide ART legislation and regulations diverge enormously, both in terms of what they regulate and how they are regulated, including, for example, the types of treatments offered and to whom. Often, these regulations are shaped in the context of local cultural values and the predominant religion (Gerrits, 2012).

## Costs

ART is an expensive technology; even if it is possible to decrease the costs considerably, funding will be needed for the building of fertility centers, running services (e.g., consumables, medication, medical interventions, staff salaries), and training of the medical, paramedical, and administrative staff. The need for funding is crucial and is likely to require input and collaboration from various role players. The medical and pharmaceutical industry can make relevant contributions such as providing inexpensive medication, manufacturing of basic ultrasound and laboratory equipment at low price, and so on. Foundations and donor agencies will have to be convinced about the value of infertility care, taking into account the growing demand from the DCs itself and the case of reproductive health rights (Ombelet, 2012).

In some DCs (e.g., Brazil, Egypt, Iran, Turkey, and Vietnam), the state, health insurance, and/or public clinics cover part of the costs of IVF and other ARTs. In most DCs, the private sector will continue to play an important role and public–private partnerships might be the answer toward sustainable fertility care delivery. For medical care providers, setting up a private fertility clinic demands a huge investment, in financial terms, in order to establish a clinic location and to buy medical instruments, materials, and medicines, but also in self-development, in order to acquire and maintain updated knowledge and skills required to provide the services of a fertility clinic, as the science changes at such a rapid pace. At the same time, though, there is no guarantee that the clinic will be successful, in the sense of achieving pregnancies, attracting sufficient clients, and being profitable. Various types of partnership models have been developed to enable the functioning of these private practices. These partnership models include, for example, a north–south partnership or an embryologist outsourcing lab services catering for more than one infertility clinic. Sometimes, highly trained foreign staff has to be recruited for competitive salaries in addition to cost and travel reimbursements (Gerrits, 2012).

## CONCLUSION

After a fascinating period of more than 30 years of IVF, millions of couples around the globe still suffer considerably from the consequences of infertility and only a small part of the population benefits from these new expensive technologies. The world has not yet recognized the right to access fertility care for couples in resource-poor countries. Time has come to start with accessible and affordable infertility centers worldwide. In Chapter 17, Willem Ombelet demonstrates that it is possible to lower the cost for IVF considerably through a combined simplification of the diagnostic phase, the ovarian stimulation protocols, and the IVF lab procedures. When these simplified procedures become operational and the world can be convinced of the reproductive rights of the millions of infertile couples living in the DCs, Bob Edwards's invention can finally be called a true success story.

## REFERENCES

Aboulghar, M. A. (2005). The importance of fertility treatment in the developing world. *BJOG*, 112, 1174–1176. doi:10.1111/j.1471–0528.2005.00705.x

Berer, M. (2003). HIV/AIDS, sexual and reproductive health: Intimately related. *Reproductive Health Matters*, 11(22), 6–11. doi:10.1016/s0968–8080(03)22108-x

Boivin, J., Bunting, L., Collins, J. A., & Nygren, K. G. (2007). International estimates of infertility prevalence and treatment-seeking: Potential need and demand for infertility medical care. *Human Reproduction*, 22, 1506–1512. doi:10.1093/humrep/dem046

Cates, W., Farley, T. M. M., & Rowe, P. J. (1985). Worldwide patterns of infertility: Is Africa different? *Lancet*, 326, 596–598. doi:10.1016/S0140–6736(85)90594-X

Collins, J. A. (2002). An international health survey of the health economics of IVF and ICSI. *Human Reproduction Update*, 8, 265–277. doi:10.1093/humupd/8.3.265

Dhont, N., Luchters, S., Muvunyi, C., Vyankandondera, J., De Naeyer, L., Temmerman, M., & van de Wijgert, J. (2011). The risk factor profile of women with secondary infertility: An unmatched case–control study in Kigali, Rwanda. *BMC Women's Health*, 11(32), 1–7. doi:10.1186/1472–6874-11–32

Dhont, N., Luchters, S., Ombelet, W., Vyankandondera, J., Gasarabwe, A., van de Wijgert, J., & Temmerman, M. (2010). Gender differences and factors associated with treatment-seeking behaviour for infertility in Rwanda. *Human Reproduction*, 25, 2024–2030. doi:10.1093/humrep/deq161

Dhont, N., Muvunyi, C., Luchters, S., Vyankandondera, J., De Naeyer, L., Temmerman, M., & van de Wijgert, J. (2011). HIV infection and sexual behaviour in primary and secondary infertile relationships: A case–control study in Kigali, Rwanda. *Sexually Transmitted Infections*, 87, 28–34. doi:10.1136/sti.2010.042879

Dhont, N., van de Wijgert, J., Coene, G., Gasarabwe, A., & Temmerman, M. (2011). "Mama and papa nothing": Living with infertility among an urban population in Kigali, Rwanda. *Human Reproduction*, 26, 623–629. doi:10.1093/humrep/deq373

Dyer, S. J. (2008). Infertility in African countries: Challenges created by the HIV epidemic. *ESHRE Monographs*, 2008(1), 48–53. doi:10.1093/humrep/den157

Dyer, S. J., Abrahams, N., Hoffman, M., & van der Spuy, Z. M. (2002). Infertility in South Africa: Women's reproductive health knowledge and treatment-seeking behaviour for involuntary childlessness. *Human Reproduction, 17*, 1657–1662. doi:10.1093/humrep/17.6.1657

Dyer, S. J., & Patel, M. (2012). The economic impact of infertility on women in developing countries—a systematic review. *Facts, Views, & Vision in ObGyn, 4*, 38–45. Retrieved from http://www.fvvo.be/archive/volume-4/number-2

Ericksen, K., & Brunette, T. (1996). Patterns and predictors of infertility among African women: A cross-national survey of twenty-seven nations. *Social Science & Medicine, 42*, 209–220. doi:10.1016/0277–9536(95)00087–9

Favot, I., Ngalula, J., Mgalla, Z., Klokke, A. H., Gumodoka, B., & Boerma, J. T. (1997). HIV infection and sexual behaviour among women with infertility in Tanzania: A hospital-based study. *International Journal of Epidemiology, 26*, 414–419. doi:10.1093/ije/26.2.414

Fritz, M. A. (2005). Female infertility. In L. Speroff & M. A. Fritz (Eds.), *Clinical gynaecologic endocrinology and infertility* (7th ed., pp. 1013–1067). Philadelphia, PA: Lippincott Williams & Wilkins.

Gerrits, T. (1997). Social and cultural aspects of infertility in Mozambique. *Patient Education & Counseling, 31*, 39–48. doi:10.1016/S0738–3991(97)01018–5

Gerrits, T. (2012). Biomedical infertility care in poor resource countries: Barriers and access: Introduction [monograph]. *Facts, Views, and Vision in ObGyn*, 1–6. Retrieved from http://www.fvvo.be/monographs/biomedical-infertility-care-in-poor-resource-countries-barriers-access-and-ethics

Habbema, J. D. F., Collins, J., Leridon, H., Evers, J. L. H., Lunenfeld, B., & te Velde, E. R. (2004). Towards less confusing terminology in reproductive medicine: A proposal. *Fertility and Sterility, 82*, 36–40. doi:10.1016/j.fertnstert.2004.04.024

Hörbst, V. (2012). "You need someone in grand boubou"—barriers and means to access ARTs in West Africa. *Facts, Views, & Vision in ObGyn*, 46–52. Retrieved from http://www.fvvo.be/assets/268/07-Horbst.pdf

Ishihara, O., Adamson, G. D., Dyer, S., de Mouzon, J., Nygren, K. G., Sullivan, E. A., . . . Mansour, R. (2015). International committee for monitoring assisted reproductive technologies: World report on assisted reproductive technologies, 2007. *Fertility and Sterility, 103*, 402–413. doi:10.1016/j.fertnstert.2014.11.004

Kamenga, M. C., De Cock, K. M., St. Louis, M. E., Touré, C. K., Zakaria, S., N'gbichi, J. M., . . . Kreiss, J. K. (1995). The impact of human immunodeficiency virus infection on pelvic inflammatory disease: A case–control study in Abidjan, Ivory Coast. *American Journal Obstetrics and Gynecology, 172*, 919–925. doi:1016/0002–9378(95)90022–5

Khalifa, D. S., & Ahmed, M. A. (2012). Reviewing infertility care in Sudan; Sociocultural, policy and ethical barriers [monograph]. *Facts, Views, & Vision in ObGyn*, 53–58. Retrieved from http://www.fvvo.be/assets/269/08-Khalifaetal.pdf

Kuku, S. F., & Osegbe, D. N. (1989). Oligo/azoospermia in Nigeria. *Archives in Andrology, 22*, 233–237. doi:10.3109/01485018908986778

Leonard, L. (2002). "Looking for children": The search for fertility among the Sara of southern Chad. *Medical Anthropology, 21*, 79–112. doi:10.1080/01459740210618

Mascarenhas, M. N., Flaxman, S. R., Boerma, T., Vanderpoel, S., & Stevens, G. A. (2012). National, regional and global trends in infertility prevalence since 1990: A systematic analysis of 277 health surveys. *PLoS Medicine, 9*(12). doi:10.1371/journal. pmed.1001356

Nachtigall, R. D. (2006). International disparities in access to infertility services. *Fertility and Sterility, 85*, 871–875. doi:10.1016/j.fertnstert.2005.08.066

Nahar, P. (2012). Invisible women in Bangladesh: Stakeholders' views on infertility services [monograph]. *Facts, Views, & Vision in ObGyn*, 30–37. Retrieved from http://www.fvvo.be/assets/266/05-Nahar.pdf

Nahar, P., Sharma, A., Sabin, K., Begum, L., Ahsan, S. K., & Baqui, A. H. (2000). Living with infertility: Experiences among urban slum populations in Bangladesh. *Reproductive Health Matters, 8*, 33–44. doi:10.1016/S0968–8080(00)90004–1

Ombelet, W. (2012). Global access to infertility care in developing countries: A case of human rights, equity and social justice. *Facts, Views, & Vision in ObGyn,* 7–16. Retrieved from http://www.fvvo.be/assets/263/02-Ombelet.pdf

Pennings, G. (2012). Ethical issues of infertility treatment in developing countries [monograph]. *Facts, Views, & Vision in ObGyn,* 17–23 . Retrieved from http://www.fvvo.be/monographs/biomedical-infertility-care-in-poor-resource-countries-barriers-access-and-ethics

Ross, A., Morgan, D., Lubega, R., Carpenter, L. M., Mayanja, B., & Whitworth, J. A. G. (1999). Reduced fertility associated with HIV: The contribution of pre-existing subfertility. *AIDS, 13,* 2133–2141. doi:10.1097/00002030–199910220-00017

Sundby, J. (1997). Infertility in the Gambia: Traditional and modern health care. *Patient Education & Counseling, 31,* 29–37. doi:10.1016/S0738–3991(97)01006–9

United Nations Population Fund. (1994). *Programme of action: Adopted at the international conference on population and development in Cairo, 1994.* Retrieved from http://www.unfpa.org/sites/default/files/event-pdf/PoA_en.pdf

United Nations UNAIDS. (2014). *Fact sheet 2014.* Retrieved from http://www.unaids.org/sites/default/files/en/media/unaids/contentassets/documents/factsheet/2014/20140716_FactSheet_en.pdf

van Balen, F., & Bos, H. M. W. (2010). The social and cultural consequences of being childless in poor-resource countries [monograph]. *Facts, Views, & Vision in ObGyn,* 11–16. Retrieved from http://www.fvvo.be/assets/126/11-van_Balen_et_al.pdf

World Bank. (2015). *Country and lending groups.* Retrieved from http://data.worldbank.org/about/country-and-lending-groups

World Health Organization (WHO). (2010). Mother or nothing: The agony of infertility. *Bulletin of the World Health Organization, 88,* 881–882. doi:10.2471/BLT.10.011210

World Health Organization (WHO). (n.d.) *Reproductive health.* Retrieved from http://www.who.int/topics/reproductive_health/en

Zaba, B., & Gregson, S. (1998). Measuring the impact of HIV on fertility in Africa. *AIDS, 12*(Suppl 1), S41–S50.

# CHAPTER 17

# EMERGING "COST-EFFECTIVE" TREATMENTS INCLUDING LOW-COST IVF

*Willem Ombelet and Nathalie Dhont*

Childlessness and infertility care are neglected aspects of family planning in resource-poor countries although the consequences of involuntary childlessness are much more dramatic and can create more wide-ranging societal problems compared with Western societies, particularly for women. Because many families in developing countries completely depend on children for economic survival, childlessness has to be regarded as a social and public health issue and not only as an individual medical problem.

According to Millennium Development Goal 5 (MDG5), universal access to reproductive care, including both contraceptive and infertility care, should be adopted by the year 2015. Until today, nothing has been done to help childless couples in developing countries. According to a recent questionnaire conducted by the Genk Institute for Fertility Technology, none of the international organizations, nongovernmental organizations, and foundations are planning to do so in the forthcoming years (Ombelet, 2011).

In the Walking Egg Project, we strive to raise awareness surrounding childlessness in resource-poor countries and to make infertility care in all its aspects, including assisted reproductive technology (ART), available and accessible for a much larger part of the world population. We hope to achieve this goal through innovation and research, advocacy and networking, training and capacity building, and service delivery.

## THE WALKING EGG PROJECT

The Walking Egg nonprofit organization has opted for a multidisciplinary and global approach toward the problem of infertility (Dhont, 2011). The main goal of the Walking Egg Project is to raise global awareness surrounding childlessness and to make infertility care in all its aspects universally available and accessible (Ombelet, 2014b). Therefore, we need to change and optimize the whole set-up of infertility care in terms of availability, affordability, and effectiveness (Ombelet & Campo, 2007).

To realize this objective, a number of actions are planned including the following: (a) to raise awareness surrounding the problem of childlessness within

(i) the donor community, politicians, funding agencies, and research organizations through lobbying and publishing; (ii) the general population through information, education, and counseling on infertility and its consequences; (b) to study the ethical, sociocultural, and economical aspects surrounding the issue of childlessness and infertility care in resource-poor countries; (c) to develop new methods to make infertility diagnosis and infertility treatment including ART accessible for a much larger part of the population by (i) simplifying the diagnostic procedures, (ii) simplifying in vitro fertilization (IVF) laboratory procedures, and (iii) modifying the ovarian stimulation protocols for IVF; and last but not least, (d) to work together with other organizations and societies working in the field of reproductive health to reach the goal of "universal access to infertility care."

In this chapter, we focus on the third planned action to meet the Walking Egg's objective, which is the development of new methods and techniques to make infertility care and treatment more affordable and accessible.

## UNIVERSAL ACCESS TO INFERTILITY CARE: CLINICAL ASPECTS

From a pure medical point of view, our first objective is the establishment of low-cost "one-stop clinics" for the diagnosis of infertility. Simplification of the ART procedures without loss of quality is our second objective. Our final goal is the implementation of "accessible" infertility services, if possible integrated within health care facilities, providing good-quality family planning services, reproductive health education, and high-standard mother care.

### The One-Stop Diagnostic Phase

Standardized investigation of the couple at minimal costs is possible and undoubtedly will enhance the likelihood that infertile couples, both men and woman, will come to the infertility centers. How to organize a one-stop diagnostic clinic has been described previously (Ombelet, Campo, Franken, Huyser, & Nargund, 2012) and is shown in Figure 17.1.

A questionnaire will be provided to both partners. This questionnaire can be adapted to the local situation in the specific locations and countries. Screening for infections and sexually transmitted infections (STI) can be done by using low-cost affordable screening tests that became recently available (Huyser, 2014; Huyser & Fourie, 2010).

Because tubal obstruction associated with previous pelvic infections is the most important reason for infertility in some developing regions in sub-Saharan Africa, hysterosalpingography and/or hysterosalpingo-contrast-sonography are affordable techniques to detect this problem, easy to perform, and without major costs. Combining these techniques with an accurate medical history will identify the majority of women's infertility causes, such as ovulatory disorders, uterine malformations, and tubal infertility. A standard gynecological and fertility ultrasound scanning of the uterus and the ovaries can easily be done. Because uterine abnormalities such as myomata and polyps are commonly observed in the Black

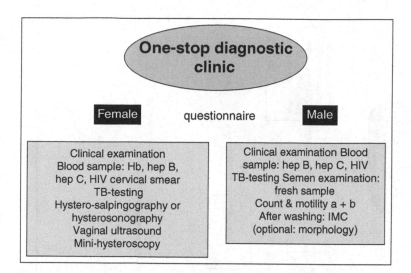

**FIGURE 17.1** One-stop diagnostic clinic for infertility workup in a resource-poor setting.

HB, hemoglobin; Hep B, hepatitis B; Hep C, hepatitis C; IMC, inseminating motile count; TB, tuberculosis.

population, diagnostic hysteroscopy is recommended. Office mini-hysteroscopy has been simplified in its instrumentation and technique, so that it can become a nonexpensive diagnostic technique accessible for every gynecologist, provided there has been appropriate training (Campo et al., 2005; Campo, Meier, Dhont, Mestdagh, & Ombelet, 2014; Ombelet & Campo, 2007).

Male factor infertility can be evaluated by a simple semen analysis (Cooper et al., 2010). Semen analyses can also be performed by well-trained paramedicals, another important advantage for developing countries. It is also important to calculate the inseminating motile count (IMC). The IMC is the total number of motile spermatozoa after a sperm-wash procedure. The IMC is very crucial in selecting patients for either intrauterine inseminations (IUI), IVF, or intracytoplasmic sperm injection (ICSI; Ombelet et al., 1997, 2012).

All the procedures of the one-day diagnostic clinic can be performed by a small team of health care providers within a short period of time in an inexpensive setting (Ombelet & Campo, 2007). A flowchart for the ᵗWE (the Walking Egg) diagnostic clinic is shown in Figure 17.2.

## Simplified Infertility Treatment and Non-IVF–Assisted Reproduction

If tubal patency is demonstrated in ovulatory women and if severe male factor subfertility has been excluded, fertility awareness programs are an inexpensive and efficient first-line approach to infertility management (Gnoth, Frank-Herrmann, & Freundl, 2002; Gnoth, Godehardt, Godehardt, Frank-Herrmann, & Freundl, 2003). Fertility awareness counseling to couples about the meaning and detection of cervical mucus secretion can be given by nurses and paramedical staff working in existing reproductive health care centers.

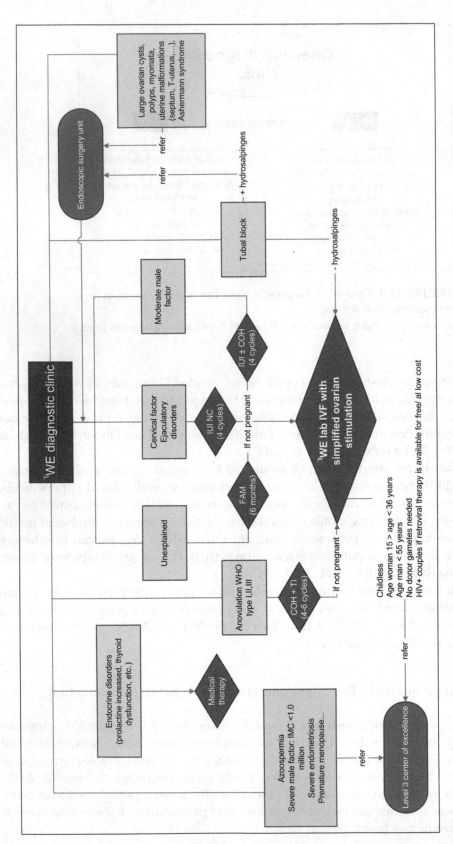

**FIGURE 17.2** Proposed flowchart for the 'WE diagnostic clinic.

COH, controlled ovarian hyperstimulation; FAM, fertility awareness methods; IMC, inseminating motile count);IUI, intrauterine insemination; NC, natural cycle; TI, timed intercourse; 'WE, the Walking Egg.

With permission of Universa Press (Ombelet & Goossens, 2014).

For ovulatory dysfunction, representing almost 20% of female infertility, clomiphene citrate (CC) is a very inexpensive and rewarding option. In case of resistance to CC, a low-dose ovarian stimulation regimen with gonadotropins aimed at monofollicular growth is advisable, although this medication is more expensive.

In case of unexplained and moderate male factor infertility and provided tubal patency has been documented, IUI with the husband's semen in natural cycles or after mild stimulation is an excellent first-line treatment without major costs and without expensive infrastructure (Ombelet et al., 2003; Veltman-Verhulst, Cohlen, Hughes, & Heineman, 2006). IUI programs can be run by well-trained paramedical staff, another advantage for resource-poor countries. Controlled ovarian hyperstimulation (COH), with or without IUI, is associated with the risk of multiple gestations, especially when gonadotropins are used (Gleicher, Oleske, Tur-Kaspa, Vidali, & Karande, 2000). Appropriate standardized protocols are available to minimize the risk of multiple pregnancies, which is even more important in developing countries because the consequences of multiple pregnancies can be devastating.

## Simplified IVF Laboratory Procedures

Another major challenge is to reduce costs of laboratory procedures, namely fertilization and culture of eggs and embryos for IVF. Different options and approaches have been developed or are presently being field-tested with promising results. As part of the Walking Egg Project and based on previous findings and experience (Swain, 2011; Van Blerkom & Manes, 1974), we developed a new simplified method of IVF culturing, called the tWE lab method. With this new system, specifically designed for low-resource settings, we can avoid the high costs of medical gases, complex incubation equipment, and infrastructure typical of IVF laboratories in high-resource settings. The method itself and the first results from a prospective trial were described by Van Blerkom et al. (2014) and are shown in Figure 17.3.

For insemination of the eggs, we only use 1,000 to 5,000 motile washed spermatozoa per oocyte, with very promising results, which makes this technique usable for more than 60% of the actual IVF/ICSI population (Ombelet, 2014a). Because development from insemination to transfer is undisturbed and is in the same tube until embryo transfer, we can avoid many problems frequently occurring in regular IVF laboratories, such as unwanted temperature changes, air-quality problems, and so on.

By April 2015, more than 30 healthy babies had been born after using this technique; some of them resulted after transferring freeze/thawed embryos (Ombelet, Van Blerkom, et al., 2014). A prospective study comparing the embryo quality and pregnancy outcome after using tWE lab versus regular IVF/ICSI procedures is still ongoing, with an aim to provide IVF for less than 20% of the actual costs of regular IVF.

## Low-Cost Ovarian Stimulation Protocols for IVF

In order to make infertility care more affordable in developing countries, effective, affordable, and safe stimulation schemes for IUI and IVF need to be established.

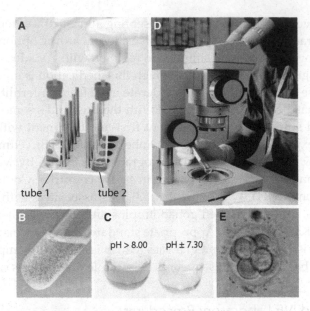

**FIGURE 17.3** ᵗWE-lab method: (A) equilibration of the culture medium in tube 2 by the $CO_2$ produced in tube 1; (B) production of $CO_2$ in the generator tube; (C) phenol red shift from dark pink (pH > 8.00) to salmon pink (pH around 7.30); (D) embryo evaluation through the glass walls of the closed tubes; (E) an embryo visualized in the ᵗWE-lab tube.

With permission of Universa Press (Klerkx et al. 2014).

A review of the literature clearly shows the value and effectiveness of mild ovarian stimulation protocols in ART settings (Verberg et al., 2009). The success rates of natural-cycle IVF can be low per cycle due to high cancelation rates because of premature luteinizing hormone (LH) rise and premature ovulation. But the use of indomethacin to block ovulation helps one to reduce cancelations. Cumulative pregnancy and live birth rates after four consecutive cycles could reach 46% and 32%, respectively, making it a cost-effective, safe, and patient-friendly option (Nargund et al., 2001). The use of CC, a very low-cost oral drug, has been proven in many studies to be an optimal alternative with acceptable results, minimal side effects, and a very low complication rate (Ingerslev, Højgaard, Hindkjær, & Kesmodel, 2001; Kato et al., 2012; Nargund et al., 2007; Verberg et al., 2009).

Monitoring of follicular development in an IVF cycle, as well as the timing of the human chorionic gonadotropin (hCG) administration, can be done solely on sonographic criteria with basic inexpensive ultrasound equipment, thereby avoiding the need of expensive endocrine investigations (Rojanasakul et al., 1994).

Nevertheless, although very promising results concerning the different steps of IVF are described, we still have to perform feasibility studies to examine the value of a one-stop diagnostic phase and to study the value of the simplified ᵗWE lab system and different low-cost ovarian stimulation protocols in resource-poor settings.

## SERVICE DELIVERY: THE IMPLEMENTATION OF 'WE PILOT CENTERS IN RESOURCE-POOR COUNTRIES

The ultimate aim of the Walking Egg Project is the implementation of good-quality but low-cost infertility centers in developing countries, preferably integrated into existing reproductive health care centers. Diagnostic and therapeutic procedures and protocols should be affordable, effective, safe, and standardized. Ideally, infertility management should be integrated into sexual and reproductive health care programs.

As developing countries differ in their status of development, three levels of assistance are suggested (Sallam, 2008). A level 1 infertility clinic is a basic infertility clinic capable of offering the following services: basic infertility workup including semen analysis, hormonal assays, follicular scanning, ovulation induction, and IUI. In level 2 infertility clinics, IVF can be performed as well.

During many meetings that included the authors and other medical and public health experts, it was decided that level 3 infertility clinics capable of offering ICSI, cryopreservation, and operative endoscopy are not part of the Walking Egg Project in the initial phase. Therefore, our first target is the implementation of good-quality level 2 centers. Table 17.1 gives an overview of the activities associated with the implementation of level 2 services.

**TABLE 17.1 Activities Needed for the Implementation of Level 2 Services**

1. *Equipping the clinics:* Infertility clinics in developing countries should be provided with low cost and easy serviceable equipment, taking into consideration the local problems often encountered (e.g., fluctuating voltage, frequent power cuts, unavailability of servicing facilities, irregular supply of consumables, etc.).

2. *Training the staff:* This includes the training of the medical, paramedical, and administrative staff. Training courses should tailor to the local conditions and the possible difficulties encountered in developing countries. Training, quality control, regular audit, and systems of accreditation and registration should be implemented in order to maintain appropriate standards of care.

3. *Educating the public:* This necessitates establishing contacts and working relationships with schools, community leaders, and traditional healers, as well as the media, producing and distributing educational materials (brochures, posters, and audiovisual material) and so on.

4. *Running the services:* This should take into consideration staff salaries, regular purchasing of consumables, cost of equipment maintenance, cost of investigations, cost of medical interventions, and the cost of medication. Special servicing contracts should be negotiated with the manufacturers. In addition, simplification of the consumables should be taken into consideration and laboratory reagents and culture media should have a long shelf life.

5. *Documentation and registration:* Within each pilot center, online data registration of all ART activities is mandatory. Administrative staff and (para) medicals have to be aware of the importance of correct and trustable data registration. The ultimate goal is to offer all pilot centers a similar registration program. Continuous monitoring of service activities will be centralized, and will provide feedback to clinics for clinical and laboratory policy adjustments, information to couples on clinic performance, and information to society.

6. *Psychological and sociocultural follow-up:* When implementing low-cost (accessible) infertility services in developing countries, it is extremely important to study social, psychological, sexual, legal, and ethical aspects of infertility and infertility treatment and take study findings into account when setting up gender- and culture-sensitive infertility services.

ART, assisted reproductive technology.
*Source:* Sallam (2008).

## Selection of Countries/Pilot Centers

Decision making on infertility treatment in developing countries assumes answers to quite a few questions: How should the infertility problem be defined? How often does infertility occur? What is the income in that specific country and what can be spent on health care? How low cost should IVF be in order to be accessible to a considerable part of the population? With what alternative health interventions should infertility treatment be compared? How cost-effective should IVF be in order to compete with other interventions? In this respect, we believe that measurements of the (utility-measure-oriented) quality of life over the infertile life course in developing countries are urgently needed.

The selection of countries where the first pilot centers are implemented will be based on (a) available data on the resources, needs, and resource gaps for infertility services on a national level; (b) percentage of gross domestic product (GDP) spent on education and health care; (c) the availability of endoscopic surgery facilities in the neighborhood; (d) a good-quality family planning unit; (e) good-quality mother care facilities; and (f) the availability of at least one experienced and dedicated gynaecologist and biologist. The community or region including the local health care authorities should be empowered to support the program from the beginning.

## Advocacy and Networking

Global access to infertility care can only be implemented and sustained if it is supported by local policy makers and the international community. Many international organizations have already expressed their desire to collaborate, including the World Health Organization (WHO), European Society of Human Reproduction and Embryology (ESHRE), and International Society for Mild Approaches in Assisted Reproduction (ISMAAR). We will also need the media, patient organizations, and interested politicians to change the existing moral and sociocultural beliefs, which are isolating and ostracizing infertile couples.

## CONCLUSION

The magnitude of childlessness in developing countries has dimensions beyond its prevalence and etiology. Differences between the developed and developing world are emerging because of the different availability in infertility care and different sociocultural value surrounding procreation and childlessness. There is a growing belief that individual health needs of impoverished people have a place next to their public health needs. Although reproductive health education and prevention of infertility are number one priorities, the need for accessible diagnostic procedures and new simplified reproductive technologies is very high. The success and sustainability of ART in resource-poor settings will depend to a large extent on our ability to optimize these techniques in terms of availability, affordability, and effectiveness. The Walking Egg nonprofit organization aims to raise awareness surrounding childlessness in resource-poor countries and to make infertility care in all its aspects, including ART, available and accessible for a much larger part of the population. By simplifying the diagnostic and IVF laboratory procedures and by modifying the ovarian stimulation protocols for IVF, assisted reproductive techniques can be offered at affordable prices. The implementation of low-cost infertility centers in resource-poor countries, if possible integrated in existing reproductive health care centers, will be a crucial step to reach the ultimate goal of "universal access to infertility care."

The selection of pilot centers will depend on different factors such as the budget for education and health care in that specific country, the availability of effective family planning and mother care facilities, and a dedicated person who can coordinate the study and shows interest for sociological support before, during, and after treatment.

Infertility will likely become one of the more predominant components of future reproductive health care practice. Taking advantage of information and communication technologies will increase the effectiveness and accessibility of health care services, as well as change patient behaviors to seek timely treatment. As evidence-based affordable solutions begin to drive global guidance within both public and private health care system solutions, access to care for the infertile couple will become one of the largest emerging fields in global medicine.

## ACKNOWLEDGMENTS

I gratefully acknowledge all the experts who were involved in the Walking Egg Project for many years (Rudi Campo, Nathalie Dhont, Eva Dierickx, Danie Franken, Trudie Gerrits, Jan Goossens, Carin Huyser, Geeta Nargund, Guido Pennings, Hassan Sallam, Frank Van Balen, Jonathan Van Blerkom, Brigitte Vandamme, Ingrid Van der Auwera, Annie Vereecken, Koen Vanmechelen, and many others).

## REFERENCES

Campo, R., Meier, R., Dhont, N., Mestdagh, G., & Ombelet, W. (2014). Implementation of hysteroscopy in an infertility clinic: The one-stop uterine diagnosis and treatment. *Facts, Views, & Vision in ObGyn, 6*, 235–239. Retrieved from http://www.fvvo.be/archive/volume-6/number-4

Campo, R., Molinas, C. R., Rombauts, L., Mestdagh, G., Lauwers, M., Braekmans, P.,...Gordts, S. (2005). Prospective multicentre randomized controlled trial to evaluate factors influencing the success rate of office diagnostic hysteroscopy. *Human Reproduction, 20*, 258–263. doi:10.1093/humrep/deh559

Cooper, T. G., Noonan, E., von Eckardstein, S., Auger, J., Baker, H. W. G., Behre, H. M.,...Vogelsong, K. M. (2010).World Health Organization reference values for human semen characteristics. *Human Reproduction Update, 16*, 231–245. doi:10.1093/humupd/dmp048

Dhont, N. (2011). The Walking Egg non-profit organisation. *Facts, Views, & Vision in ObGyn, 3*, 253–255. Retrieved from http://www.fvvo.be/archive/volume-3/number-4

Gleicher, N., Oleske, D. M., Tur-Kaspa, I., Vidali, A., & Karande, V. (2000). Reducing the risk of high-order multiple pregnancy after ovarian stimulation with gonadotropins. *New England Journal of Medicine, 343*, 2–7. doi:10.1056/NEJM200007063430101

Gnoth, C., Frank-Herrmann, P., & Freundl, G. (2002). Opinion: Natural family planning and the management of infertility. *Archives of Gynecology and Obstetrics, 267*, 67–71. doi:10.1007/s00404-002-0293-8

Gnoth, C., Godehardt, D., Godehardt, E., Frank-Herrmann, P., & Freundl, G. (2003). Time to pregnancy: Results of the German prospective study and impact on the management of infertility. *Human Reproduction, 18*, 1959–1966. doi:10.1093/humrep/deg366

Huyser, C. (2014). Prevention of infections in an ART laboratory: A reflection on simplistic methods. *Facts, Views, & Vision in ObGyn, 6*, 231–234. Retrieved from http://www.fvvo.be/archive/volume-6/number-4

Huyser, C., & Fourie, J. (2010). SPERM ONLY PLEASE: Prevention of infections in an assisted reproduction laboratory in a developing country [monograph]. *Facts, Views, & Vision in ObGyn*, 97–106. Retrieved from http://www.fvvo.be/monographs/artificial-insemination-an-update

Ingerslev, H. J., Højgaard, A., Hindkjær, J., & Kesmodel, A. (2001). A randomized study comparing IVF in the unstimulated cycle with IVF following clomiphene citrate. *Human Reproduction, 16*, 696–702. doi:10.1093/humrep/16.4.696

Kato, K., Takehara, Y., Segawa, T., Kawachiya, S., Okuno, T., Kobayashi, T.,...Kato, O. (2012). Minimal ovarian stimulation combined with elective single embryo transfer policy: Age-specific results of a large, single-centre, Japanese cohort. *Reproductive Biology and Endocrinology, 10*, 35. doi:10.1186/1477-7827-10-35

Klerkx, E., Janssen, M., Van der Auwera, I., Campo, R., Goossens, J., Vereecken, A., & Ombelet, W. (2014). The Walking Egg Project: A simplified IVF laboratory method. *Facts, Views, & Vision in ObGyn*, Monograph, 4–5.

Nargund, G., Fauser, B. C. J. M., Macklon, N. S., Ombelet, W., Nygren, K., & Frydman, R. (2007). The ISMAAR proposal on terminology for ovarian stimulation for IVF. *Human Reproduction, 22*, 2801–2804. doi:10.1093/humrep/dem285

Nargund, G., Waterstone, J., Bland, J. M., Philips, Z., Parsons, J., & Campbell, S. (2001). Cumulative conception and live birth rates in natural (unstimulated) IVF cycles. *Human Reproduction, 16*, 259–262. doi:10.1093/humrep/16.2.259

Ombelet, W. (2011). Global access to infertility care in developing countries: A case of human rights, equity and social justice. *Facts, Views, & Vision in ObGyn, 3*, 257–266. Retrieved from http://www.fvvo.be/archive/volume-3/number-4

Ombelet, W. (2014a). *Genk*. Unpublished raw data.

Ombelet, W. (2014b). Is global access to infertility care realistic? The Walking Egg Project. *Reproductive Biomedicine Online, 28*, 267–272. doi:10.1016/j.rbmo.2013.11.013

Ombelet W., & Campo, R. (2007). Affordable IVF for developing countries. *Reproductive Biomedicine Online, 15*, 257–265. doi:10.1016/S1472-6483(10)60337-9

Ombelet, W., Campo, R., Franken, D., Huyser, C., & Nargund, G. (2012). The Walking Egg Project: An example of medical education and training [monograph]. *Facts, Views, & Vision in ObGyn*, 66–75. Retrieved from http://www.fvvo.be/assets/255/15-Ombelet_et_al.pdf

Ombelet, W., Deblaere, K., Bosmans, E., Cox, A., Jacobs, P., Janssen, M., & Nijs, M. (2003). Semen quality and intrauterine insemination. *Reproductive Biomedicine Online, 7*, 485–492. doi:10.1016/S1472-6483(10)61894-9

Ombelet, W., & Goossens, J. (2014). The Walking Egg Project: How to start a TWE center? *Facts, Views, & Vision in ObGyn*, Monograph, 39–43.

Ombelet, W., Van Blerkom, J., Klerkx, E., Janssen, M., Dhont, N., Mestdagh, G.,...Campo, R. (2014). The (t)WE lab simplified IVF procedure: First births after freezing/thawing. *Facts, Views, & Vision in ObGyn, 6*, 45–49. Retrieved from http://www.fvvo.be/archive/volume-6/number-1

Ombelet, W., Vandeput, H., Van de Putte, G., Cox, A., Janssen, M., Jacobs, P.,...Kruger, T. (1997). Intrauterine insemination after ovarian stimulation with clomiphene citrate:

Predictive potential of inseminating motile count and sperm morphology. *Human Reproduction, 12,* 1458–1463. doi:10.1093/humrep/12.7.1458

Rojanasakul, A., Choktanasiri, W., Suchartwatanachai, C., Srisombut, C., Chinsomboon, S., & Chatasingh, S. (1994). "Simplified IVF": Program for developing countries. *Journal of the Medical Association of Thailand, 77*(1), 12–18.

Sallam, H. N. (2008). Infertility in developing countries: Funding the project [monograph]. *Human Reproduction, 2008*(1), 97–101. doi:10.1093/humrep/den144

Swain, J. E. (2011). A self-contained culture platform using carbon dioxide produced from a chemical reaction supports mouse blastocyst development in vitro. *Journal of Reproduction and Development, 57,* 551–555. doi:10.1262/jrd.11–022M

Van Blerkom, J., & Manes, C. (1974). Development of preimplantation rabbit embryos in vivo and in vitro: II. A comparison of qualitative aspects of protein synthesis. *Developmental Biology, 40,* 40–51. doi:10.1016/0012–1606(74)90105–5

Van Blerkom, J., Ombelet, W., Klerkx, E., Janssen, M., Dhont, N., Nargund, G., & Campo, R. (2014). First births with a simplified culture system for clinical IVF and embryo transfer. *Reproductive Biomedicine Online, 28,* 310–320. doi:10.1016/j.rbmo.2013.11.012

Veltman-Verhulst, S. M., Cohlen, B. J., Hughes, E., & Heineman, M. J. (2006). Intra-uterine insemination for unexplained subfertility. *Cochrane Database of Systematic Reviews, 4,* CD001838. doi:10.1002/14651858.CD001838.pub3

Verberg, M. F. G., Macklon, N. S., Nargund, G., Frydman, R., Devroey, P., Broekmans, F. J., & Fauser, B. C. J. M. (2009). Mild ovarian stimulation for IVF. *Human Reproduction Update, 15,* 13–29. doi:10.1093/humupd/dmn056

# CHAPTER 18

# DEFINING INFERTILITY: GLOBAL VIEWS ON TIMING OF IVF AND THE ABILITY TO ACCESS CARE

*Irma Scholten and Ben W. Mol*

A common accepted definition of infertility is "the inability to conceive after 12 months of unprotected intercourse" (Zegers-Hochschild et al., 2009, p. 1522). However, the word *infertility* suggests an absolute inability to conceive. This is not true, per se, for all couples that meet the definition of infertility. Although some couples will never conceive due to double-sided tubal pathology, very poor sperm quality, or anovulation not responding on ovulation induction, many others conceive spontaneously during fertility workup, while on a waiting list to start treatment, or even after treatments. The term *subfertility* better expresses the state of these couples.

A challenge in reproductive medicine is to distinguish couples who have a low probability to conceive naturally from couples with a high probability. Although the first category would benefit from effective treatments, the latter group may be better off awaiting natural conception for a defined period of time that extends beyond the conventional "1 year" time frame. These couples are particularly at risk for earlier than necessary intervention, which not only puts them at risk for side effects from in vitro fertilization (IVF) but also has an impact on the availability of care for those who really need treatment. The equitable and appropriate use of resources would best treat both cohorts. Therefore, this chapter focuses on the identification of couples with good natural fertility chances and couples with a lower risk of natural conception.

## NATURAL COURSE OF CONCEPTION

Several cohort studies have examined the natural course of couples trying to conceive (Brandes, Hamilton, de Bruin, Nelen, & Kremer, 2010; Collins, Burrows, & Wilan, 1995; Eimers et al., 1994; Gnoth, Godehardt, Godehardt, Frank-Herrmann, & Freundl, 2003; Snick, Snick, Evers, & Collins, 1997; van der Steeg et al., 2007). Although pregnancy rates differ between studies, likely caused by differences in populations, the bigger picture between studies is similar. Approximately 80% of the couples who plan a pregnancy conceive within the first 6 months of unprotected well-timed intercourse, whereas 50% of those who did not conceive in the first 6 months will conceive in the second 6 months, resulting in a cumulative conception rate of 90% (Gnoth et al., 2003). Similarly, half of those not pregnant after 1 year of well-timed intercourse will conceive in the next year, followed by another 14% in the third year (te Velde, Eijkemans, & Habbema, 2000). Thus, infertility is not synonymous with an absolute need for treatment and subfertility is a more appropriate term in these couples.

## FERTILITY WORKUP AND DIAGNOSES

Based on the commonly used definition of *infertility*, couples can turn to a fertility specialist after a year of nonconceiving, unless their medical history gives rise to an earlier review; for example, in the case of known anovulation (National Institute for Health and Care Excellence, 2013; Practice Committee of the American Society for Reproductive Medicine, 2013). The usual first step is a fertility workup. Some couples are able to be given a clear diagnosis, for which targeted treatment is an appropriate solution to the underlying condition: about 5% of the couples are diagnosed with double-sided tubal factor for which IVF is the best treatment, 10% are diagnosed with severe semen impairment needing intracytoplasmic sperm injection (ICSI), whereas an additional 20% suffers an ovulation disorder, for which ovulation induction is the treatment of first choice. The other 65% of couples, however, are found to have no absolute factor explaining their infertility, with either unexplained infertility (30%), or a relative limiting factor such as a cervical factor, one-sided tubal pathology, or mild male subfertility (35%; Brandes et al., 2010; Hull et al., 1985).

## EFFECTIVENESS OF TREATMENT

When considering whether to treat subfertile couples, it is important to consider the effectiveness of the available treatment, particularly for those couples in whom the underlying cause of infertility is poorly understood. There is no dispute on how to treat the 15% of couples found to have an absolute infertility factor such as double-sided tubal pathology or severe semen impairment. The birth of Louise Brown in 1978, the world's first IVF baby, provided hope for couples who suffered from tubal pathology (Steptoe & Edwards, 1978). ICSI, introduced in addition to IVF in early 1990s, provided an effective treatment alternative for couples suffering from severe semen impairment, which was not treatable until that time (Palermo, Joris, Devroey, & Van Steirteghem, 1992). Currently, IVF and ICSI are still the preferred treatments for these couples. However, only the minority of treatment cycles with IVF and IVF–ICSI are performed in couples with tubal pathology or severe male subfertility (Macaldowie, Wang, Chambers, & Sullivan, 2012), as these treatments are increasingly used for other indications including unexplained subfertility.

The optimal treatment for couples with unexplained subfertility is less clear. A first step in treatment of these couples is often intrauterine insemination (IUI).

Although applied for more than four decades, the number of studies comparing IUI to no treatment is limited. Investigators performed a randomized clinical trial in which immediate start of IUI was compared with expectant management for 6 months in couples with unexplained subfertility and a prognosis for spontaneous conception in the next year of 30% to 40%. After 6 months, ongoing pregnancy rates were comparable between groups. After 3 years, pregnancy rates both in the early and the delayed treatment group were close to 80% (Custers et al., 2012; Steures et al., 2006). Similarly, a trial by Bhattacharya et al. (2008) showed no benefit of either IUI without ovarian stimulation or treatment with clomiphene citrate over no treatment.

As randomization for treatment versus no treatment in couples with long-standing infertility is difficult, our group performed a retrospective cohort study comparing treatment with several cycles of IUI to no treatment, using couples who stopped treatment after one or two cycles as controls. Over a 36-month period, we found no difference in cumulative pregnancy rates with the IUI group as compared with the no treatment group. Only when IVF was added did the pregnancy rate of the IVF group become significantly better (Scholten et al., 2013).

These data question the effectiveness of treatment with IUI. Still, the Cochrane Review on this topic concludes that IUI with mild ovarian stimulation with gonadotropins increases the live birth rate compared with IUI without stimulation. However, the studies underlying these meta-analyses report on a limited number of treatment cycles. Although hyperstimulation resulting in multifactorial growth might increase pregnancy (and multiple!) rates over a short number of cycles, its effectiveness over a longer period of years is unclear. Yet, a statement on the effectiveness of IUI compared with no intervention could not be given, implicating that the real effectiveness of the treatment remains unclear (Veltman-Verhulst, Cohlen, Hughes, & Heineman, 2012).

A following step in the treatment cascade of unexplained subfertile couples is usually IVF. One trial compared live birth rate after IVF to expectant management in couples with nontubal infertility, in which couples with 3 years of unexplained subfertility formed only a small subgroup ($n = 51$; original group $n = 149$; Hughes et al., 2004). This trial showed one pregnancy in the control group (4%) versus a 46% pregnancy rate in the IVF group. The subsequent Cochrane review judging the effectiveness of IVF in couples with unexplained subfertility concludes that IVF may be more effective than IUI with stimulation. Due to paucity of data from trials, they could not conclude on the effectiveness of IVF relative to expectant management (Pandian, Gibreel, & Bhattacharya, 2012). However, a recent trial compared IUI with mild ovarian stimulation to immediate treatment with IVF in couples with unexplained subfertility and a poor prognosis for spontaneous conception in the following year. It found that treatment with IVF was not superior to treatment with IUI. Pregnancy rates for couples treated with six cycles of IUI versus with three cycles of IVF were compared at 12 months after randomization. After 12 months, there were comparable pregnancy rates between groups, with no substantial difference in multiple pregnancies (Bensdorp et al., 2015).

Thus, although IVF treatment is effective in couples who try to conceive for 3 years or more, its effectiveness is unknown in couples who try to conceive for a shorter period of time.

## SAFETY

Another critical aspect to be cognizant of when considering treatment of couples is the safety of the treatment. Fertility treatments are not without drawbacks. Couples undergoing fertility treatments experience the treatment to be stressful, and 30% of couples end IVF treatment prematurely because of the psychological burden (Boivin, Griffiths, & Venetis, 2011). In addition to the psychological impact, there are also physical considerations. Case series describe the incidental occurrence of maternal death after IVF treatment, caused by ovarian hyperstimulation syndrome (OHSS), pulmonary embolism, and sepsis after oocyte retrieval (Braat, Schutte, Bernardus, Mooij, & van Leeuwen, 2010; Venn, Hemminki, Watson, Bruinsma, & Healy, 2001). However, the largest incidence of adverse events is seen in pregnancies due to fertility treatments, not in treatment itself. Due to ovarian stimulation and transfer of multiple embryos, IVF bears the risk of multiple and higher order pregnancies, which are known to be high-risk pregnancies with poorer pregnancy and neonate outcomes (Pinborg, 2005).

Single embryo transfer (SET) was introduced to lower the incidence of multiple pregnancies after IVF due to a new technology available (Gerris & Van Royen, 2000; Maheshwari, Griffiths, & Bhattacharya, 2011). Even when singleton pregnancies can be achieved via IVF, it does not eliminate the increased risk that exists to IVF pregnancies in general. When controlling for gestational size, pregnancies conceived after IVF have higher rates of poor perinatal outcomes including preterm birth, low birth weight, small for gestational age, congenital abnormalities, and perinatal mortality—independent of being a singleton or multiple pregnancy (Ceelen, van Weissenbruch, Vermeiden, van Leeuwen, & Delemarre-van de Waal, 2008a; Davies et al., 2012; Helmerhorst, Perquin, Donker, & Keirse, 2004; Jackson, Gibson, Wu, & Croughan, 2004; Pandey, Shetty, Hamilton, Bhattacharya, & Maheshwari, 2012; Pinborg et al., 2013).

In addition to poor perinatal outcomes, there are indications that children born after IVF are at increased risk of health problems including elevated blood pressure, impaired glucose tolerance, increased preclinical atherosclerosis, generalized endothelial dysfunction, increased arterial stiffness and decreased cardiac function, altered pubertal maturation, altered cortisol, and increased body fat (Belva et al., 2007, 2013; Belva, Painter, et al., 2012; Belva, Roelants, et al., 2012; Ceelen et al., 2007; Ceelen, van Weissenbruch, Vermeiden, van Leeuwen, & Delemarre-van de Waal, 2008b; Scherrer et al., 2012; Valenzuela-Alcaraz et al., 2013). Several leaders in the field have also postulated that because early present cardiometabolic risk factors are known to have an influence later in life, alterations may lead to increased rates of actual cardiometabolic diseases in IVF offspring in the future (Hayman et al., 2007; Williams et al., 2002). Current findings on the effects of children conceived by IVF procedures are conflicting, indicating the need for additional research in this area.

## IMPLICATIONS FOR TREATMENT USAGE

In the absence of data on the long-term safety of IVF and in view of the continuing rise in cost associated with these technologies, providers should be careful when making the decision to utilize IVF versus considering allowing additional time for spontaneous conception. If we are able to better understand the prospects of the couples presenting in our clinics, we might be able to make more substantiated decisions on whether and when treatment would be helpful. Prediction models, incorporating several patient characteristics, might be helpful in this. The dilemma for treatment gets more complex when women at older ages are confronted with infertility. For older women in whom ovarian reserve is a consideration, waiting bears the risk of compromising their already diminished fertile capacity. On the other hand, IVF and ICSI are treatments that are proven to be effective when egg and sperm cannot meet. IVF and ICSI by itself do not provide a solution for the "old" egg.

An important question is why the number of couples with unexplained subfertility being treated with IUI and IVF continue to increase? One explanation for this increase is that providers caring for these couples genuinely want to help achieve the goal of parenthood. Patients seek a solution when they are unable to achieve a pregnancy and want to be treated, even if a definitive diagnosis is not present. Therefore, providers feel compelled to treat, even if it may be prudent and appropriate to consider no treatment. Furthermore, providers believe that treatment is the right thing to do for their patients. Often providers do not weigh the perinatal and health risks and increased cost as heavy when their desire is to achieve a pregnancy and feel that the best approach is to use the available treatment. Another significant variable that may drive provider decisions is the financial side of infertility care. Reproductive medicine is, probably more than any other specialty, money-driven. In many countries, services are paid by patients out of pocket, ensuring reliable reimbursement for services. Providers may have a financial incentive to start treatment as well, even when not completely sure of the effectiveness. Additionally, pharmaceutical companies benefit from an increase in fertility treatment by selling more of their products, as most infertility treatments are largely supported by multiple, expensive medications. Information on the effectiveness of these treatments may therefore be unilateral or incomplete, making physicians believe that they are doing the right thing when starting the treatment.

## CONCLUSION

In conclusion, the timing of care for couples with fertility challenges and appropriate utilization of technology currently available is most relevant to couples with unexplained subfertility. Lacking an absolute cause for not conceiving, these couples cannot be offered a treatment that will definitely overcome their problem, and yet, they very often are treated as though there was a definitive diagnosis. A more prudent approach may be a "wait and see" approach, giving couples who fall into this category an opportunity to be able to spontaneously conceive. It is imperative for those in the reproductive field to question who is the most appropriate to start medically assisted reproduction treatments such as IVF and when the optimal time is to begin this treatment. More research is needed in this area, such as trials that compare IUI and IVF to expectant management in couples with unexplained subfertility, to better understand the appropriate use of treatment. Simply initiating treatment because that is what the patients desire is not appropriate. Providers have an ethical obligation to consider the possible associated risks in balance with the effectiveness of the treatment in these couples when developing safe, effective treatment plans.

# REFERENCES

Belva, F., Henriet, S., Liebaers, I., Van Steirteghem, A., Celestin-Westreich, S., & Bonduelle, M. (2007). Medical outcome of 8-year-old singleton ICSI children (born >or=32 weeks' gestation) and a spontaneously conceived comparison group. *Human Reproduction, 22*(2), 506–515. doi:10.1093/humrep/del372

Belva, F., Painter, R., Bonduelle, M., Roelants, M., Devroey, P., & De Schepper, J. (2012). Are ICSI adolescents at risk for increased adiposity? *Human Reproduction, 27*, 257–264. doi:10.1093/humrep/der375

Belva, F., Painter, R. C., Schiettecatte, J., Bonduelle, M., Roelants, M., Roseboom, T. J.,...De Schepper, J. (2013). Gender-specific alterations in salivary cortisol levels in pubertal intracytoplasmic sperm injection offspring. *Hormone Research in Paediatrics, 80*, 350–355. doi:10.1159/000355515

Belva, F., Roelants, M., Painter, R., Bonduelle, M., Devroey, P., & De Schepper, J. (2012). Pubertal development in ICSI children. *Human Reproduction, 27*, 1156–1161. doi:10.1093/humrep/des001

Bensdorp, A. J., Tjon-Kon-Fat, R. I., Bossuyt, P. M. M., Koks, C. A. M., Oosterhuis, G. J. E., Hoek, A.,...Mol, B. W. J. (2015). Prevention of multiple pregnancies in couples with unexplained or mild male subfertility: Randomised controlled trial of in vitro fertilisation with single embryo transfer or in vitro fertilisation in modified natural cycle compared with intrauterine insemination with controlled ovarian hyperstimulation. *British Medical Journal, 350*, g7771. doi:10.1136/bmj.g7771

Bhattacharya, S., Harrild, K., Mollison, J., Wordsworth, S., Tay, C., Harrold, A.,...Templeton, A. (2008). Clomifene citrate or unstimulated intrauterine insemination compared with expectant management for unexplained infertility: Pragmatic randomised controlled trial. *British Medical Journal, 33*, a716. doi: http://dx.doi.org/10.1136/bmj.a716

Boivin, J., Griffiths, E., & Venetis, C. A. (2011). Emotional distress in infertile women and failure of assisted reproductive technologies: Meta-analysis of prospective psychosocial studies. *British Medical Journal, 342*, d223. doi:10.1136/bmj.d223

Braat, D. D. M., Schutte, J. M., Bernardus, R. E., Mooij, T. M., & van Leeuwen, F. E. (2010). Maternal death related to IVF in the Netherlands 1984–2008. *Human Reproduction, 25*, 1782–1786. doi:10.1093/humrep/deq080

Brandes, M., Hamilton, C. J. C. M., de Bruin, J. P., Nelen, W. L. D. M., & Kremer, J. A. M. (2010). The relative contribution of IVF to the total ongoing pregnancy rate in a subfertile cohort. *Human Reproduction, 25*, 118–126. doi:10.1093/humrep/dep341

Ceelen, M., van Weissenbruch, M. M., Roos, J. C., Vermeiden, J. P. W., van Leeuwen, F. E., & Delemarre-van de Waal, H. A. (2007). Body composition in children and adolescents born after in vitro fertilization or spontaneous conception. *Journal of Clinical Endocrinology & Metabolism, 92*, 3417–3423. doi:10.1210/jc.2006–2896

Ceelen, M., van Weissenbruch, M. M., Vermeiden, J. P. W., van Leeuwen, F. E., & Delemarre-van de Waal, H. A. (2008a). Growth and development of children born after in vitro fertilization. *Fertility and Sterility, 90*, 1662–1673. doi: 10.1016/j.fertnstert.2007.09.005

Ceelen, M., van Weissenbruch, M. M., Vermeiden, J. P. W., van Leeuwen, F. E., & Delemarre-van de Waal, H. A. (2008b). Cardiometabolic differences in children born after in vitro fertilization: Follow-up study. *Journal of Clinical Endocrinology & Metabolism, 93*, 1682–1688. doi:10.1210/jc.2007–2432

Collins, J. A., Burrows, E. A., & Wilan, A. R. (1995). The prognosis for live birth among untreated infertile couples. *Fertility and Sterility, 64*, 22–28.

Custers, I. M., van Rumste, M. M. E., van der Steeg, J. M., vanWely, M., Hompes, P. G. A., Bossuyt, P.,...CECERM. (2012). Long-term outcome in couples with unexplained subfertility and an intermediate prognosis initially randomized between expectant management and immediate treatment. *Human Reproduction, 27*, 444–450. doi:10.1093/humrep/der389

Davies, M. J., Moore, V. M., Willson, K. J., Van Essen, P., Priest, K., Scott, H.,...Chan, A. (2012). Reproductive technologies and the risk of birth defects. *New England Journal of Medicine, 366*, 1803–1813. doi:10.1056/NEJMoa1008095

Eimers, J. M., te Velde, E. R., Gerritse, R., Vogelzang, E. T., Looman, C. W., & Habbema, J. D. (1994). The prediction of the chance to conceive in subfertile couples. *Fertility and Sterility, 61*, 44–52.

Gerris, J., & Van Royen, E. (2000). Avoiding multiple pregnancies in ART: A plea for single embryo transfer. *Human Reproduction, 15*, 1884–1888. doi:10.1093/humrep/15.9.1884

Gnoth, C., Godehardt, D., Godehardt, E., Frank-Herrmann, P., & Freundl, G. (2003). Time to pregnancy: Results of the German prospective study and impact on the management of infertility. *Human Reproduction, 18*, 1959–1966. doi:10.1093/humrep/deg366

Hayman, L. L, Meininger, J. C., Daniels, S. R., McCrindle, B. W., Helden, L., Ross, J.,...Williams, C. L. (2007). Primary prevention of cardiovascular disease in nursing practice: Focus on children and youth: A scientific statement from the American Heart Association Committee on Atherosclerosis, Hypertension, and Obesity in Youth of the Council on Cardiovascular Disease in the Young, Council on Cardiovascular Nursing, Council on Epidemiology and Prevention, and Council on Nutrition, Physical Activity, and Metabolism. *Circulation, 116*, 344–357. doi:10.1161/CIRCULATIONAHA.107.184595

Helmerhorst, F. M., Perquin, D. A. M., Donker, D., & Keirse, M. J. N. C. (2004). Perinatal outcome of singletons and twins after assisted conception: A systematic review of controlled studies. *British Medical Journal, 328*, 261. doi:10.1136/bmj.37957.560278.EE

Hughes, E. G., Beecroft, M. L., Wilkie, V., Burville, L., Claman, P., Tummon, I.,...Thorpe, K. (2004). A multicentre randomized controlled trial of expectant management versus IVF in women with fallopian tube patency. *Human Reproduction, 19*, 1105–1109. doi:10.1093/humrep/deh209

Hull, M. G., Glazener, C. M., Kelly, N. J., Conway, D. I., Foster, P. A., Hinton, R. A.,...Desai, K. M. (1985). Population study of causes, treatment, and outcome of infertility. *British Medical Journal, 291*, 1693–1697. doi:10.1136/bmj.291.6510.1693

Jackson, R. A., Gibson, K. A., Wu, Y. W., & Croughan, M. S. (2004). Perinatal outcomes in singletons following in vitro fertilization: A meta-analysis. *Obstetrics & Gynecology, 103*, 551–563. doi:10.1097/01.AOG.0000114989.84822.51

Macaldowie, A., Wang, Y. A., Chambers, G. M., & Sullivan, E. A. (2012). *Assisted reproductive technology in Australia and New Zealand 2010.* Retrieved from http://www.aihw.gov.au/WorkArea/DownloadAsset.aspx?id=10737423255

Maheshwari, A., Griffiths, S., & Bhattacharya, S. (2011). Global variations in the uptake of single embryo transfer. *Human Reproduction Update, 17*, 107–120. doi:10.1093/humupd/dmq028

National Institute for Health and Care Excellence. (2013). *Fertility: Assessment and treatment for people with fertility problems.* Retrieved from https://www.nice.org.uk/guidance/cg156

Palermo, G., Joris, H., Devroey, P., & Van Steirteghem, A. C. (1992). Pregnancies after intracytoplasmic injection of single spermatozoon into an oocyte. *Lancet, 340*(8810), 17–18. doi:10.1016/0140–6736(92)92425-F

Pandey, S., Shetty, A., Hamilton, M., Bhattacharya, S., & Maheshwari, A. (2012). Obstetric and perinatal outcomes in singleton pregnancies resulting from IVF/ICSI: A systematic review and meta-analysis. *Human Reproduction Update, 18,* 485–503. doi:10.1093/humupd/dms018

Pandian, Z., Gibreel, A., & Bhattacharya, S. (2012). In vitro fertilisation for unexplained subfertility. *Cochrane Database of Systematic Reviews, 4,* CD003357. doi:10.1002/14651858.CD003357.pub3

Pinborg, A. (2005). IVF/ICSI twin pregnancies: Risks and prevention. *Human Reproduction Update, 11,* 575–593. doi:10.1093/humupd/dmi027

Pinborg, A., Wennerholm, U. B., Romundstad, L. B., Loft, A., Aittomaki, K., Söderström-Anttila, V.,...Bergh, C. (2013). Why do singletons conceived after assisted reproduction technology have adverse perinatal outcome? Systematic review and meta-analysis. *Human Reproduction Update, 19,* 87–104. doi:10.1093/humupd/dms044

Practice Committee of the American Society for Reproductive Medicine. (2013). Definitions of infertility and recurrent pregnancy loss : A committee opinion. *Fertility and Sterility, 99,* 63. doi:10.1016/j.fertnstert.2012.09.023

Scherrer, U., Rimoldi, S. F., Rexhaj, E., Stuber, T., Duplain, H., Garcin, S.,...Sartori, C. (2012). Systemic and pulmonary vascular dysfunction in children conceived by assisted reproductive technologies. *Circulation, 125,* 1890–1896.

Scholten, I., Moolenaar, L. M., Gianotten, J., van der Veen, F., Hompes, P. G. A., Mol, B. W. J., & Steures, P. (2013). Long term outcome in subfertile couples with isolated cervical factor. *European Journal of Obstetrics & Gynecology and Reproductive Biology, 170,* 429–433. doi:10.1016/j.ejogrb.2013.06.042

Snick, H. K., Snick, T. S., Evers, J. L., & Collins, J. A. (1997). The spontaneous pregnancy prognosis in untreated subfertile couples: The Walcheren primary care study. *Human Reproduction, 12,* 1582–1588. doi:10.1093/humrep/12.7.1582

Steptoe, P. C., & Edwards, R. G. (1978). Birth after the reimplantation of a human embryo. *Lancet, 312*(8085), 366. doi:10.1016/S0140-6736(78)92957-4

Steures, P., van der Steeg, J. W., Hompes, P. G. A., Habbema, J. D. F., Eijkemans, M. J. C., Broekmans, F. J.,...Mol, B. W. J. (2006). Intrauterine insemination with controlled ovarian hyperstimulation versus expectant management for couples with unexplained subfertility and an intermediate prognosis: A randomised clinical trial. *Lancet, 368,* 216–221. doi:10.1016/S0140-6736(06)69042-9

te Velde, E. R., Eijkemans, R., & Habbema, H. D. (2000). Variation in couple fecundity and time to pregnancy, an essential concept in human reproduction. *Lancet, 355,* 1928–1929. doi:10.1016/S0140-6736(00)02320-5

Valenzuela-Alcaraz, B., Crispi, F., Bijnens, B., Cruz-Lemini, M., Creus, M., Sitges, M.,...Gratacós, E. (2013). Assisted reproductive technologies are associated with cardiovascular remodeling in utero that persists postnatally. *Circulation, 128,* 1442–1450. doi:10.1161/CIRCULATIONAHA.113.002428

van der Steeg, J. W., Steures, P., Eijkemans, M. J. C., Habbema, J. D. F., Hompes, P. G. A., Broekmans, F. J.,...Mol, B. W. J. (2007). Pregnancy is predictable: A large-scale prospective external validation of the prediction of spontaneous pregnancy in subfertile couples. *Human Reproduction, 22,* 536–542. doi:10.1093/humrep/del378

Veltman-Verhulst, S. M., Cohlen, B. J., Hughes, E., & Heineman, M. J. (2012). Intra-uterine insemination for unexplained subfertility. *Cochrane Database of Systematic Reviews, 9,* CD001838. doi:10.1002/14651858.CD001838.pub4

Venn, A., Hemminki, E., Watson, L., Bruinsma, F., & Healy, D. (2001). Mortality in a cohort of IVF patients. *Human Reproduction, 16,* 2691–2696. doi:10.1093/humrep/16.12.2691

Williams, C. L., Hayman, L. L., Daniels, S. R., Robinson, T. N., Steinberger, J., Paridon, S., & Bazzarre, T. (2002). Cardiovascular health in childhood: A statement for health professionals from the Committee on Atherosclerosis, Hypertension, and Obesity in the Young (AHOY) of the Council on Cardiovascular Disease in the Young, American Heart Association. *Circulation, 106,* 143–160. doi:10.1161/01.CIR.0000019555.61092.9E

Zegers-Hochschild, F., Adamson, G. D., de Mouzon, J., Ishihara, O., Mansour, R., Nygren, K. G.,...Vanderpoel, S. (2009). International Committee for Monitoring Assisted Reproductive Technology (ICMART) and the World Health Organization (WHO) revised glossary of ART terminology, 2009. *Fertility and Sterility, 92,* 1520–1524. doi:10.1016/ j.fertnstert.2009.09.009

# CHAPTER 19

# CHANGING TIMES: HOW IS SAME-SEX RELATIONSHIP EQUALITY IMPACTING THE FERTILITY CARE LANDSCAPE?

*Bethany G. Everett, Oluwatitofunmi O. Apatira, and Katharine McCabe*

In recent years, the United States and many other countries (e.g., Canada, the United Kingdom, and Norway) have seen radical changes in both cultural and social acceptance of same-sex couples and sexual minorities (lesbian, gay, bisexual, and transgender persons [LGBT]). These changes are reflected not only in increasing acceptance of sexual minorities at the population level, but also in new state and federal policies that legally recognize same-sex relationships and sexual minorities. As of early 2015, 37 states in the United States legally recognize same-sex relationships, and internationally, 18 countries legally recognize same-sex marriage. Other legal standings are changing in the United States and elsewhere that ban medical care providers from denying the use of assisted reproductive technology (ART) services that include the use of donor sperm to sexual minorities (Mishra, 2014). Several countries (e.g., Israel, Canada, and the United Kingdom) provide full coverage for the use of ART for men and women under a certain age, including sexual minorities. More children than ever before will be raised by sexual minority parents: In the United States alone, almost 3 million sexual minorities have had a child at some point in their lives, and as many as 6 million American children and adults have a sexual minority parent (Gates, 2013).

Overwhelmingly, research shows no differences in multiple developmental and health-related outcomes between children raised by heterosexual parents and those raised by same-sex parents (for a review see Manning, Fettro, & Lamidi, 2014). The lack of negative effects of being raised in a same-sex family has bolstered legal arguments that advocate for protections for and recognition of sexual minority parents (Robertson, 2004). The Ethics Committee of the American Society for Reproductive Medicine (2013) has supported the push for legal recognition and equal access to ART and concluded in their official 2013 recommendation that fertility programs "should treat all requests for assisted reproduction equally without regard to marital/partner status or sexual orientation" (p. 1524).

Increases in legal recognition of same-sex relationships have also changed the expectation for parenthood among sexual minorities (Jennings, Mellish, Tasker,

Lamb, & Golombok, 2014): A study of child intentions among young gay men and women showed that 86% of men and 91% of women saw themselves raising children in the future (D'Augelli, Rendina, Sinclair, & Grossman, 2007). Relatedly, the number of sexual minority men and women using medically assisted reproduction (MAR) to form their families has also increased (Farr & Patterson, 2013; Riggs & Due, 2014). Although LGBT persons and heterosexuals share many fertility and reproductive care–related concerns, sexual minorities often face unique challenges in the fertility care landscape. In this chapter, we focus primarily on sexual minority women's (SMW) experiences with fertility including the decision-making process to have children, deciding which MAR method to use, issues surrounding choosing sperm donors, experiences in health care settings and interacting with fertility and reproduction care providers, and fertility outcomes. Additionally, we discuss how sexual minority men's decision to parent impacts the fertility landscape via the use of surrogacy, and present the limited data available to date on transgender individuals' fertility experiences.

## SMW AND ART METHOD CHOICE

Advances in MAR methods have increased the number of methods from which SMW may choose to become parents, including vaginal insemination, intrauterine insemination, and in vitro fertilization (IVF). One major distinction between SMW and heterosexual women is that SMW's use of fertility services may not be the result of medically related difficulties in conceiving, but rather the sex of their partner. The second major distinction is that, historically, lesbians trying to conceive have been excluded from fertility care settings and the use of ART both formally and informally (Mamo, 2007). As a result, SMW approach fertility care from a different perspective and with different needs.

The historical exclusion of lesbians from formal reproductive care settings meant that parenthood for many was negotiated outside the context of mainstream fertility care settings and instead was the result of informal negotiations between friends, acquaintances, and networks within the LGB community (Mamo, 2007). In these contexts, artificial insemination largely reflected a "do it yourself" ethos, a rejection of the medical community from which they were excluded, and embraced their ability to negotiate parenthood outside of traditional norms and expectations (Dunne, 2000; Mamo, 2007). Although these fertility strategies were often subject to several logistical and legal obstacles, for many women, the independence from the medical community in the context of fertility was liberating and produced a celebratory space for women to form families on their own terms (Dunne, 2000; Mamo, 2007). Furthermore, avoiding clinical settings also allowed SMW to avoid potentially homophobic and discriminatory interactions (Hayman, Wilkes, Halcomb, & Jackson, 2014; Hayman, Wilkes, Jackson, & Halcomb, 2013). To this day, in-home insemination is the preferred method by many women who do not have any medically related barriers to conception; thus, they are able to avoid clinical settings altogether (Hayman et al., 2014).

Inside the context of fertility clinics, MAR methods that are least invasive are preferred (Hayman et al., 2014). In a recent study of lesbians using MAR methods, it was found that although some women chose intrauterine insemination as their first method of choice, no women chose IVF as their first choice as a method of conception due to the high costs and invasiveness of the procedure (Hayman et al. 2014). Additionally, because many SMW have experienced rejection from biological family members and formed nonbiological kinship networks, some research has found that some SMW feel that biological ties to their children are less a priority than their heterosexual counterparts and if they experience difficulty conceiving, they are more likely than heterosexuals to turn to adoption as an alternative (Jennings et al., 2014).

Lesbian women may also choose to use IVF with reception of oocytes from partners, a method that allows both mothers to share kinship by allowing one mother to carry a fetus that was conceived with the other partner's eggs. In previous decades, this method was particularly legally useful, as it allowed both parents' legal guardian status (Mamo, 2007). Several countries including Italy, Germany, and Austria have recently adopted policies that ban the reception of oocytes from partners as an MAR method. These changes may disproportionately hinder lesbian couples' ability to form families in their preferred way and decrease legal protections for both mothers.

## CHOOSING A SPERM DONOR

The process of choosing a donor can be a daunting experience for SMW using MAR. Using a known donor outside of the clinical context may be desirable to lesbian couples as it significantly reduces the cost of insemination and increases the odds of insemination success, because fresh sperm is associated with higher fecundity rates than frozen sperm (Markus, Weingarten, Duplessi, & Jones, 2010). In addition, some lesbians express an interest in personally selected donors playing a role in their child's life (McManus, Hunter, & Renn, 2006), and women who select open-identity donors within clinical settings have an interest in the child having some information about his genetic and biological origins (Goldberg, 2006).

Alternatively, women who do not have the economic means to access MAR in a clinical setting may use informal networks, including sexual intercourse with acquaintances, to achieve pregnancy (Reed, Miller, & Timm, 2011). Informal donor relationships may result in complicated negotiations surrounding the role of the donor-father in the life of the child (Dempsey, 2012). Furthermore, informal sexual relationships may put women at risk for sexually transmitted infections, and some women report that such encounters can be psychologically disturbing events (Baetens & Brewaeys, 2001). Another work has shown that SMW who conceive via heterosexual sex have higher rates of reporting unmet medical health services (Steele, Ross, Epstein, Strike, & Goldfinger, 2008). Thus, increasing access to MAR methods may be an important facet of reproductive justice, in particular for SMW of color or women with low socioeconomic status (SES).

Inside the clinical setting, some SMW express personal preferences for biogenetic links to their children (Dunne, 2000). Petra Norqvist's work on lesbian mothers in the United Kingdom shows that traditional notions of kinship (e.g., biological ties to family) influence not only the selection of donors who physically resemble themselves or their partners, but also can result in women selecting the same donor when they plan to have more children, increasing the odds that siblings will have a shared life trajectory based on genetic, physical, and personality affinities (Nordqvist, 2012, 2014; Raes et al., 2014). However, because of the costs associated with MAR, which often exclude women with lower SES and women of color, oftentimes the profiles of donors in clinics largely reflect the desired traits of Caucasian middle-class women: their own. As a result, racial/ethnic minority women have reported dissatisfaction of a lack of ethnocultural diversity among donor options, which presents barriers to traditional notions of kinship based on physical resemblance for non-White groups (Ross, Steele, & Epstein, 2006).

Due to the small sample sizes of studies that look at MAR usage among lesbians, it is difficult to generalize about their preferences for a known versus anonymous or unknown donor. However, in one of the largest studies of its kind, Gartrell, Bos, Goldberg, Deck, and van Rijn-van Gelderen (2015) found, in their sample of 129 lesbian families, that 36.4% were conceived using known donors, 24.7% through open-identity donors, and 39% through unknown donors. Preferences for an unknown donor may be rooted in concerns about protecting the legal constitution of the family as defined by the mothers (Goldberg, 2006; Nordqvist, 2012). Indeed, one of the greatest concerns in lesbian donor insemination is the parental rights of the known donors (McManus et al., 2006). Considerable care is often taken by lesbian couples who chose to use a known donor as they consider options such as obtaining legal counsel and establishing a contract with their donor setting the conditions of parental involvement (Ross et al., 2006). Among Goldberg's sample of 29 lesbian couples, she found that a number of women who had initially expressed a desire for a known donor were persuaded otherwise after talking with friends and lawyers about the legal risks (2006). Thus, the fertility clinic itself can provide a space where health care providers act as witnesses to the insemination process, thereby protecting lesbian couples from paternity claims by known donors (Brill, 2006).

## CARE EXPERIENCES IN REPRODUCTIVE CARE SETTINGS

Although most same-sex couples who seek fertility care to achieve pregnancy report overall positive experiences with medical care providers and staff, there is much empirical evidence to suggest that they also experience stigmatizing interactions in care settings (Hammond, 2014; Lee, Taylor, & Raitt, 2011; Ross et al., 2006; Wilton & Kaufmann, 2001). Many studies have documented that lesbians prefer being treated "normally" or no differently than heterosexual couples during the fertility and pregnancy process (Dahl, Fylkesnes, Sørlie, & Malterud, 2013; Wilton & Kaufmann, 2001). And most of the negative encounters that SMW and co-mothers face in fertility and maternity care settings are nuanced. For instance, body language, lack of eye contact, and physical distance counter co-mothers' expectations regarding provider–patient communication and signal provider discomfort (Dahl et al., 2013; Larsson & Dykes, 2009). Some women, however, reported more blatant discriminatory interactions such as inappropriate questions regarding sexual orientation and off-color humor about sexuality are perceived as insensitive (Dahl et al., 2013; Lee et al., 2011; Wilton & Kaufmann, 2001).

Health care providers, however, should be aware that SMW and co-mothers may have different similar needs and desires to that of hetero-fathers including wanting to be involved as a support person to the carrying mother, as a copartner when making medical decisions, and in the bonding process after the infant is born (Cherguit, Burns, Pettle, & Tasker, 2013). In fact, excluding, ignoring, or otherwise not appropriately acknowledging the noncarrying co-mother was one of the most prevalent findings of discriminatory or stigmatizing behavior by medical staff across studies (Dahl et al., 2013; Hayman et al., 2013; Larsson & Dykes, 2009; O'Neill, Hamer, & Dixon, 2013). Noncarrying mothers reported facing bureaucratic exclusion and challenges to their authenticity as parents (Brennan & Sell, 2014; Hayman et al., 2013; Rondahl, 2009). For example, in a study of 20 noncarrying mothers, Brennan and Sell (2014) found that many women reported being mistaken for sisters or friends during medical visits. Other research has shown that some noncarrying mothers report being formally excluded from appointments because they were not male partners (Hayman et al., 2013).

Acknowledging the specific needs and desires of lesbian couples is crucial to creating a nonhostile and trusting care environment (Ross et al., 2006; Wilton & Kaufmann, 2001). For noncarrying mothers, integration into the planning and birthing process is imperative. This includes participating in insemination, attending all appointments, and maintaining an active role in all decision-making processes throughout the pregnancy and the birth (Hayman et al., 2013). Other studies have shown that medical providers' use of terms like *mommies* or *mothers* when interacting with both birth and nonbirth mothers and changing official forms to include the term *partner* rather than *father* are ways to improve the experiences of same-sex parents (Brennan & Sell, 2014; Cherguit et al., 2013).

Less research has examined how bisexual women experience fertility care and what specific needs this population may have. The few studies that have considered bisexual women's reproductive experiences have documented that bisexual women with male partners report concerns about their sexual orientation becoming "invisible," especially if they are perceived as heterosexual due to the sex of their partner and their status as pregnant women (Ross, Siegel, Dobinson, Epstein, & Steele, 2012). Taken together, research on lesbian and bisexual women suggests that recognition and validation of their sexual orientation identity by health care providers is critical for both bisexual and lesbian women in fertility care settings.

## MATERNAL AND FETAL OUTCOMES

New research on a sample of women in Sweden using donor insemination or embryo transfer after IVF showed no differences in live birth rates between heterosexual and lesbian identified women (Nordqvist et al., 2014). Furthermore, despite the additional burdens and stressors that same-sex couples encounter as consumers in the fertility industry, most evidence to date suggests that lesbian couples trying to conceive experience few to no negative mental health outcomes relative to their heterosexual counterparts (Borneskog, Lampic, Sydsjö, Bladh, & Svanberg, 2014; Borneskog, Sydsjö, Lampic, Bladh, & Svanberg, 2013). In fact, a series of studies carried out by Swedish researcher Borneskog and her research team demonstrate that, relative to heterosexual couples who utilize fertility services, lesbian couples experience lower levels of depression and stress (Borneskog et al., 2013), lower levels of parenting stress after the infant is born, and higher levels of partner satisfaction (Borneskog et al., 2014).

Lack of social support from the medical community, family, and/or friends, however, has been shown to be important predictors of postpartum depression among SMW (Alang & Fomotar, 2015; Goldberg & Smith, 2011). Furthermore, because the process of having a child—from the decision to conceive up to childbirth—is one that is deliberately planned and meticulously carried out, reproductive loss among lesbians has been found to be particularly a psychologically disturbing event for both carrying and noncarrying mothers (Black & Fields, 2014; Peel, 2010), which can be worsened by the perception of a lack of support from family and peers (Black & Fields, 2014; Wojnar, 2007). Recognizing the unique loss experiences of lesbians trying to conceive is an important area for future research in order to develop appropriate care responses and services to this population.

## SURROGACY AND GAY MEN

As parenthood becomes increasingly seen as desirable and feasible for men in same-sex relationships, the demand or market for surrogate mothers has increased (Berkowitz & Marsiglio, 2007). Because male same-sex couples do not have the option of having one partner carry the pregnancy, surrogacy is often the preferred method of forming families with biological ties to their children (Berkowitz & Marsiglio, 2007). For many men, the total costs for surrogacy are often prohibitively expensive, resulting in a stratified system of family formation among gay men, whereby high SES men are able to realize their preferred family forms and lower SES men are not. Furthermore, in several countries, surrogacy arrangements are banned or do not provide adequate legal protections for gay males who wish to form families (Dana, 2011). As a result of bans and/or the high costs associated with surrogacy in many developed countries, the use of surrogates by gay males has become concentrated in countries where the process remains legal and/or more affordable, primarily India and Asian countries (Smerdon, 2008). The trend toward international surrogacy has been the subject of much debate and criticism, as businesses offering surrogacy have emerged in developing countries. These businesses have been framed either as providing women opportunities to earn an income and support their own families, or as exploitative systems of oppression whereby largely White and middle-income men form their ideal families using the bodies of women with limited alternative economic options (Riggs, Due, & Power, 2015). More research is needed not only on how gay males negotiate parenthood and their mental health during the process of surrogacy, but also on the repercussions of the increasing demand of surrogate mothers in international settings.

## TRANSGENDER EXPERIENCES IN FERTILITY CARE SETTINGS

Very few studies to date have considered the fertility care experiences of transgender or gender variant men and women, that is, men and women whose gender presentation does not align with their biological sex at birth. Many female-born transgender men may not elect to have surgical or hormonal changes made to their reproductive organs, resulting in them not only being capable of becoming pregnant and becoming biological parents (Ellis, Wojnar, & Pettinato, 2015), but also desiring pregnancy (Light, Obedin-Maliver, Sevelius, & Kerns, 2014). The existing research that has considered transgender men's experience during pregnancy has found that they experience distress surrounding gender identity disclosure, concerns about being seen as a "woman" while identifying as male, and high levels of loneliness and social isolation, from peer and family networks and within medical settings (Ellis et al., 2015). For transgender men, the decision to carry a fetus was overwhelmingly seen as undesirable, but due to economic constraints, it was often the easiest and most affordable way to achieve parenthood. Advances in reproductive technologies may also mean that transgender women may be capable of carrying a pregnancy with the use of uterus transplantation (Murphy, 2014). As the number of transgender men and women who desire to become pregnant increases, more research on this population is needed and improved cultural competency among health care providers is imperative. More research is also needed to understand the effects of hormone therapy undergone by transgender men on parent, fetus, and developing child.

## RECOMMENDATIONS FOR HEALTH CARE PROVIDERS AND FUTURE DIRECTIONS

The growing literature on LGBT persons' experiences with reproductive care has improved our understanding of the experiences and unique challenges faced by LGBT persons as they engage with health care providers (McManus et al., 2006). However, these findings also provide insights into ways that care can be improved. Indeed, as the number of LGBT-headed families increases, so does the need to address and improve their care experiences. Sensitivity and cultural competency training for health care providers on LGBT families and their fertility care needs is an important first step for improving provider–patient interactions (Goldberg, 2006; Malmquist & Zetterqvist Nelson, 2014; O'Neill et al., 2013; Rozental & Malmquist, 2015). For many providers, training in appropriate language and terminology for interacting with LGBT parents could improve the experiences of LGBT patients. Providing health care providers with materials that not only include definitions, but also incorporate findings about the health and well-being of children of same-sex parents, may help to reduce stigma and discriminatory attitudes among providers. Changes to health care forms to include gender-neutral or inclusive language (e.g., partner or co-parent) or letting patients fill in the role themselves and use their preferred term (e.g., nonbirth mother, mather, or other mother) will also improve the care experiences of LGBT parents and reduce the frequency of unintentional discriminatory interactions.

Furthermore, the fertility industry and care providers within it should consider the unique needs of lesbian and other LBGT couples in order to reduce the undue burden and emotional strain they encounter. For example, because the majority of lesbian couples do not seek care for infertility issues, communication about options, informational pamphlets, testing procedures, and counseling services should not center solely on issues of infertility (Ross et al., 2006; Rozental & Malmquist, 2015). However, when lesbian couples do experience infertility, it is important to present nonhetero specific options, for example, discussing the possibility of switching the carrying mother and the additional emotional and legal challenges that may develop as a consequence.

## CONCLUSION

Changes in social and cultural attitudes toward sexual minority persons and their civil and reproductive rights have precipitated numerous transformations to the legal, technological, and medical fields. New international, domestic, and biomedical markets have opened up to serve LGBT families and innovations in the area of MAR have accelerated to meet the unique needs of sexual minority mothers and fathers. However, within this rapidly changing context, we must still contend with and more effectively address lingering remnants of bias and exclusion that prospective sexual minority parents face in clinical settings. More research is needed to understand the unique experiences of bisexual and transgender men and women, as well as the fertility care experiences of sexual minorities in countries where same-sex marriage remains illegal or same-sex sex is a criminal offense. Furthermore, improving access to MAR for sexual minorities with low SES is critical for facilitating family formation among this population.

## REFERENCES

Alang, S. M., & Fomotar, M. (2015). Postpartum depression in an online community of lesbian mothers: Implications for clinical practice. *Journal of Gay & Lesbian Mental Health, 19*, 21–39. doi:10.1080/19359705.2014.910853

Baetens, P., & Brewaeys, A. (2001). Lesbian couples requesting donor insemination: An update of the knowledge with regard to lesbian mother families. *Human Reproduction Update, 7*, 512–519. doi:10.1093/humupd/7.5.512

Berkowitz, D., & Marsiglio, W. (2007). Gay men: Negotiating procreative, father, and family identities. *Journal of Marriage and Family, 69*, 366–381. doi:10.1111/j.1741–3737.2007.00371.x

Black, B. P., & Fields, W. S. (2014). Contexts of reproductive loss in lesbian couples. *MCN: The American Journal of Maternal/Child Nursing, 39*, 157–162. doi:10.1097/NMC.0000000000000032

Borneskog, C., Lampic, C., Sydsjö, G., Bladh, M., & Svanberg, A. S. (2014). Relationship satisfaction in lesbian and heterosexual couples before and after assisted reproduction: A longitudinal follow-up study. *BMC Women's Health, 14*, 154. doi:10.1186/s12905–014–0154–1

Borneskog, C., Sydsjö, G., Lampic, C., Bladh, M., & Svanberg, A. S. (2013). Symptoms of anxiety and depression in lesbian couples treated with donated sperm: A descriptive study. *BJOG: An International Journal of Obstetrics & Gynaecology, 120*, 839–846. doi:10.1111/1471–0528.12214

Brennan, R., & Sell, R. L. (2014). The effect of language on lesbian nonbirth mothers. *Journal of Obstetric, Gynecologic, & Neonatal Nursing, 43*, 531–538. doi:10.1111/1552–6909.12471

Brill, S. (2006). *The new essential guide to lesbian conception, pregnancy, and birth*. New York, NY: Alyson Books.

Cherguit, J., Burns, J., Pettle, S., & Tasker, F. (2012). Lesbian co-mothers' experiences of maternity healthcare services. *Journal of Advanced Nursing, 69*, 1269–1278.

Dahl, B., Fylkesnes, A. M., Sørlie, V., & Malterud, K. (2013). Lesbian women's experiences with healthcare providers in the birthing context: A meta-ethnography. *Midwifery, 29*, 674–681. doi:10.1016/j.midw.2012.06.008

Dana, A. R. (2011). The state of surrogacy laws: Determining legal parentage for gay fathers. *Duke Journal of Gender Law & Policy, 18*, 353–390. Retrieved from http://scholarship.law .duke.edu/djglp/vol18/iss2/5

D'Augelli, A. R., Rendina, H. J., Sinclair, K. O., & Grossman, A. H. (2007). Lesbian and gay youth's aspirations for marriage and raising children. *Journal of LGBT Issues in Counseling, 1*, 77–98. doi:10.1300/J462v01n04_06

Dempsey, D. (2012). More like a donor or more like a father? Gay men's concepts of relatedness to children. *Sexualities, 15*, 156–174. doi:10.1177/1363460711433735

Dunne, G. A. (2000). Opting into motherhood: Lesbians blurring the boundaries and transforming the meaning of parenthood and kinship. *Gender & Society, 14*, 11–35. doi:10.1177/089124300014001003

Ellis, S. A., Wojnar, D. M., & Pettinato, M. (2015). Conception, pregnancy, and birth experiences of male and gender variant gestational parents: It's how we could have a family. *Journal of Midwifery & Women's Health, 60*, 62–69. doi:10.1111/jmwh.12213

Ethics Committee of the American Society for Reproductive Medicine. (2013). Access to fertility treatment by gays, lesbians, and unmarried persons: A committee opinion. *Fertility and Sterility, 100*, 1524–1527. doi:10.1016/j.fertnstert.2013.08.042

Farr, R. H., & Patterson, C. J. (2013). Lesbian and gay adoptive parents and their children. In A. E. Goldberg & K. R. Allen (Eds.), *LGBT-parent families: Innovations in research and implications for practice* (pp. 39–55). New York, NY: Springer.

Gartrell, N. K., Bos, H., Goldberg, N. G., Deck, A., & van Rijn-van Gelderen, L. (2015). Satisfaction with known, open-identity, or unknown sperm donors: Reports from lesbian mothers of 17-year-old adolescents. *Fertility and Sterility, 103*, 242–248. doi:10.1016/ j.fertnstert.2014.09.019

Gates, G. J. (2013). *LGBT parenting in the United States.* Retrieved from http://williamsinstitute.law.ucla.edu/wp-content/uploads/LGBT-Parenting.pdf

Goldberg, A. E. (2006). The transition to parenthood for lesbian couples. *Journal of GLBT Family Studies, 2*, 13–42. doi:10.1300/J461v02n01_02

Goldberg, A. E., & Smith, J. Z. (2011). Stigma, social context, and mental health: Lesbian and gay couples across the transition to adoptive parenthood. *Journal of Counseling Psychology, 58*, 139–150. doi:10.1037/a0021684

Hammond, C. (2014). Exploring same sex couples' experiences of maternity care. *British Journal of Midwifery, 22*, 495–500. doi:10.12968/bjom.2014.22.7.495

Hayman, B., Wilkes, L., Halcomb, E., & Jackson, D. (2015). Lesbian women choosing motherhood: The journey to conception. *Journal of GLBT Family Studies, 11*(4), 395–409.

Hayman, B., Wilkes, L., Jackson, D., & Halcomb, E. (2013). De novo lesbian families: Legitimizing the other mother. *Journal of GLBT Family Studies, 9*, 273–287. doi:10.1080/1 550428X.2013.781909

Jennings, S., Mellish, L., Tasker, F., Lamb, M., & Golombok, S. (2014). Why adoption? Gay, lesbian, and heterosexual adoptive parents' reproductive experiences and reasons for adoption. *Adoption Quarterly, 17*(3), 205–226. doi:10.1080/10926755.2014.891549

Larsson, A.-K., & Dykes, A.-K. (2009). Care during pregnancy and childbirth in Sweden: Perspectives of lesbian women. *Midwifery, 25*, 682–690. doi:10.1016/j .midw.2007.10.004

Lee, E., Taylor, J., & Raitt, F. (2011). "It's not me, it's them": How lesbian women make sense of negative experiences of maternity care: A hermeneutic study. *Journal of Advanced Nursing, 67*, 982–990. doi:10.1111/j.1365-2648.2010.05548.x

Light, A. D., Obedin-Maliver, J., Sevelius, J. M., & Kerns, J. L. (2014). Transgender men who experienced pregnancy after female-to-male gender transitioning. *Obstetrics & Gynecology, 124*, 1120–1127. doi:10.1097/AOG.0000000000000540

Malmquist, A., & Zetterqvist Nelson, K. (2014). Efforts to maintain a "just great" story: Lesbian parents' talk about encounters with professionals in fertility clinics and maternal and child healthcare services. *Feminism & Psychology, 24*, 56–73. doi:10.1177/0959353513487532

Mamo, L. (2007). *Queering reproduction: Achieving pregnancy in the age of technoscience.* Durham, NC: Duke University Press.

Manning, W. D., Fettro, M. N., & Lamidi, E. (2014). Child well-being in same-sex parent families: Review of research prepared for American Sociological Association Amicus Brief. *Population Research and Policy Review, 33*, 485–502. doi:10.1007/s11113–014-9329–6

Markus, E. B., Weingarten, A., Duplessi, Y., & Jones, J. (2010). Lesbian couples seeking pregnancy with donor insemination. *Journal of Midwifery & Women's Health, 55*, 124–132. doi:10.1016/j.jmwh.2009.09.014

McManus, A. J., Hunter, L. P., & Renn, H. (2006). Lesbian experiences and needs during childbirth: Guidance for health care providers. *Journal of Obstetric, Gynecologic, & Neonatal Nursing, 35*, 13–23. doi:0.1111/j.1552–6909.2006.00008.x

Mishra, S. K. (2014). An insight into access to fertility treatment by gays, lesbians, and unmarried persons: Changing nature of reproduction and family. *International Journal of Reproduction Fertility Sex Health, 1*, 14–19. Retrieved from http://www.scidoc.org.cp-13.webhostbox.net/articlepdfs/IJRFSH/IJRFSH-01-301.pdf

Murphy, T. F. (2015). Assisted gestation and transgender women. *Bioethics, 29*(6), 389–397.

Nordqvist, P. (2012). Origins and originators: Lesbian couples negotiating parental identities and sperm donor conception. *Culture, Health & Sexuality, 14*, 297–311. doi:10.1080/1369 1058.2011.639392

Nordqvist, P. (2014). Bringing kinship into being: Connectedness, donor conception and lesbian parenthood. *Sociology, 48*, 268–283. doi: 10.1177/0038038513477936

Nordqvist, S., Sydsjö, G., Lampic, C., Åkerud, H., Elenis, E., & Svanberg, A. S. (2014). Sexual orientation of women does not affect outcome of fertility treatment with donated sperm. *Human Reproduction, 29*, 704–711. doi:10.1093/humrep/det445

O'Neill, K. R., Hamer, H. P., & Dixon, R. (2013). Perspectives from lesbian women: Their experiences with healthcare professionals when transitioning to planned parenthood. *Diversity and Equality in Health and Care, 10*, 213–222.

Peel, E. (2010). Pregnancy loss in lesbian and bisexual women: An online survey of experiences. *Human Reproduction, 25*, 721–727. doi 10.1093/humrep/dep441

Raes, I., Van Parys, H., Provoost, V., Buysse, A., De Sutter, P., & Pennings, G. (2014). Parental (in)equality and the genetic link in lesbian families. *Journal of Reproductive and Infant Psychology, 32*, 457–468. doi:10.1080/02646838.2014.947473

Reed, S. J., Miller, R. L., & Timm, T. (2011). Identity and agency: The meaning and value of pregnancy for young black lesbians. *Psychology of Women Quarterly, 35*, 571–581. doi:10.1177/0361684311417401

Riggs, D. W., & Due, C. (2014). Gay fathers' reproductive journeys and parenting experiences: A review of research. *Journal of Family Planning and Reproductive Health Care, 40*, 289–293. doi:10.1136/jfprhc-2013–100670

Riggs, D. W., Due, C., & Power, J. (2015). Gay men's experiences of surrogacy clinics in India. *Journal of Family Planning and Reproductive Health Care, 41*, 48–53. doi:10.1136/jfprhc-2013–100671

Robertson, J. A. (2004). Gay and lesbian access to assisted reproductive technology. *Case Western Reserve Law Review, 55*, 323–372. Retrieved from http://www.utexas.edu/law/faculty/jrobertson/robertson.DARBY.pdf

Rondahl, G. (2009). Students' inadequate knowledge about lesbian, gay, bisexual and transgender persons. *International Journal of Nursing Education Scholarship, 6,* 1548–923X. doi:10.2202/1548–923X.1718

Ross, L. E., Siegel, A., Dobinson, C., Epstein, R., & Steele, L. S. (2012). "I don't want to turn totally invisible": Mental health, stressors, and supports among bisexual women during the perinatal period. *Journal of GLBT Family Studies, 8,* 137–154. doi:10.1080/1550428X.2012.660791

Ross, L. E., Steele, L. S., & Epstein, R. (2006). Lesbian and bisexual women's recommendations for improving the provision of assisted reproductive technology services. *Fertility and Sterility, 86,* 735–738. doi:10.1016/j.fertnstert.2006.01.049

Rozental, A., & Malmquist, A. (2015). Vulnerability and acceptance: Lesbian women's family-making through assisted reproduction in Swedish public health care. *Journal of GLBT Family Studies, 11,* 127–150. doi:10.1080/1550428X.2014.891088

Smerdon, U. R. (2008). Crossing bodies, crossing borders: International surrogacy between the United States and India. *Cumberland Law Review, 39*(1), 15–85.

Steele, L. S., Ross, L. E., Epstein, R., Strike, C., & Goldfinger, C. (2008). Correlates of mental health service use among lesbian, gay, and bisexual mothers and prospective mothers. *Women & Health, 47,* 95–112. doi:10.1080/03630240802134225

Wilton, T., & Kaufmann, T. (2001). Lesbian mothers' experiences of maternity care in the UK. *Midwifery, 17,* 203–211. doi:10.1054/midw.2001.0261

Wojnar, D. (2007). Miscarriage experiences of lesbian couples. *The Journal of Midwifery & Women's Health, 52,* 479–485. doi:10.1016/j.jmwh.2007.03.015

# CHAPTER 20

# *Exemplar:* A GENETICALLY AT-RISK COUPLE CONSIDERS THE USE OF PREIMPLANTATION GENETIC DIAGNOSIS IN THE UNITED STATES

*Patricia E. Hershberger*

Sickle cell disease affects millions of individuals throughout the world (Centers for Disease Control and Prevention, 2011). In the United States, about 70,000 to 100,000 Americans are diagnosed with sickle cell disease and another estimated 1 to 3 million Americans have the sickle cell trait (American Society of Hematology, 2015a, 2015b). Sickle cell disease and sickle cell trait are common among African Americans; however, sickle cell disease and sickle cell trait can also be found among Hispanics, South Asians, Caucasians, and individuals from Middle Eastern countries (American Society of Hematology, 2015a; John, 2010).

Sickle cell disease is an inherited autosomal recessive disorder. As such, two recessive copies of the sickle hemoglobin gene mutation (e.g., HgS and HgC) must be present in order for the disease to develop in an individual (Rees, Williams, & Gladwin, 2010). Although there are several types of sickle cell disease and clinical manifestations vary, sickle cell disease in the severe form (i.e., sickle cell anemia) occurs when an individual inherits two copies of the HgS mutation, one from each parent. Clinical features and complications of sickle cell disease can be classified into three categories (i.e., vaso-occlusive, hemolysis, and infectious; Rees et al., 2010; Steinberg, 1999). The complications often lead to progressive damage to most body organs including the brain, kidneys, lungs, bones, and cardiovascular system (Rees et al., 2010; Steinberg, 1999). In 1994, a National Institutes of Health sponsored study reported the median survival for individuals with sickle cell anemia (i.e., HgS/S) was 42 years for men and 48 years for women (Platt et al., 1994), although more recent data indicate that survival rates are climbing (Quinn, Rogers, & Buchanan, 2004).

Unlike individuals who have sickle cell disease, individuals with sickle cell trait have inherited one copy of a normal hemoglobin gene from one parent and one copy of a sickle hemoglobin gene mutation from the other parent and are typically healthy (John, 2010). However, individuals with sickle cell trait can pass on the mutated copy of the sickle hemoglobin gene to their children. In instances where both reproductive partners have sickle cell trait, each of the couples' future children is at a 25% risk for acquiring sickle cell disease.

Advances in assisted reproductive technology and genetic sciences have resulted in the reproductive option of preimplantation genetic diagnosis (PGD) to prevent the transmission of known genetic disorders such as cystic fibrosis to future child(ren) (Hershberger, Schoenfeld, & Tur-Kaspa, 2011; Tur-Kaspa, Jeelani, & Doraiswamy, 2014). In 1999, Xu, Shi, Veeck, Hughes, and Rosenwaks reported the first successful pregnancy using PGD to prevent the transmission of sickle cell disease to a future child. Since the initial report, other scientists have continued to advance the genetic and procedural techniques of PGD to prevent the transmission of sickle cell disease for other at-risk couples (De Rycke et al., 2001).

The decision to undergo PGD is not taken lightly by genetically at-risk couples (Hershberger et al., 2012). The PGD procedure is complex and requires couples to undergo in vitro fertilization (IVF). As with many of the assisted reproductive technologies, couples consider multiple factors, such as the human risks, costs, accuracy, and moral implications of using PGD (Hershberger & Pierce, 2010). In the following, a hypothetical case exemplar is provided to demonstrate the experiences of couples who are considering the use of IVF+PGD.

## CASE STUDY

B.E. is a 29-year-old African American woman and E.E. is a 30-year-old African American man. B.E. is an elementary school teacher and E.E. teaches math at the local high school near the couple's home. B.E. and E.E. have been married for 3 years and are in the process of starting a family. B.E. has met with her nurse practitioner to receive preconception health care. Both partners are aware that they have sickle cell trait (both have one copy of the HbS gene mutation and one copy of a normal hemoglobin gene) and are aware of their risk of having a child that has sickle cell disease. The possibility of having a child with sickle cell disease is of significant concern to B.E., as her mother had sickle cell disease. For as long as B.E. can remember, she saw her mother experience multiple episodes of illness and pain as a result of sickle cell disease. Witnessing the personal experiences of her mother left B.E. with a hope that her future children would be spared from having sickle cell disease. Contributing to her experience is that B.E had promised her mother, who passed away 2 years ago from complications of sickle cell disease, that she would do everything possible to prevent her future children from having sickle cell disease. B.E. is deeply religious; and while she had thought about becoming pregnant and then having prenatal genetic testing to determine whether her fetus had sickle cell disease, she felt a strong religious objection to personally terminating a pregnancy.

B.E. found information on the Internet about PGD, including the need to undergo IVF; the financial cost, estimated at about US$8,000 to US$12,400 for IVF and an additional US$3,200 for PGD (American Society for Reproductive Medicine, 2015; RESOLVE: The National Infertility Association, 2006); and the accuracy of the PGD testing, estimated at about 98% for recessive disorders (Lewis, Pinêl, Whittaker, & Handyside, 2001). For a variety of reasons including B.E's good health, she does not have supplemental or other means of financial support to cover the cost of the IVF+PGD procedures. The couple currently reside just outside of St. Louis, Missouri, a state that was scored a grade of "F" on a grading scale of

"A to F," with an "A" grade demonstrating the best state policies available for fertility health care (RESOLVE: The National Infertility Association, 2015). B.E. has "looked into" relocating to Illinois, an "A" graded state, where insurance coverage is more amenable to assisted reproductive technologies (RESOLVE: The National Infertility Association, 2015). However, E.E. is not as comfortable with the idea of moving to a different location, although he is supportive of B.E. in her choice to use PGD.

## Sample Discussion Questions

1. What larger issues, such as societal and political issues, does the use of PGD for B.E and E.E encompass, if any?
2. What strategies might B.E and E.E. consider regarding the financing of the IVF+PGD procedure?
3. Should the use of PGD be a couple's, governmental, or a societal decision? Or combination of those? And why?

## REFERENCES

American Society for Reproductive Medicine. (2015). *Q6: Is in vitro fertilization expensive?* Retrieved from http://www.asrm.org/detail.aspx?id=3023
American Society of Hematology. (2015a). *Sickle cell anemia.* Retrieved from http://www.hematology.org/Patients/Anemia/Sickle-Cell.aspx
American Society of Hematology. (2015b). *Sickle cell trait.* Retrieved from http://www.hematology.org/Patients/Anemia/Sickle-Cell-Trait.aspx
Centers for Disease Control and Prevention. (2011). *Sickle cell disease: Data & statistics.* Retrieved from http://www.cdc.gov/ncbddd/sicklecell/data.html
De Rycke, M., Van de Velde, H., Sermon, K., Lissens, W., De Vos, A., Vandervorst, M.,...Liebaers, I. (2001). Preimplantation genetic diagnosis for sickle-cell anemia and for beta-thalassemia. *Prenatal Diagnosis, 21*(3), 214–222. doi:10.1002/1097–0223 (200103)21:3<214::AID-PD51>3.0.CO;2–4
Hershberger, P. E., Gallo, A. M., Kavanaugh, K., Olshansky, E., Schwartz, A., & Tur-Kaspa, I. (2012). The decision-making process of genetically at-risk couples considering preimplantation genetic diagnosis: Initial findings from a grounded theory study. *Social Science & Medicine, 74*, 1536–1543. doi:10.1016/j.socscimed.2012.02.003
Hershberger, P. E., & Pierce, P. F. (2010). Conceptualizing couples' decision making in PGD: Emerging cognitive, emotional, and moral dimensions. *Patient Education and Counseling, 81*, 53–62. doi: 10.1016/j.pec.2009.11.017
Hershberger, P. E., Schoenfeld, C., & Tur-Kaspa, I. (2011). Unraveling preimplantation genetic diagnosis for high-risk couples: Implications for nurses at the front line of care. *Nursing for Women's Health, 15*, 36–45. doi: 10.1111/j.1751–486X.2011.01609.x
John, N. (2010). A review of clinical profile in sickle cell traits. *Oman Medical Journal, 25*, 3–8. doi:10.5001/omj.2010.2
Lewis, C. M., Pinêl, T., Whittaker, J. C., & Handyside, A. H. (2001). Controlling misdiagnosis errors in preimplantation genetic diagnosis: A comprehensive model encompassing extrinsic and intrinsic sources of error. *Human Reproduction, 16*, 43–50. doi:10.1093/humrep/16.1.43
Platt, O. S., Brambilla, D. J., Rosse, W. F., Milner, P. F., Castro, O., Steinberg, M. H., & Klug, P. P. (1994). Mortality in sickle cell disease. Life expectancy and risk factors for early death. *New England Journal of Medicine, 330*, 1639–1644. doi:10.1056/NEJM199406093302303

Quinn, C. T., Rogers, Z. R., & Buchanan, G. R. (2004). Survival of children with sickle cell disease. *Blood, 103*, 4023–4027. doi:10.1182/blood-2003-11-3758

Rees, D. C., Williams, T. N., & Gladwin, M. T. (2010). Sickle-cell disease. *Lancet, 376*, 2018–2031. doi:10.1016/S0140–6736(10)61029-X

RESOLVE: The National Infertility Association. (2006). *The costs of infertility treatment.* Retrieved from http://www.resolve.org/family-building-options/making-treatment-affordable/the-costs-of-infertility-treatment.html

RESOLVE: The National Infertility Association. (2015). *State fertility scorecard*. Retrieved from http://familybuilding.resolve.org/fertility-scorecard

Steinberg, M. H. (1999). Management of sickle cell disease. *New England Journal of Medicine, 340*, 1021–1030. doi:10.1056/NEJM199904013401307

Tur-Kaspa, I., Jeelani, R., & Doraiswamy, P. M. (2014). Preimplantation genetic diagnosis for inherited neurological disorders. *Nature Reviews Neurology, 10*, 417–424. doi:10.1038/nrneurol.2014.84

Xu, K., Shi, Z. M., Veeck, L. L., Hughes, M. R., & Rosenwaks, Z. (1999). First unaffected pregnancy using preimplantation genetic diagnosis for sickle cell anemia. *JAMA, 281*, 1701–1706.

# PART IV

## PRACTICE: IMPROVING THE DELIVERY OF CARE IN THE ART SETTING

Since 1978 when Louise Brown was conceived via in vitro fertilization (IVF), care of infertile individuals has been the centerpiece of the science that drives our knowledge about this area forward (Johnson, 2011). Everything we do "behind the scenes" from theory development, to the expansion of the science and development of technology, to the policy that allows access, ultimately impacts how we care for those who have fertility challenges.

This final part of the book approaches many of the care aspects surrounding safe and efficacious health care for this population. Stevenson provides an overview of treatment options with assisted reproductive technologies (ARTs) for those with fertility challenges, whereas Abdalmageed, Eaton, and Hurd delve deeper into polycystic ovarian syndrome, a disease that is challenging to understand and treat. Essential to superior care delivery is effective communication among the health care team members and Leonard and Stevenson examine the care team and team communication in fertility clinics. Moody provides insight into an emerging role for nurses in the United Kingdom that allows expansion of care providers to help meet the needs of patients, and McEleny provides an overview of caring for men diagnosed with infertility, a patient population more often neglected in the literature.

## REFERENCE

Johnson, M. H. (2011). Robert Edwards: The path to IVF. *Reproductive Biomedicine Online, 23,* 245–262. doi:10.1016/j.rbmo.2011.04.010

# PRACTICE IMPROVING THE DELIVERY OF CARE IN THE ART SETTING

# ASSISTED REPRODUCTIVE TECHNOLOGY TREATMENT OPTIONS FOR COUPLES WITH FERTILITY ISSUES

## *Eleanor L. Stevenson*

The process of bearing children is a significant experience for most individuals; however, many struggle to achieve a pregnancy. Infertility is estimated to affect between 37 and 70 million couples around the world (Boivin, Bunting, Collins, & Nygren, 2007). In the United States, there are approximately 2 million infertile couples, which is about 9% of the married couples with female partners aged 15 to 44 years (Chandra, Copen, & Stephen, 2013). According to the 2010 National Survey of Family Growth, while infertility rates have actually dropped in the United States from 8.5% in 1982 to 6% in 2010, the ability to become pregnant or carry a pregnancy to term has actually risen from 11% to 12% during the same time period (Chandra et al., 2013).

Parallel with this upward trend in infertility, increased numbers of people are seeking treatment from health care professionals. Although an estimated 12% (7.4 million) of American women aged 15 to 44 years have received infertility services at some point during their lifetime (Chandra et al., 2013), this represents only half the number of women who actually need infertility services. Although some women and men do seek care (or service) for infertility, not all move forward and undergo recommended treatment (Jain, 2006; Kessler, Craig, Plosker, Reed, & Quinn, 2013).

In this chapter, we have a brief discussion of the etiology of infertility and lower-level treatment, with a particular focus on assisted reproductive technology (ART) as a treatment option. Although the focus of this chapter is on heterosexual couples, couples in same-sex relationships and those without partners will share many of the same challenges as well as additional ones that are beyond the scope of this chapter.

## ETIOLOGY OF INFERTILITY

Equal distribution of the causes of infertility occurs between women and men. According to the American Society for Reproductive Medicine (2012), in 40% of infertile couples, the female partner is either the sole or a contributing cause of infertility, in 40% the male partner is either the sole or a contributing cause of infertility, and the remaining 20% of couples have no identifiable reasons and are labeled as unexplained infertile.

## Contributors to Female Infertility

A number of key causes for female-related infertility are addressed. *Advancing age* is a significant contributor to female infertility. In the United States, the age at which women will have their first child has increased in the past decades (Finer & Philbin, 2014), with similar trends in many European countries (Kohler & Ortega, 2002). Aging leads to declining fertility because of diminishing ovarian reserves and increasing chromosomal problems with the oocytes. Although the pool of available oocytes decline with age (Seifer & Naftolin, 1998), the primary reason for age-related decline in fertility is the exponential rise in oocyte aneuploidy, in which there is a deviation in the normal number of chromosomes (Hunt & Hassold, 2010). Even though many women will often have regular menstrual cycles past the age of 35 years, the actual percentage of ovulatory cycles decreases significantly (Small et al., 2006). Despite the regularity of menstrual cycles, a decline in ovarian reserve is reflected by changing hormones that indicate a woman is nearing perimenopause; thus, many women falsely believe that the continued presence of a normal menstrual cycle indicates that they are still fertile (Small et al., 2006).

*Endometriosis* affects 10% to 15% of all women of reproductive age and greater than 30% of the infertile women. Uterine fibroids, such as leiomyomas or myomas, affect more than three quarters of women in the reproductive age, of whom 20% to 50% are symptomatic (Ciarmela, Critchley, Christman, & Reis, 2013). These conditions may have a direct impact on fertility, as well as quality of life due to dysfunctional uterine bleeding and pelvic pain. Both endometriosis and fibroids require surgery, and the socioeconomic cost is significant. One study found that U.S. women diagnosed with endometriosis incur a loss of 10.8 hours (SD ± 12.2) of work per week as well as a decline in the overall quality of life (Nnoaham et al., 2011).

*Tubal blockage* is another significant contributor to female infertility. Because fertilization occurs in the fallopian tubes, when they become damaged or blocked, primarily through scarring, a physical barrier prevents sperm from meeting the oocytes. The biggest contributor to tubal blockage is pelvic inflammatory disease, which is a serious complication of sexually transmitted infections (STIs), such as chlamydia and gonorrhea. The incidence of pelvic inflammatory disease is 1% to 2% annually in sexually active women younger than 25 years. Risk factors for pelvic inflammatory disease include the history of an STI, young sexual debut, multiple sexual partners, inconsistent condom use, vaginal douching, smoking, alcohol use, and exchange of sex for drugs or money (Crossman, 2006). It is estimated that fallopian tube abnormalities account for 30% to 40% of female infertility. In addition to tubal blockages contributing to infertility, another complication that women, with a history of pelvic inflammatory disease, face is the 12% to 15% increased risk of ectopic pregnancy, should a spontaneous pregnancy occur (Steinkeler, Woodfield, Lazarus, & Hillstrom, 2009).

*Hormonal imbalances* also contribute to female infertility. Polycystic ovary syndrome is the most common endocrine disorder of reproductive-aged women, affecting from 5% to 10% of women aged 15 to 44 years (4 million) in the United States

(Sirmans & Pate, 2014). Risk factors for polycystic ovarian syndrome in adults include both type 1 and type 2 diabetes and gestational diabetes. Insulin resistance affects 50% to 70% of women with polycystic ovary syndrome and can lead to comorbidities including hypertension, glucose intolerance, metabolic syndrome, dyslipidemia, and diabetes. It also has a negative cardiovascular impact including increased coronary artery calcium scores and increased carotid intima-media thickness. Additionally, women with ovary syndrome are at increased risk of mental health disorders, including depression, anxiety, bipolar disorder, and binge eating disorder (Sirmans & Pate, 2014).

## Contributors to Male Infertility

About 7% of all men are affected by infertility (Krausz, 2011), and can be placed into two different categories, acquired and congenital conditions. Recent evidence also indicates a worldwide temporal decline in sperm parameters, thought to be due to environmental effects (Rolland, Le Moal, Wagner, Royère, & DeMouzon, 2013).

*Acquired conditions* are often caused by acquired factors including infection/ inflammation, immunoinfertility, trauma, and surgical insult to the reproductive organs, as well as exposure to toxic environmental chemicals. The degradation of sperm quality can result from infection and can be the result of conditions including prostatitis and genital tuberculosis. Because testicles need to be two degrees cooler than the body temperature, situations in which there is increased heat to the scrotum can be a factor in proper spermatogenesis. Immunological factors are typically secondary to trauma. Sperm is not formed until puberty; therefore, they are normally considered "foreign" and kept in an immune-protected environment via the blood–testicular barrier. Disruption of this barrier, via trauma or surgery, leads to the development of antisperm antibodies (Collins, Burrows, Yeo, & YoungLai, 1993). These incidents can include accidental ligation of the vas deferens during hernia repair, testicular cancer, and previous cryptorchidism, as well as trauma and surgical insult (Wald, 2005). Finally, men taking testosterone supplements, either given for bodybuilding or for men with mildly deficient testosterone levels, can experience a side effect of sperm count drops (MacIndoe et al., 1997).

*Congenital conditions* are those that are present from birth and cannot be modifiable. One such congenital condition is a varicocele, which is surgically correctable. Men who were born with undescended testicles can also have infertility, and the older the age at time of repair directly impacts the reversibility of infertility (Kolon et al., 2014). Other congenital conditions are endocrine abnormalities of the hypothalamic–pituitary–gonadal axis. They are usually caused by defects in genes encoding modulators of sexual development and function. Finally, other genetic causes can include Klinefelter syndrome and other gene abnormalities in chromosome Y (Lamb & Lipshultz, 2000; Wald, 2005). About 1% to 2% of male infertility can be attributed to congenital bilateral absence of the vas deferens seen in men who are cystic fibrosis carriers (Hotaling, 2014). It is critical for these men to receive genetic counseling if this abnormality is discovered. For many of the congenital conditions described, ART will be necessary to achieve a pregnancy, as often only small numbers of sperm are needed for certain procedures, giving hope to many men who previously had no options.

# TREATMENT OPTIONS

Treatment options are grouped into two broad categories: in vivo fertilization, namely fertilization that occurs naturally within the fallopian tube, or in vitro fertilization (IVF), namely fertilization that occurs in the laboratory. Any procedure, such as IVF, that requires the egg and sperm to be outside the body is classified under the broad heading of ART. Most patients will be offered in vivo fertilization or IVF treatment plans and typically after implementation, different procedures are selected based on the couples' diagnosis and previous treatment. In vivo fertilization cycles have an approximate pregnancy success rate of 5% to 15%, depending on the age of the woman (Schorsch et al., 2013). In the United States, the success rates or live birth rates for couples undergoing IVF is about 29% (Centers for Disease Control and Prevention, 2014). Although there are many treatment options associated with in vivo fertility treatment, the next sections focus on those that typically follow the unsuccessful use of in vivo techniques, broadly classed as ART, which include such technologies as IVF and intracytoplasmic sperm injection (ICSI), among others.

## Assisted Reproductive Technology

### In Vitro Fertilization

IVF involves the extraction of oocytes from the ovaries so that fertilization can occur in the lab. To ensure a greater number of oocytes, and thus increase success rates, very often, higher doses of gonadotrophin drugs are prescribed. During the IVF cycle, the typical process includes performing a baseline pelvic ultrasound, ovarian stimulation with injectable gonadotropins, regular monitoring of follicle development with ultrasounds and serum hormonal levels, injectable human chorionic gonadotropin (hCG) administration timed precisely before the oocyte retrieval, transvaginal oocyte retrieval, fertilization of the retrieved oocytes in the laboratory, and transfer of select embryo back into the uterus. Many women will also receive progesterone supplementation via daily intramuscular injections or vaginal suppositories and be followed with hormonal and pregnancy testing (Society for Assisted Reproductive Technology, n.d.).

The process is time intensive and requires women having IVF to essentially be "on-call" as monitoring schedules and medication dosages change based on follicular and hormonal development. Oocytes are retrieved typically under general anesthesia or conscious sedation; therefore, women must miss work or other obligations on the day of retrieval. In traditional IVF cycles, fertilization in the laboratory occurs by placing the oocytes and sperm together and allowing fertilization to occur without additional assistance, with transfer back into the uterus occurring approximately 3 to 5 days following retrieval and fertilization. In the past, bed rest was prescribed anywhere from 1 hour to several days following embryo transfer, though recent research suggests that there is no need for any bed rest following embryo transfer (Gaikwad, Garrido, Cobo, Pellicer, & Remohi, 2013). About 10 days after embryo transfer, the monitoring of beta-hCG levels occurs, which indicate pregnancy, and a clinical pregnancy is confirmed via ultrasound. Any confirmed pregnancy will be frequently monitored in the first weeks. During this time, women are still under the care of the infertility clinic staff. If the pregnancy is proceeding without problems, women are released into obstetrical care for the remainder of the pregnancy, which is usually around 45 to 50 days after the ovulation surge (Practice Committee of the American Society for Reproductive Medicine; Practice Committee of the Society for Assisted Reproductive Technology, 2014).

## Intracytoplasmic Sperm Injection

There are additional technologies that have been developed and that can be offered during the IVF cycle. ICSI is a procedure that was introduced in the early 1990s that involves the isolation of one spermatozoon that is then injected directly into the oocyte. This procedure has been useful for couples in which there is diagnosed male infertility (Lanzendorf et al., 1988; Palermo, Joris, Devroey, & Van Steirteghem, 1992), although other uses are evolving. This technique has given hope to many men, particularly those with extremely low sperm counts. There are potential risks associated with ICSI to be considered in the treatment decision-making process, including an increased risk of abnormalities of the genitourinary system (Seggers et al., 2015).

## Preimplantation Genetic Diagnosis/Screening

Preimplantation genetic diagnosis (PGD) and preimplantation genetic screening (PGS) are procedures performed during the process of IVF where genetic material from developing embryos is tested before the transfer of the embryo back into the uterus. PGD allows couples with a known genetic predisposition such as cystic fibrosis to select unaffected embryos to be transferred back into the uterus. PGS is similar to PGD in that it also uses IVF; however, with PGS the purpose of testing is for the diagnosis of aneuploidy in the embryo. Aneuploidy is more common with advanced maternal age, a history of recurrent miscarriage, a history of repeated implantation failure, or severe male fertility problems.

One of the benefits of PGS is the ability to identify embryos that are more likely to result in a viable pregnancy and a healthy baby. In the past, no definitive means were available to determine which embryos would result in successful pregnancies. In order to balance the achievement of a successful pregnancy with multiple gestation, two or more embryos were transferred into the uterus. This resulted in the likelihood of a 30% multiple gestation rate, which can have a significant effect on the pregnancy, including preeclampsia and gestational hypertension, which can lead to prematurity and low birth weight (Bensdorp et al., 2009; Fauser, Devroey, & Macklon, 2005; Gleicher, Oleske, Tur-Kaspa, Vidali, & Karande, 2000). With the implementation of PGS, more cycles can use a single-embryo transfer approach with the goal of increased chance of a single gestation (Forman, Hong, Franasiak, & Scott, 2014). It is unclear, though if PGS technology improves outcomes (Chen, Yu, Soong, & Lee, 2014). Another recent technology, comprehensive chromosomal screening, is similar to PGS and is showing promise for those at higher risk of aneuploidy in reducing first trimester pregnancy loss (Scott, Werner, & Scott, 2013).

## Gamete Donation

There are some situations in which couples cannot use their own gametes, such as in the case of a premature ovarian failure, previous cancer treatment, and azoospermia. In these cases, they can choose oocytes or sperm from a donor. Sperm donation can be with either a known, designated sperm donor or an anonymous donor where couples can make choices based on reported characteristics of the donor. Oocyte donation, however, presents additional challenges. Although oocyte donors can still be identified via known or anonymous sources like sperm donors, the donor typically must go through the stimulation phase of the IVF cycle and usually have her cycle coordinated with the recipient's to allow for precisely timed embryo transfer, though the recent availability of oocyte cryopreservation may allow donor oocyte banking, thus eliminating the need to coordinate the cycles between the donor and the intended parent. This process can only be accomplished within a cycle of IVF (Sidebotham, 2003).

## Gestational Carrier

When women cannot carry pregnancy due to an underlying medical condition or in the case of a gay couple, there is an option of usage of a gestational carrier in which the embryo(s) are transferred into a woman who will carry the pregnancy for the intended parents. In most instances, the gestational carrier is not genetically related to the fetus. Use of a gestational carrier can be complicated as state laws vary regarding the legality of this process. Additionally, psychological and economic ramifications need to be considered. Gestational carriers must go through a battery of physical and emotional testing before undergoing IVF in order to achieve a pregnancy and must be fully informed of the risks of the process and of pregnancy. Additionally, they should receive psychological evaluation and counseling and should have independent legal counsel. The economic burden on the intended parents is significant; in addition to the cost of the IVF cycle and possibly an oocyte donor, the compensation for a gestational carrier can be prohibitive (Ethics Committee of the American Society for Reproductive Medicine, 2013), with some sources indicating the process to be in excess of US$100,000 (Herron, n.d.).

All of the ART treatments that are available are complex and require couples to have a good understanding of their treatment options in making informed decisions about their treatment. This technical process is one that needs comprehensive discussion by an interdisciplinary health care team (Table 21.1).

## Mitochondrial Transfer

Mitochondrial diseases occur when there are mutations in the nuclear and mitochondrial DNA (mtDNA). Maternally inherited mtDNA mutations are a frequent cause of severe disease with an incidence of 0.5% of the population (Elliott, Samuels, Eden, Relton, & Chinnery, 2008). This disease is passed on maternally; previously, the treatment options for patients who have mitochondrial

**TABLE 21.1** In Vitro Fertilization (IVF) and Intracytoplasmic Sperm Injection (ICSI): Indications, Advantages, and Disadvantages

| Indications for IVF/ICSI | • Low sperm<br>• Blocked tubes<br>• During preimplantation genetic diagnosis (PGD) procedure–single gene/translocation<br>• Diminished ovarian reserve with time constraints that make in vivo fertilization less optimal treatment<br>• Failed prior treatment |
| --- | --- |
| Advantages of IVF/ICSI | • Early genetic screening<br>• Higher success rates than intrauterine insemination<br>• Fertility preservation for those who need to preserve/delay childbearing (e.g., diagnosis of cancer) |
| Disadvantages of IVF/ICSI | • Invasive<br>• Expensive<br>• Risk of ovarian hyperstimulation syndrome (OHSS)<br>• Potential negative outcomes (e.g., some health risks for women, long term, are unknown) |

disease were limited. Because there is no reliable and predictable way to identify mitochondrial disease using existing diagnostics for embryos and oocytes, an alternative approach to this problem is emerging in which there is a partial or complete replacement of defective mtDNA with healthy mtDNA through embryo manipulations from donor embryos (Yabuuchi et al., 2012). Having cleared some of the governmental hurdles, the United Kingdom is very likely going to be the world's first country to begin clinical trials by the end of 2015 of mitochondrial donation in couples known to be at high risk of passing on mitochondrial diseases to their children. Two techniques that show promise are the nuclear transfer from the affected zygote to an enucleated donor zygote with healthy mitochondria and maternal meiotic spindle transfer in which the meiotic spindle from the affected oocyte is transferred into a healthy donor oocyte after its spindle has been removed; fertilization with the partner's sperm would occur after the transfer. Currently, neither technique is permissible worldwide, and countries such as the United States are examining the ethical questions surrounding these techniques.

## TREATMENT CONSIDERATIONS

Treatment for infertility provides hope for many couples desiring family building. By the time most couples are offered ART, they have been a part of the health care team for a considerable amount of time. The testing and treatment alone can be complex for couples, especially as the science continues to advance at such a rapid pace. Every step in the process is perceived as significant and may impact future decision making (Williams, Green, & Roberts, 2010). In order to help couples best navigate the process, there are many care needs and considerations for those seeking ART.

## Educational Needs

The rate of multiple gestation increases with the use of in vitro fertility treatments; 43% of higher order multiple gestations are a result of IVF and ART (Fong et al., 2011). The challenge comes when patients express a desire to increase the number of embryos transferred with the belief of increasing their odds of success with their ART cycle. It is imperative that when couples are being counseled about these therapies, they must be well educated and thoroughly informed about the possibility of a multiple gestation and the risk to the pregnancy. Although many patients perceive a twin outcome as desirable, it is imperative for them to understand the significant increase in morbidity and mortality over singletons (Pinborg, 2005).

## Psychosocial Needs

Research indicates that the process of infertility treatment can be stressful, and has a negative impact on the psychological well-being and sexual relationships of couples (Luk &Loke, 2014) and infertile women have more unfavorable mental health sequalae (Hasanpour, Bani, Mirghafourvand, & Yahyavi Kochaksarayie, 2014). As couples navigate this process of testing and treatment, the complexity and time commitment increases; this places additional demands on themselves and their relationships. The process has been found to be stressful (Brucker & McKenry, 2004).

## Socioeconomic Considerations

The average cost of IVF in the United States approaches $25,000 per cycle (Katz et al., 2011), and in addition to the actual monetary cost of these services, there are other costs to consider. The cost alone may already be prohibitive for many in the United States (Drazba, Kelley, & Hershberger, 2014); however, the time spent in seeking infertility care is an additional source of potential financial burden due to lost wages and other economic hardships. Time spent on care may also have a significant mental and social burden. One study found that over a period of 18 months, on average 125 hours (translating to 15 working days) were spent on fertility care (Wu, Elliott, Katz, & Smith, 2013). Although many countries do offer coverage for ART, these are often limited and dependent on the couple meeting certain criteria.

## Physiological Considerations

Ovarian hyperstimulation syndrome (OHSS) can occur in the days and weeks following the IVF process. The key feature is an increase in vascular permeability of the ovaries under the influence of hCG, resulting in leaking fluid into the abdomen and the swelling of the ovaries (Steward et al., 2014). OHSS is not uncommon, with some studies reporting the incidence of moderate or severe forms in up to 10% of all IVF cycles, and more recently an incidence of 1% to 5%, though the true incidence is probably much higher (Mocanu, Redmond, Hennelly, Collins, & Harrison, 2007; Papanikolaou et al., 2006).

The risk factors for OHSS syndrome include lean body habitus, young age, polycystic ovarian syndrome, the use of high-dose gonadotropin treatment, high-serum E2 levels during treatment, luteal-phase hCG supplementation, and pregnancy (Forman, Frydman, Egan, Ross, & Barlow, 1990; MacDougall, Tan, & Jacobs, 1992). Mild symptoms may include palpable ovaries, moderate symptoms may include abdominal distension and nausea, and, if OHSS advances to severe, symptoms can include oliguria, renal failure, tense ascites, and acute respiratory distress syndrome (Budev, Arroliga, & Falcone, 2005). Treatment is largely supportive, and education about early identification of symptoms is critical so supportive therapies can be implemented in a timely fashion to prevent the advancement to severe symptomology.

## Couple and Individual Partner Concerns

An important aspect of comprehensive fertility care pertains to the emerging, and at times conflicting, evidence about potential risks of these advanced procedures. Some studies suggest that the prevalence of birth defects is increased for pregnancies conceived via IVF, suggesting that gastrointestinal, cardiovascular, and musculoskeletal anomalies occur more in children conceived through IVF than the general population (El-Chaar et al., 2009; Shankaran, 2014). On the other hand, a recent systematic review of research examining child neurodevelopment found that children born following ART were comparable to spontaneous conceived children (Bay, Mortensen, & Kesmodel, 2013). Although additional research will continue to comprehensively evaluate the outcomes of babies born after IVF, health care providers need to continue to advocate for and stay current of evidence to be able to best inform couples as they make care choices. Clinicians in need of additional resources to guide caring for couples can use those listed in Box 21.1.

## BOX 21.1 ADDITIONAL RESOURCES

| | |
|---|---|
| American Association of Reproductive Medicine | http://www.asrm.org |
| Basic Infertility Diagnostic and Treatment Algorithm | http://www.guideline.gov/ algorithm/3764/NGC-3764_2.pdf |
| RESOLVE, the National Infertility Association | http://resolve.org |
| Society for Assisted Reproductive Technology | http://www.sart.org |

## CONCLUSION

When couples experience difficulty conceiving, the path to diagnosis and treatment is not always linear. The many different contributing factors associated with infertility often make identifying a cause challenging, as are the appropriate treatment options. The health care team is positioned to interact and care for the couple going through fertility treatment at many care points. The science that supports infertility, specifically ART, continues to evolve at a rapid pace. Those who work in the specialty area of reproductive endocrinology will have an opportunity to have frequent and meaningful interactions throughout the care process when advanced treatments are needed. It is imperative that the care team continue to keep current with new and emerging technologies and be able to support couples appropriately, regardless of the care setting; the needs of couples during the evaluation and care are multifaceted and complex. The health care team must act as a collaborative unit as they work with the couple navigating this complicated and often stressful process as they work toward biological parenthood, adoption, or childfree living.

## REFERENCES

American Society for Reproductive Medicine. (2012). *Infertility: An overview*. Retrieved from http://www.asrm.org/Booklet_Infertility_An_Overview

Bay, B., Mortensen, E. L., & Kesmodel, U. S. (2013). Assisted reproduction and child neurodevelopmental outcomes: A systematic review. *Fertility and Sterility, 100*(3), 844–853. doi:10.1016/j.fertnstert.2013.05.034

Bensdorp, A. J., Slappendel, E., Koks, C., Oosterhuis, J., Hoek, A., Hompes, P., . . . van Wely, M. (2009). The INeS study: Prevention of multiple pregnancies: A randomised controlled trial comparing IUI COH versus IVF e SET versus MNC IVF in couples with unexplained or mild male subfertility. *BMC Women's Health, 9*, 35.

Boivin, J., Bunting, L., Collins, J. A., & Nygren, K. G. (2007). International estimates of infertility prevalence and treatment-seeking: Potential need and demand for infertility medical care. *Human Reproduction, 22*(6), 1506–1512. doi:10.1093/humrep/dem046

Brucker, P. S., & McKenry, P. C. (2004). Support from health care providers and the psychological adjustment of individuals experiencing infertility. *Journal of Obstetric, Gynecologic, and Neonatal Nursing, 33*, 597–603. doi:10.1177/0884217504268943

Budev, M. M., Arroliga, A. C., & Falcone, T. (2005). Ovarian hyperstimulation syndrome. *Critical Care Medicine, 33*(10 Suppl), S301–S306. doi:10.1097/01.CCM.0000182795.31757.CE

Centers for Disease Control and Prevention, American Society for Reproductive Medicine, Society for Assisted Reproductive Technology. (2014). *2012 Assisted Reproductive Technology National Summary Report*. Retrieved from http://www.cdc.gov/art/pdf/2012-report/national-summary/art_2012_national_summary_report.pdf

Chandra, A., Copen, C. E., & Stephen, E. H. (2013). *Infertility and impaired fecundity in the United States, 1982–2010: Data from the National Survey of Family Growth*. National Health Statistics Report (Report No. 67). Retrieved from http://www.cdc.gov/nchs/data/nhsr/nhsr067.pdf

Chen, C. K., Yu, H. T., Soong, Y. K., & Lee, C. L. (2014). New perspectives on preimplantation genetic diagnosis and preimplantation genetic screening. *Taiwanese Journal of Obstetrics & Gynecology, 53*(2), 146–150. doi:10.1016/j.tjog.2014.04.004

Ciarmela, P., Critchley, H., Christman, G. M., & Reis, F. M. (2013). Pathogenesis of endometriosis and uterine fibroids. *Obstetrics and Gynecology International, 2013*, 656571. doi:10.1155/2013/656571

Collins, J. A., Burrows, E. A., Yeo, J., & YoungLai, E. V. (1993). Frequency and predictive value of antisperm antibodies among infertile couples. *Human Reproduction, 8*(4), 592–598.

Crossman, S. H. (2006). The challenge of pelvic inflammatory disease. *American Family Physician, 73,* 859–864. Retrieved from http://www.aafp.org/afp/2006/0301

Drazba, K. T., Kelley, M. A., & Hershberger, P. E. (2014). A qualitative inquiry of the financial concerns of couples opting to use preimplantation genetic diagnosis to prevent the transmission of known genetic disorders. *Journal of Genetic Counseling, 23*(2), 202–211. doi:10.1007/s10897-013-9638-7

El-Chaar, D., Yang, Q., Gao, J., Bottomley, J., Leader, A., Wen, S. W., & Walker, M. (2009). Risk of birth defects increased in pregnancies conceived by assisted human reproduction. *Fertility and Sterility, 92*(5), 1557–1561. doi:10.1016/j.fertnstert.2008.08.080

Elliott, H. R., Samuels, D. C., Eden, J. A., Relton, C. L., & Chinnery, P. F. (2008). Pathogenic mitochondrial DNA mutations are common in the general population. *American Journal of Human Genetics, 83*(2), 254–260. doi:10.1016/j.ajhg.2008.07.004

Ethics Committee of the American Society for Reproductive Medicine. (2013). Consideration of the gestational carrier: A committee opinion. *Fertility and Sterility, 99,* 1838–1841. doi:10.1016/j.fertnstert.2013.02.042

Fauser, B. C., Devroey, P., & Macklon, N. S. (2005). Multiple birth resulting from ovarian stimulation for subfertility treatment. *Lancet, 365*(9473), 1807–1816. doi:10.1016/s0140-6736(05)66478-1

Finer, L. B., & Philbin, J. M. (2014). Trends in ages at key reproductive transitions in the United States, 1951–2010. *Women's Health Issues, 24,* e271–e279. doi:10.1016/j.whi.2014.02.002

Fong, S. A., Palta, V., Oh, C., Cho, M. M., Loughlin, J. S., & McGovern, P. G. (2011). Multiple pregnancy after gonadotropin-intrauterine insemination: An unavoidable event? *ISRN Obstetrics and Gynecology, 2011*(465483), 1–5. doi:10.5402/2011/465483

Forman, E. J., Hong, K. H., Franasiak, J. M., & Scott, R. T. (2014). Obstetrical and neonatal outcomes from the BEST Trial: Single embryo transfer with aneuploidy screening improves outcomes after in vitro fertilization without compromising delivery rates. *American Journal of Obstetrics and Gynecology, 210*(2), 157.e1–157.e6. doi:10.1016/j.ajog.2013.10.016

Forman, R. G., Frydman, R., Egan, D., Ross, C., & Barlow, D. H. (1990). Severe ovarian hyperstimulation syndrome using agonists of gonadotropin-releasing hormone for in vitro fertilization: A European series and a proposal for prevention. *Fertility and Sterility, 53*(3), 502–509.

Gaikwad, S., Garrido, N., Cobo, A., Pellicer, A., & Remohi, J. (2013). Bed rest after embryo transfer negatively affects in vitro fertilization: A randomized controlled clinical trial. *Fertility and Sterility, 100*(3), 729–735. doi:10.1016/j.fertnstert.2013.05.011

Gleicher, N., Oleske, D. M., Tur-Kaspa, I., Vidali, A., & Karande, V. (2000). Reducing the risk of high-order multiple pregnancy after ovarian stimulation with gonadotropins. *The New England Journal of Medicine, 343*(1), 2–7. doi:10.1056/nejm200007063430101

Hasanpour, S., Bani, S., Mirghafourvand, M., & Yahyavi Kochaksarayie, F. (2014). Mental health and its personal and social predictors in infertile women. *Journal of Caring Sciences, 3*(1), 37–45. doi:10.5681/jcs.2014.005

Herron, J. (n.d.). *The costs of adoption vs. surrogacy.* Retrieved from http://www.bankrate.com/finance/smart-spending/costs-adoption-vs-surrogacy.aspx

Hotaling, J. M. (2014). Genetics of male fertility. *Urologic Clinics of North America, 41,* 1–17. doi:10.1016/j.ucl.2013.08.009

Hunt, P., & Hassold, T. (2010). Female meiosis: Coming unglued with age. *Current Biology: CB, 20*(17), R699–R702. doi:10.1016/j.cub.2010.08.011

Jain, T. (2006). Socioeconomic and racial disparities among infertility patients seeking care. *Fertility and Sterility, 85*(4), 876–881. doi:10.1016/j.fertnstert.2005.07.1338

Katz, P., Showstack, J., Smith, J. F., Nachtigall, R. D., Millstein, S. G., Wing, H.,…Adler, N. (2011). Costs of infertility treatment: Results from an 18-month prospective cohort study. *Fertility and Sterility, 95*(3), 915–921. doi:10.1016/j.fertnstert.2010.11.026

Kessler, L. M., Craig, B. M., Plosker, S. M., Reed, D. R., & Quinn, G. P. (2013). Infertility evaluation and treatment among women in the United States. *Fertility and Sterility, 100*(4), 1025–1032. doi:10.1016/j.fertnstert.2013.05.040

Kohler, H.-P., & Ortega, J. A. (2002). Tempo-adjusted period parity progression measures, fertility postponement and completed cohort fertility. *Demographic Research, 6*(6), 91–144. doi:10.4054/DemRes.2002.6.6

Kolon, T. F., Herndon, C. D., Baker, L. A., Baskin, L. S., Baxter, C. G., Cheng, E. Y.,...Barthold, J. S. (2014). Evaluation and treatment of cryptorchidism: AUA guideline. *The Journal of Urology, 192*, 337–345. doi:10.1016/j.juro.2014.05.005

Krausz, C. (2011). Male infertility: Pathogenesis and clinical diagnosis. *Best Practice & Research. Clinical Endocrinology & Metabolism, 25*(2), 271–285. doi:10.1016/j.beem.2010.08.006

Lamb, D. J., & Lipshultz, L. I. (2000). Male infertility: Recent advances and a look towards the future. *Current Opinion in Urology, 10*, 359–362. doi:10.1097/00042307–200007000–00011

Lanzendorf, S. E., Maloney, M. K., Veeck, L. L., Slusser, J., Hodgen, G. D., & Rosenwaks, Z. (1988). A preclinical evaluation of pronuclear formation by microinjection of human spermatozoa into human oocytes. *Fertility and Sterility, 49*(5), 835–842.

Luk, B. H.-K., & Loke, A. Y. (2014). The impact of infertility on the psychological well-being, marital relationships, sexual relationships, and quality of life of couples: A systematic review. *Journal of Sex & Marital Therapy*. Advance online publication. doi:10.1080/00926 23x.2014.958789

MacDougall, M. J., Tan, S. L., & Jacobs, H. S. (1992). In-vitro fertilization and the ovarian hyperstimulation syndrome. *Human Reproduction, 7*(5), 597–600.

MacIndoe, J. H., Perry, P. J., Yates, W. R., Holman, T. L., Ellingrod, V. L., & Scott, S. D. (1997). Testosterone suppression of the HPT axis. *Journal of Investigative Medicine, 45*(8), 441–447.

Mocanu, E., Redmond, M. L., Hennelly, B., Collins, C., & Harrison, R. (2007). Odds of ovarian hyperstimulation syndrome (OHSS)—time for reassessment. *Human Fertility, 10*(3), 175–181. doi:10.1080/14647270701194143

Nnoaham, K. E., Hummelshoj, L., Webster, P., d'Hooghe, T., de Cicco Nardone, F., de Cicco Nardone, C.,...Zondervan, K. T.; World Endometriosis Research Foundation Global Study of Women's Health consortium. (2011). Impact of endometriosis on quality of life and work productivity: A multicenter study across ten countries. *Fertility and Sterility, 96*(2), 366–373.e8. doi:10.1016/j.fertnstert.2011.05.090

Palermo, G., Joris, H., Devroey, P., & Van Steirteghem, A. C. (1992). Pregnancies after intracytoplasmic injection of single spermatozoon into an oocyte. *Lancet, 340*(8810), 17–18. doi:10.1016/0140–6736(92)92425-F

Papanikolaou, E. G., Pozzobon, C., Kolibianakis, E. M., Camus, M., Tournaye, H., Fatemi, H. M.,...Devroey, P. (2006). Incidence and prediction of ovarian hyperstimulation syndrome in women undergoing gonadotropin-releasing hormone antagonist in vitro fertilization cycles. *Fertility and Sterility, 85*(1), 112–120. doi:10.1016/j .fertnstert.2005.07.1292

Pinborg, A. (2005). IVF/ICSI twin pregnancies: Risks and prevention. *Human Reproduction Update, 11*(6), 575–593. doi:10.1093/humupd/dmi027

Practice Committee of the American Society for Reproductive Medicine; Practice Committee of the Society for Assisted Reproductive Technology. (2014). Role of assisted hatching in in vitro fertilization: A guideline. *Fertility and Sterility, 102*, 348–351. doi:10.1016/j .fertnstert.2014.05.034

Rolland, M., Le Moal, J., Wagner, V., Royère, D., & De Mouzon, J. (2013). Decline in semen concentration and morphology in a sample of 26,609 men close to general population between 1989 and 2005 in France. *Human Reproduction, 28*(2), 462–470. doi:10.1093/ humrep/des415

Schorsch, M., Gomez, R., Hahn, T., Hoelscher-Obermaier, J., Seufert, R., & Skala, C. (2013). Success rate of inseminations dependent on maternal age? An analysis of 4246 insemination cycles. *Geburtshilfe und Frauenheilkunde, 73*(8), 808–811. doi:10.1055/s-0033-1350615

Scott, K. L., Werner, M. D., & Scott, R. T., Jr., (2013). Comprehensive chromosomal screening (CCS) dramatically reduces the age related increase in 1st trimester clinical losses, but has only minimal impact on biochemical losses. *Fertility and Sterility, 100*(Suppl.), S20–S21. doi: 10.1016/j.fertnstert.2013.07.186

Seggers, J., de Walle, H. E., Bergman, J. E., Groen, H., Hadders-Algra, M., Bos, M. E.,...Haadsma, M. L. (2015). Congenital anomalies in offspring of subfertile couples: A registry-based study in the northern Netherlands. *Fertility and Sterility, 103*(4), 1001–1010.e3. doi:10.1016/j.fertnstert.2014.12.113

Seifer, D. B., & Naftolin, F. (1998). Moving toward an earlier and better understanding of perimenopause. *Fertility and Sterility, 69*(3), 387–388. doi:10.1016/S0015–0282(97)00564–5

Shankaran, S. (2014). Outcomes from infancy to adulthood after assisted reproductive technology. *Fertility and Sterility, 101,* 1217–1221. doi:10.1016/j.fertnstert.2014.03.049

Sidebotham, M. (2003). Egg and sperm donation: An issue for health care professionals? *The Journal of Family Health Care, 13*(5), 134–136.

Sirmans, S. M., & Pate, K. A. (2014). Epidemiology, diagnosis, and management of polycystic ovary syndrome. *Clinical Epidemiology, 2014*(6), 1–13. doi:10.2147/CLEP.S37559

Small, C. M., Manatunga, A. K., Klein, M., Feigelson, H. S., Dominguez, C. E., McChesney, R., & Marcus, M. (2006). Menstrual cycle characteristics: Associations with fertility and spontaneous abortion. *Epidemiology, 17*(1), 52–60. doi:10.1097/01.ede.0000190540.95748.e6

Society for Assisted Reproductive Technology. (n.d.). *ART: Step-by-step guide.* Retrieved from http://www.sart.org/detail.aspx?id=1903

Steinkeler, J. A., Woodfield, C. A., Lazarus, E., & Hillstrom, M. M. (2009). Female infertility: A systematic approach to radiologic imaging and diagnosis. *Radiographics: A Review Publication of the Radiological Society of North America, Inc, 29*(5), 1353–1370. doi:10.1148/rg.295095047

Steward, R. G., Lan, L., Shah, A. A., Yeh, J. S., Price, T. M., Goldfarb, J. M., & Muasher, S. J. (2014). Oocyte number as a predictor for ovarian hyperstimulation syndrome and live birth: An analysis of 256,381 in vitro fertilization cycles. *Fertility and Sterility, 101*(4), 967–973. doi:10.1016/j.fertnstert.2013.12.026

Wald, M. (2005). Male infertility: Causes and cures. *Sexuality, Reproduction & Menopause, 3,* 83–87. doi:10.1016/j.sram.2005.09.006

Williams, M., Green, L., & Roberts, K. (2010). Exploring the needs and expectations of women presenting for hysterosalpingogram examination following a period of subfertility: A qualitative study. *International Journal of Clinical Practice, 64*(12), 1653–1660. doi:10.1111/j.1742–1241.2010.02431.x

Wu, A. K., Elliott, P., Katz, P. P., & Smith, J. F. (2013). Time costs of fertility care: The hidden hardship of building a family. *Fertility and Sterility, 99*(7), 2025–2030. doi:10.1016/j.fertnstert.2013.01.145

Yabuuchi, A., Beyhan, Z., Kagawa, N., Mori, C., Ezoe, K., Kato, K.,...Kato, O. (2012). Prevention of mitochondrial disease inheritance by assisted reproductive technologies: Prospects and challenges. *Biochimica Et Biophysica Acta, 1820*(5), 637–642. doi:10.1016/j.bbagen.2011.10.014

# CHAPTER 22

# POLYCYSTIC OVARY SYNDROME: REPRODUCTIVE AND PSYCHOLOGICAL IMPLICATIONS

*Osama S. Abdalmageed, Jennifer L. Eaton, and William W. Hurd*

Dramatic advances have been made over the past several decades in the diagnosis and treatment of infertility. Many of these advances were made possible as a result of assisted reproductive technologies (ART), particularly in vitro fertilization (IVF). The benefits of ART are obvious for the treatment of infertile couples with blocked tubes or extremely low sperm counts. Less apparent are the benefits of ART for treatment of women with ovulatory dysfunction, the most common single cause of female infertility. The most common, and perhaps the most challenging, cause of ovulatory dysfunction is polycystic ovary syndrome (PCOS).

PCOS is a surprisingly prevalent endocrine disorder in women, affecting approximately 10% of reproductive-aged women in the United States (Okoroh, Hooper, Atrash, Yusuf, & Boulet, 2012). Women with this syndrome typically present with irregular or absent menses associated with increased hair grown on the face, chest, and lower abdomen. Most of these women will also demonstrate ultrasonographic evidence of polycystic ovary morphology (Franks, 1995; Setji & Brown, 2014). In addition, the majority of women with PCOS are obese and approximately 70% struggle with infertility (Franks, 1995). Infertility is usually the result of oligo- or anovulation and can be difficult to treat, particularly in women with PCOS who are obese and/or suffer from insulin resistance.

This review addresses the current information about diagnosis, treatment, and medical conditions associated with PCOS. Special emphasis is placed on the reproductive and psychosocial health implications of PCOS.

## DIAGNOSIS

### Clinical Presentation

Women with PCOS most commonly present to a health care provider with menstrual irregularity, hirsutism, and/or infertility. These symptoms can appear in

**TABLE 22.1 Rotterdam Criteria**

| POLYCYSTIC OVARIAN SYNDROME IS DIAGNOSED WHEN TWO OF THE FOLLOWING THREE CRITERIA ARE MET |
| --- |
| • Ovulatory dysfunction |
| • Clinical and/or biochemical signs of hyperandrogenism |
| • Polycystic ovary morphology determined by ultrasonography |

Source: The Rotterdam ESHRE/ASRM-Sponsored PCOS Consensus Workshop Group (2004).

some combination or individually. The presentation can vary greatly depending on the woman's age, ethnicity, and racial background (Fauser et al., 2012).

Menstrual irregularity, manifesting as either oligo- or amenorrhea, is the most common presenting symptom of women with PCOS. Menstrual irregularity is the result of anovulation or oligoovulation. PCOS is the most common diagnosis among nonpregnant reproductive-aged women presenting with oligomenorrhea or amenorrhea (Brassard, AinMelk, & Baillargeon, 2008).

## Diagnostic Criteria

The diagnosis of PCOS is most commonly based on the Rotterdam criteria (Fauser et al., 2012), whereby two of the following must be met: (a) ovulatory dysfunction, (b) clinical and/or biochemical signs of hyperandrogenism, and (c) polycystic ovary morphology determined by ultrasonography (Table 22.1; Rotterdam ESHRE/ASRM-Sponsored PCOS Consensus Workshop Group, 2004). Additionally, other conditions that mimic PCOS should be excluded (Franks, 1995). The advantage of this relatively inclusive diagnostic criteria set is that it includes women with many of the associated conditions and risk factors of PCOS but do not necessarily have both ovulatory dysfunction and hyperandrogenism. The disadvantage of the Rotterdam criteria is that it includes a relatively broad, heterologous group, which can make it more difficult to study in a research setting.

Ovulatory dysfunction is diagnosed when a woman has fewer than nine menses per year or menstrual cycles are more than 35 days in length. Because many adolescent women will have irregular menses, this criterion should be used with caution in very young women (Murphy, Hall, Adams, Lee, & Welt, 2006).

Hyperandrogenism can be diagnosed by either laboratory tests or clinical signs. Laboratory evidence of hyperandrogenism includes increased testosterone (free or total) or dehydroepiandrosterone sulfate (DHEAS). The most common clinical signs of hyperandrogenism are hirsutism and acne. Hirsutism refers to increased growth of thick, long, and dark "terminal hair" in women located in areas where hair follicles are sensitive to androgens. The most common areas women with PCOS complain about increased hair grown are in the midline, including the upper lip, chin, chest, and lower abdomen. Increased hair can also occur on the sides of the face and the thighs.

Polycystic ovarian morphology is determined by transvaginal or transabdominal ultrasound. It is defined by the presence of either 12 or more antral follicles in one or both ovaries measuring 2 to 9 mm in diameter, or a total ovarian volume of

TABLE 22.2 Conditions and Screening Tests to Exclude in Women Presumed to Have Polycystic Ovary Syndrome

| CONDITION | SCREENING TESTS |
| --- | --- |
| Nonclassical congenital adrenal hyperplasia | 17-hydroxyprogesterone |
| Hypothyroidism | Thyroid-stimulating hormone |
| Hyperprolactinemia | Prolactin |
| Ovarian tumors | Total testosterone |
| Adrenal tumors | DHEAS |
| Cushing's syndrome[a] | 24-hour urinary free cortisol |

[a]Screen only in women with physical findings suggestive of this condition.
DHEAS, dehydroepiandrosterone sulfate.

more than 10 cc. One problem with using ovarian morphology as a diagnostic criterion is that many young women without PCOS have polycystic-appearing ovaries. In one study, 33.3% of women younger than 30 years of age were found to meet the criteria for polycystic ovarian morphology (Lauritsen et al., 2014).

## Differential Diagnosis

The most important step in diagnosing PCOS is to exclude other medical conditions that can result in hyperandrogenism and/or anovulation (Table 22.2). Relatively common conditions that can be mistaken for PCOS include nonclassical congenital adrenal hyperplasia (CAH), hypothyroidism, hyperprolactinemia, and Cushing's syndrome (Goodarzi & Azziz, 2006). Less common conditions that should also be excluded are androgen-secreting tumors of the ovary and the adrenal glands.

Screening tests should be performed in all women suspected of having PCOS to exclude these conditions. These include basal serum 17-hydroxyprogesterone (nonclassical CAH), hypothyroidism (TSH), prolactin (hyperprolactinemia), total testosterone (ovarian tumors), and DHEAS (adrenal tumors). Women with physical findings suggestive of Cushing's syndrome, such as abdominal striae or dorsocervical fat pad, should be screened by measuring 24-hour urinary-free cortisol levels (Setji & Brown, 2014).

## REPRODUCTIVE IMPACT

Decreased or absent menstruation is the most frequent presenting symptom of PCOS, occurring in 70% to 80% of women with PCOS (Norman, Dewailly, Legro, & Hickey, 2007). Women with oligomenorrhea often have menorrhagia as well, caused by irregular endometrial shedding related to unopposed prolonged estrogen exposure (Stabile et al., 2014). The underlying cause of menstrual abnormalities in women with PCOS is anovulation; thus, the majority of women with PCOS will have difficulty conceiving.

In many women with PCOS, menstrual irregularity begins at puberty. In other women, the disturbance in the menstruation may start in association with weight gain. The link between the weight gain and menstrual disturbances in PCOS appears to be related to insulin resistance. In support of this is the finding that in many obese women with PCOS, regular menstrual cycles will resume after either therapy with an insulin sensitizer (e.g., metformin) or after weight reduction (Pasquali, Casimirri, & Vicennati, 1997).

Another consequence of chronic anovulation is an increased risk of endometrial cancer (Barry, Azizia, & Hardiman, 2014). It is believed that chronic unopposed estrogen exposure of the endometrium induces endometrial hyperplasia and eventually endometrial cancer. Women with PCOS appear to be at an almost threefold risk for endometrial hyperplasia and endometrial cancer (Barry et al., 2014). Although long-term treatment with oral progestins (e.g., oral contraceptives) is likely to reduce this risk, the effectiveness of this treatment approach has never been examined in prospective studies.

## INFERTILITY

Infertility, while not one of the diagnostic criteria for PCOS, is one of the most common presenting symptoms and affects at least 70% of women with PCOS (Brassard et al., 2008). Most women with PCOS and infertility will have irregular or absent menses and polycystic ovarian morphology on ultrasound. However, some infertile women with PCOS have regular menses and only subtle findings of hyperandrogenemia and/or polycystic ovary morphology on ultrasound (Messinis, Messini, Anifandis, & Dafopoulos, 2015).

### Infertility Treatments

Anovulation is the primary cause in at least 40% of women with infertility, and PCOS is the underlying etiology in the vast majority of these women. As a result, a number of treatment approaches have been developed to correct or counteract the effects of PCOS (Table 22.3). These treatment approaches are usually applied serially, beginning with the least expensive and safest treatments, and only progressing to the more expensive and risky treatments when required.

### Weight Loss

Approximately 50% of women with PCOS are overweight or obese (Pelletier & Baillargeon, 2010). For these women, the first line of therapy is lifestyle modification consisting of a healthy weight-reducing diet and regular exercise in an effort to lose weight. Studies have shown that weight reduction by as little as 5% will often result in the reinstitution of ovulatory cycles in women with PCOS, presumably by decreasing insulin levels (Kiddy et al., 1992). However, like weight loss efforts in general, sustained weight loss is often difficult and only 20% of women with PCOS will be able to sustain a more than 10% loss for 3 or more years (Pelletier &

TABLE 22.3 Fertility Treatment Approaches for Women With PCOS

| TREATMENT | RISKS AND DISADVANTAGES |
|---|---|
| Weight loss | Difficult to achieve and sustain |
| | Takes years |
| Metformin | Gastrointestinal side effects |
| **Ovulation Induction Techniques** | |
| Oral clomiphene | Inexpensive |
| | Low multiple pregnancy rates |
| Combination oral and injectable | Less expensive than injectables alone |
| | Multiple pregnancy rates: intermediate |
| Injectable gonadotropins | Relatively expensive |
| | Increased multiple pregnancy rates |
| Ovarian drilling | Requires laparoscopic surgery |
| | Risk of ovarian scarring |
| | Effect lasts only 6–12 months |
| In vitro fertilization | Very expensive |
| | Risk of ovarian hyperstimulation syndrome |

PCOS, polycystic ovary syndrome.

Baillargeon, 2010). Interestingly, even in women with PCOS who are unable to maintain substantial weight loss, a continued exercise program has been shown to improve their metabolic status (Setji & Brown, 2014).

## Metformin

Metformin inhibits hepatic gluconeogenesis and makes the body's tissues more sensitive to insulin. It is often used in women with PCOS who are trying to achieve pregnancy and are believed to be insulin resistant. Metformin administration has been shown to increase the chances of ovulation in women with PCOS and insulin resistance, and appears to enhance the ability of clomiphene to induce ovulation (Vandermolen et al., 2001).

Metformin is currently approved by the U.S. Food and Drug Administration (FDA) for the treatment of women with type 2 diabetes. Although a number of other insulin sensitizers have been developed for the treatment of type 2 diabetes, metformin has gained widespread use for treatment of women with PCOS because of its safety and relatively mild side-effect profile. In women with PCOS who are insulin resistant, metformin decreases circulating levels of insulin with little risk of hypoglycemia (Vandermolen et al., 2001).

Unfortunately, there are no standard methods for screening for insulin resistance in women with PCOS (Abdel-Rahman et al., 2011). Clearly, women with

PCOS who have diabetes or prediabetes are insulin resistant and thus candidates for metformin therapy. Obese women with PCOS are also good candidates, because approximately 90% of these women are also insulin resistant. Only about 25% of nonobese women with PCOS will be found to be insulin resistant, and so the benefit of treating women in this group is more variable.

The ability of metformin to decrease insulin levels in insulin-resistant women with PCOS has been shown to have several beneficial effects. Metformin use is associated with modest weight loss (usually < 10 pounds) in obese women with PCOS (Nieuwenhuis-Ruifrok, Kuchenbecker, Hoek, Middleton, & Norman, 2009). However, it is suggested that metformin can increase spontaneous ovulation and the chances of ovulation and pregnancy, particularly when used in conjunction with clomiphene (Vandermolen et al., 2001).

Metformin has been shown to be safe in pregnancy, and is thus a Category B drug. It can be used during pregnancy (Vandermolen et al., 2001). However, it is not clear that metformin decreases the risk or severity of gestational diabetes, and for this reason many obstetricians discontinue it after the first trimester of pregnancy (Ghazeeri, Nassar, Younes, & Awwad, 2012).

Metformin is not without side effects and risks. The most common metformin side effect is gastrointestinal intolerance in the form of diarrhea or abdominal discomfort, which occurs in up to 17% of women when first taking metformin (Refuerzo et al., 2015). Fortunately, this side effect resolves in a matter of weeks in many of them. An extremely rare complication of metformin is potentially fatal lactic acidosis. For this reason, it should not be used in women with renal or liver disease.

## Ovulation Induction With Oral Medications

The most common treatment for infertile women with PCOS is ovulation induction after other causes of infertility have been excluded and/or treated. Oral medications for ovulation induction are attempted first as they are the least expensive and have the least risk of multiple pregnancies. Ovulation induction can be combined with intrauterine insemination where high concentrations of washed sperm are placed through the cervix into the uterus, because this relatively inexpensive and low-risk process increases per cycle pregnancy rates.

The only oral medication approved by the FDA for ovulation induction is clomiphene (Vandermolen et al., 2001). This nonsteroidal estrogen receptor antagonist is given for 5 days early in the menstrual cycle and blocks the negative feedback of estrogen primarily on the hypothalamus. This results in increased circulating levels of follicle-stimulating hormone (FSH) and luteinizing hormone (LH), which will trigger ovulation in the majority of women with PCOS.

Common side effects of clomiphene include hot flushes, nausea, and vague feelings of anxiety or irritability. Clinically, the antiestrogen effects of clomiphene sometimes result in endometrial thinning as evidenced by transvaginal ultrasound.

Approximately 75% of women with PCOS treated with clomiphene will ovulate; of these, approximately 50% will become pregnant within the first three to six cycles (Imani et al., 2002). Of these pregnancies, approximately 10% will be twins, compared with a rate of 2% twins for women who achieved pregnancy spontaneously

(Goodarzi, Dumesic, Chazenbalk, & Azziz, 2011). Triplets are very uncommon with clomiphene treatment, but certainly more common than would be expected after spontaneous ovulation.

Letrozole is a relatively new oral medication used "off label" to induce ovulation (Legro et al., 2014). This aromatase inhibitor is approved by the FDA for use in postmenopausal women to treat breast cancer (Franik, Kremer, Nelen, & Farquhar, 2014). The FDA and the manufacturer both state that it is contraindicated in premenopausal women and that it not be used for ovulation induction because early studies suggested that its use was associated with an increased risk of congenital anomalies. Later studies have not demonstrated an increased risk compared with clomiphene, and most studies have found that it is slightly more effective than clomiphene and appears to have fewer side effects (Franik et al., 2014; Legro et al., 2014). Letrozole is sometimes successful in inducing ovulation when clomiphene is not.

## Ovarian Drilling

Ovarian drilling is a laparoscopic procedure in which electrical current is used via a needle placed into the ovaries to destroy some of the hormone-producing ovarian cortex. Afterward, the majority of women with PCOS will ovulate spontaneously for a number of months, and approximately half will become pregnant (Mitra, Nayak, & Agrawal, 2015). The disadvantages, in addition to risks inherent to laparoscopic surgery, are a small risk of ovarian scarring and the fact that the effect is temporary, rarely lasting more than 6 to 12 months. The advantages are that this treatment approach is often paid for by insurance and does not increase the risk of multiple pregnancies.

## Ovulation Induction With Injectable Gonadotropins

In the past, ovulation induction using injectable FSH with or without LH was the most common next step for women with PCOS for whom oral ovulation induction was not successful. This relatively expensive method is more effective than oral medications for inducing ovulation and achieving pregnancy (Homburg & Howles, 1999). With careful monitoring, the risk of twins and higher order multiple pregnancies (i.e., triples or more) is only slightly greater than with oral ovulation induction medications. However, higher order multiple pregnancies occur in at least 5% of cycles (Dickey et al., 2001). The cost of three to four cycles of ovulation induction with injectable medications can be similar to the cost of an IVF cycle (Allen, Adashi, & Jones, 2014).

## In Vitro Fertilization

IVF is recommended for women with PCOS who do not conceive after three or more cycles of ovulation induction with oral medications. Although much more expensive than ovarian drilling or ovulation induction with injectable medications, it avoids the primary disadvantages of these two approaches. The primary advantage of IVF is that the number of embryos transferred into the uterus can be limited to minimize the risk of multiple pregnancies. Expense remains a major disadvantage for women whose insurance does not cover the procedures, which is the most common situation in most states where laws do not require coverage.

The process for IVF has evolved over the past 30 years to include stimulation of the ovaries to produce large follicles with large doses of injectable FSH and LH while monitoring closely with periodic transvaginal ultrasound. Injections of a gonadotropin-releasing hormone (GnRH) agonist or antagonist are used to prevent premature ovulation. When the ovarian follicles reach a size consistent with mature oocytes, the ovulation process is triggered, most commonly with an injection of hCG and the oocytes retrieved with a transvaginal needle before being released during ovulation. The oocytes are fertilized in vitro, and one or more embryos are transferred into the uterus 3 to 5 days after fertilization (Allen et al., 2014).

Live birth rates for women younger than 35 years of age are more than 40% per cycle with modern IVF. The implantation rate per embryo remains frustratingly low particularly in women older than 35 years of age. For this reason, more than one embryo is usually transferred into the uterus during a cycle. National guidelines for the number of embryos to transfer based on age and quality of the embryos has resulted in a twin rate of approximately 25% and higher order multiple pregnancy rate of less than 2% in this country (Allen et al., 2014).

It is well appreciated that multiple pregnancies put the infants at increased risk of permanent disabilities, primarily as a result of premature birth. Additionally, maternal complications such as gestational diabetes and preeclampsia are more common with multiple gestations. For this reason, efforts continue to be made to develop strategies to decrease the multiple pregnancy rates even further. The ultimate goal is single embryo transfer with an excellent pregnancy rate, as this would result in a twin rate close to the natural rate of 2% and theoretically avoid higher order multiples.

## PCOS and Pregnancy

Women with PCOS who do become pregnant are at an increased risk for a number of problems, including miscarriages, gestational diabetes, and difficulty in breastfeeding after delivery. Surprisingly, little progress has been made in understanding or decreasing these risks in the past several decades.

Women with PCOS appear to be at an increased risk for early miscarriage, which can occur in more than 30% of their conceptions (Thatcher & Jackson, 2006). Although the reason for this increase remains unclear, miscarriages in women with PCOS are associated with obesity, hyperinsulinemia, hyperandrogenism, and elevated LH levels. (Thatcher & Jackson, 2006).

Women with PCOS appear to be at an increased risk for other pregnancy and neonatal complications as well. These conditions include gestational diabetes (40%–50%), pregnancy-induced hypertension and preeclampsia (5%), and fetal intrauterine growth restriction (10%–15%; Fauser et al., 2012). Their babies are at an increased risk of neonatal complications such as prematurity and perinatal mortality with higher rate of admission to neonatal ICU. Although the specific etiologies of these increased risks remain unclear, they appear to be associated with obesity, insulin resistance, and underlying hypertension often found in women with PCOS.

# MEDICAL CONDITIONS ASSOCIATED WITH PCOS

In addition to the impact on reproduction, PCOS is associated with several medical conditions, most notably obesity, impaired glucose tolerance, hyperlipidemia, and hypertension. It is likely that the prolonged metabolic dysfunction associated with PCOS increases the risk for cardiovascular disease (CVD) with aging. The risk for CVD is augmented by vascular and endothelial dysfunction in women with PCOS (Kao, Chiu, Hsu, & Chen, 2013). Prevention of and early identification of these conditions are important to the overall health of women with PCOS, as well as optimizing health during fertility care and pregnancy.

## Obesity

More than 50% of women with PCOS are obese, compared with less than 20% of the general population (Lim, Davies, Norman, & Moran, 2012). If obese women with PCOS lose a significant amount of weight through diet, exercise, or surgery, insulin resistance will often improve. Many of these women will resume normal menstruation and ovulation and, over time, see improvements in hirsutism (Gambineri, Pelusi, Vicennati, Pagotto, & Pasquali, 2002; Lim et al., 2012). However, it important for clinicians to keep in mind that approximately one third of women with PCOS are not obese.

## Glucose Intolerance and Diabetes Mellitus

Insulin resistance, defined as the decreased ability of insulin to increase glucose uptake and utilization, is present in more than half of all women with PCOS. Insulin resistance is associated with obesity, and approximately 90% of obese women with PCOS are insulin resistant. However, it is often unclear which of these conditions is causal. In some women with PCOS, there appears to be a defect in insulin metabolism or effect unrelated to obesity, particularly in the 25% of normal weight women with PCOS found to have insulin resistance (Jamil, Alalaf, Al-Tawil, & Al-Shawaf, 2015).

Regardless of the etiology, women with PCOS who are insulin resistant have a five- to tenfold higher risk of developing glucose intolerance and type 2 diabetes mellitus than the general population, and often at an earlier age. For this reason, it is recommended that women with PCOS should be tested regularly for early detection of abnormal glucose tolerance (Joham, Ranasinha, Zoungas, Moran, & Teede, 2014).

Recommendations for the most appropriate method for screening for abnormal glucose tolerance in women with PCOS continue to evolve. Fasting glucose has been shown to be relatively insensitive with women with PCOS, and the 2-hour oral glucose tolerance test has been recommended as the standard screening (Legro, Kunselman, Dodson, & Dunaif, 1999). More recently, hemoglobin A1C has become the recommended screening test for the general population. However, the effectiveness of this test for screening women with PCOS remains unclear (Hurd et al., 2011).

## Metabolic Syndrome

Metabolic syndrome is diagnosed in patients with some combination of increased waist circumference (central obesity), dyslipidemia, and hypertension, and/or glucose intolerance (Ford, Giles, & Dietz, 2002; National Center for Health Statistics, 1994). Women with PCOS are twice as likely to have metabolic syndrome as unaffected women. The underlying cause of metabolic syndrome is believed to be insulin resistance. Women with metabolic syndrome are known to be at an increased risk for coronary heart disease.

## PSYCHOSOCIAL IMPLICATIONS OF PCOS

The clinical characteristics commonly found in women with PCOS can threaten her self-image and body image in terms of both femininity and sexuality. Most important among these characteristics appear to be obesity, signs of hyperandrogenism (i.e., hirsutism and acne) and infertility. As a result, more than half of women with PCOS will experience significant psychological distress, and as many as 15% will have moderate to severe depression (Barry, Kuczmierczyk, & Hardiman, 2011; Deeks, Gibson-Helm, & Teede, 2010). In addition to anxiety and depression, psychological stress related to PCOS can manifest as social maladjustment, impaired sexual functioning, or marital issues. Other subtle manifestations can include difficulty in concentrating, fatigue, and mood swings. It is important to remember that these effects tend to be more common in younger women, who can be more psychological vulnerable to the effect of PCOS on appearance and infertility (Barry et al., 2011).

It is well appreciated that obesity in women is commonly associated with both anxiety and depression. Because as many as 70% of women with PCOS are obese, it is not surprising that weight problems are a common cause of psychological stress in these women. Of all the symptoms of PCOS, weight problems appear to have the greatest negative impact on quality of life for these women (Álvarez-Blasco, Luque-Ramírez, & Escobar-Morreale, 2010).

Regardless as to whether obesity is the cause or the effect of PCOS in any individual women, efforts at weight loss are an important treatment goal for these women. The results of medical treatment with drugs including metformin and oral contraceptives have been disappointing. The most effective treatment approach has been a combination of decreased caloric intake, particularly of carbohydrates (i.e., a diabetic diet), and increased physical activity (Ujvari et al., 2014). Counseling from a dietician and psychological support appear to improve the chances of long-term adherence to these lifestyle changes. In selected cases, antiobesity drugs and bariatric surgery have been shown to be effective for sustained weight loss in women with PCOS.

Many of the psychological symptoms associated with PCOS are related to hyperandrogenism, most notably hirsutism and acne. Surprisingly, while obesity has consistently been shown to increase the risk of anxiety and depression in these women, hirsutism and acne have been linked to increased psychological distress in some studies but not in others (Bazarganipour et al., 2013). Clearly, multiple factors contribute to the high prevalence of both anxiety and depression in women with PCOS (Dilbaz, Cinar, Özkaya, Tonyali, & Dilbaz, 2012).

Although it is not clear that the physical stigmata of hyperandrogenism are related to psychological stress, medical treatment of hyperandrogenism appears to effectively decrease both depression and psychological distress (Rasgon et al., 2003). In women with PCOS who are not trying to become pregnant, oral contraceptives are the cornerstone of treatment.

At least 70% of women with PCOS will have some degree of infertility, and concerns about infertility are an important contributor to decreased quality of life for these women. The inability to have children is often a life crisis that can cause substantial stress to both the women with PCOS and their partners. Infertility and its treatment can lead to episodic increased levels of anxiety and depression and can be associated with feelings of grief, loss, sadness, and anger (Benyamini, Gozlan, & Kokia, 2009).

Reduction of emotional stress might also increase the chances of becoming pregnant. Emotional stress can be reduced by individual, couple, or group therapeutic approaches (Benyamini et al., 2009). Although studies have shown mixed results, it appears that psychological therapy increases pregnancy rates for women undergoing treatment with ART (Hämmerli, Znoj, & Barth, 2009). It is hypothesized that stress reduction might reverse subtle effects of stress on ovulation or gamete and embryo transportation that decrease fertility. The effects of stress reduction on IVF are more difficult to demonstrate (Hämmerli et al., 2009).

## LONG-TERM TREATMENT OF PCOS

Treatment of each woman with PCOS must be tailored to fit her symptoms and desired outcomes. Although women with PCOS share a number of clinical features as discussed earlier, they can be relatively heterologous in terms of physical characteristics and underlying metabolic disturbances. More than one treatment approach is often used simultaneously, and many treatments can have positive effects on more than one clinical feature.

### Weight Loss

As previously stated, obesity is common in women with PCOS. In some women, it is likely that the underlying metabolic abnormalities associated with PCOS result in obesity and make weight loss difficult (Lim et al., 2012). Obesity, in turn, intensifies hormonal and clinical features of PCOS and puts the women at increased risk for type 2 diabetes, hyperlipidemia, endometrial cancer, and psychological issues. Lifestyle interventions, including activity and dietary modifications, are first lines in management to both prevent weight gain and induce weight loss. In women who do not respond to these measures and develop significant comorbidities, various medications and/or bariatric surgery are often used (Turkmen, Andreen, & Cengiz, 2015; Vosnakis et al., 2013).

## Oral Contraceptives

In those not trying to become pregnant, oral contraceptives containing both estrogen and progestin have become the treatment cornerstone. This combination of hormones treats two of the most common symptoms of women with PCOS: irregular menses and hirsutism.

The progestin component of oral contraceptives is an effective treatment for irregular menses in women with PCOS, who ovulate infrequently or not at all. Anovulation results in prolonged stimulation of the endometrium to unopposed estrogen without the cyclic exposure to progesterone related to ovulation. Oral contraceptives provide daily exposure of the endometrium to progesterone for 21 or more days per month, which tends to stabilize and thin the endometrium. A hormone-free period at the end of each month usually results in normal menses as a result of progestin withdrawal. This progestin exposure decreases the risk of irregular menses and possibly endometrial cancer later in life.

The estrogen component of oral contraceptives is present primarily to minimize irregular uterine bleeding as a result of the thinning effect of progestin on the endometrium. However, in women with PCOS the estrogen component has the added benefit of stimulating the liver to produce an increased amount of sex hormone binding globulin (SHBG). This circulating glycoprotein binds testosterone, effectively decreasing free testosterone (the hormonally active form) by an average of 39% (Zimmerman et al., 2015). This often has an immediate positive effect on acne and a slow effect on hirsutism. Unfortunately, the terminal hair already present in women with hirsutism is unaffected. Because the female hair growth cycle is 2 to 4 years, only the hair that grows in over the next 6 to 12 months will come in finer and shorter with the decreased androgen stimulation (Azziz, Carmina, & Sawaya, 2000).

For many women with PCOS, it is advantageous to remain on oral contraceptives until pregnancy is desired (Vitek & Hoeger, 2014). If menses in these women do not result within 2 to 3 months of oral contraceptive cessation, ovulation induction is indicated. After delivery, once breastfeeding is established, oral contraceptive pill use remains an excellent method for preventing and treating many of the negative long-term effects of PCOS. Ideally, oral contraceptives can be continued until menopause.

## Metformin

As discussed earlier, metformin is an insulin sensitizer approved for the treatment of type 2 diabetes mellitus. It is commonly used in women with PCOS and diabetes. It can also be considered for the treatment of women with PCOS who are prediabetic, because it has been shown to decrease both weight and the risk of developing diabetes in prediabetic women (Lily, Lilly, & Godwin, 2009). It should be considered as a second-line therapy, however, as it is less effective than lifestyle modification with diet and exercise (Knowler et al., 2002). Metformin has also been found to help in the treatment of hirsutism, although it is not recommended for that indication (Blumer et al., 2013; Buzney, Sheu, Buzney, & Reynolds, 2014; Knowler et al., 2002). Its long-term use in women with PCOS who are not diabetic, prediabetic, or hirsute and who are not attempting pregnancy remains to be demonstrated.

## Treatments for Hirsutism

Excessive hair growth on the upper lip, chin, cheeks, chest, and lower abdomen is a troublesome symptom for many women with PCOS. The quickest treatment approach is hair removal such as shaving, plucking, waxing, and bleaching, although most of these treatments are temporary and must be repeated. Hair removal methods are often used in conjunction with medical treatments.

For patients who desire medical therapy for hirsutism, oral contraceptives are considered first line (Buzney et al., 2014). If patients do not experience sufficient improvement with oral contraceptives alone, spironolactone can be added. Spironolactone is an androgen receptor antagonist that has relatively few risks and side effects. For more severe cases, a number of more potent anti-androgens are also available. As many of these drugs are known to be teratogenic, women using them require effective contraception.

## Psychological Support

Recognizing and treating the potential psychological issues of women with PCOS is important. Women with PCOS should be monitored on a regular basis for signs of anxiety, depression, low self-esteem, negative body image, and sexual dysfunction. Appropriate treatment and follow-up are essential for some women with PCOS.

## CONCLUSION

PCOS is a relatively common cause of infertility that appears to be increasing in incidence. Rather than a simple unidimensional problem, PCOS is a complex syndrome that can affect women in a number of ways. Effective treatment requires a comprehensive understanding of the condition and its potentially associated problems. The reproductive and psychological health of women with PCOS can be optimized by comprehensive evaluation and monitoring coupled with appropriate treatment interventions as needed.

## REFERENCES

Abdel-Rahman, M. Y., Abdellah, A. H., Ahmad, S. R., Ismail, S. A., Frasure, H., & Hurd, W. W. (2011). Prevalence of abnormal glucose metabolism in a cohort of Arab women with polycystic ovary syndrome. *International Journal of Gynecology and Obstetrics: The Official Organ of the International Federation of Gynaecology and Obstetrics, 114*(3), 288–289. doi:10.1016/j.ijgo.2011.03.019

Allen, B. D., Adashi, E. Y., & Jones, H. W. (2014). On the cost and prevention of iatrogenic multiple pregnancies. *Reproductive Biomedicine Online, 29*(3), 281–285. doi:10.1016/j.rbmo.2014.04.012

Álvarez-Blasco, F., Luque-Ramírez, M., & Escobar-Morreale, H. F. (2010). Obesity impairs general health-related quality of life (HR-QoL) in premenopausal women to a greater extent than polycystic ovary syndrome (PCOS). *Clinical Endocrinology, 73*(5), 595–601. doi:10.1111/j.1365-2265.2010.03842.x

Azziz, R., Carmina, E., & Sawaya, M. E. (2000). Idiopathic hirsutism. *Endocrine Reviews, 21*(4), 347–362. doi:10.1210/edrv.21.4.0401

Barry, J. A., Azizia, M. M., & Hardiman, P. J. (2014). Risk of endometrial, ovarian and breast cancer in women with polycystic ovary syndrome: A systematic review and meta-analysis. *Human Reproduction Update, 20*(5), 748–758. doi:10.1093/humupd/dmu012

Barry, J. A., Kuczmierczyk, A. R., & Hardiman, P. J. (2011). Anxiety and depression in polycystic ovary syndrome: A systematic review and meta-analysis. *Human Reproduction, 26*(9), 2442–2451. doi:10.1093/humrep/der197

Bazarganipour, F., Ziaei, S., Montazeri, A., Foroozanfard, F., Kazemnejad, A., & Faghihzadeh, S. (2013). Psychological investigation in patients with polycystic ovary syndrome. *Health and Quality of Life Outcomes, 11*, 141. doi:10.1186/1477-7525-11-141

Benyamini, Y., Gozlan, M., & Kokia, E. (2009). Women's and men's perceptions of infertility and their associations with psychological adjustment: A dyadic approach. *British Journal of Health Psychology, 14*(Pt 1), 1–16. doi:10.1348/135910708X279288

Blumer, I., Hadar, E., Hadden, D. R., Jovanovic, L., Mestman, J. H., Murad, M. H., & Yogev, Y. (2013). Diabetes and pregnancy: An endocrine society clinical practice guideline. *The Journal of Clinical Endocrinology and Metabolism, 98*(11), 4227–4249. doi: 10.1210/jc.2013-2465

Brassard, M., AinMelk, Y., & Baillargeon, J. P. (2008). Basic infertility including polycystic ovary syndrome. *The Medical Clinics of North America, 92*(5), 1163–1192, xi. doi:10.1016/j.mcna.2008.04.008

Buzney, E., Sheu, J., Buzney, C., & Reynolds, R. V. (2014). Polycystic ovary syndrome: A review for dermatologists: Part II. Treatment. *Journal of the American Academy of Dermatology, 71*(5), 859.e1–859.e15; quiz 873. doi:10.1016/j.jaad.2014.05.009

Deeks, A. A., Gibson-Helm, M. E., & Teede, H. J. (2010). Anxiety and depression in polycystic ovary syndrome: A comprehensive investigation. *Fertility and Sterility, 93*(7), 2421–2423. doi:10.1016/j.fertnstert.2009.09.018

Dickey, R. P., Taylor, S. N., Lu, P. Y., Sartor, B. M., Rye, P. H., & Pyrzak, R. (2001). Relationship of follicle numbers and estradiol levels to multiple implantation in 3,608 intrauterine insemination cycles. *Fertility and Sterility, 75*(1), 69–78. doi:10.1016/S0015-0282(00)01631-9

Dilbaz, B., Cinar, M., Özkaya, E., Tonyali, N. V., & Dilbaz, S. (2012). Health related quality of life among different PCOS phenotypes of infertile women. *Journal of the Turkish German Gynecological Association, 13*(4), 247–252. doi:10.5152/jtgga.2012.39

Fauser, B. C., Tarlatzis, B. C., Rebar, R. W., Legro, R. S., Balen, A. H., Lobo, R.,... Barnhart, K. (2012). Consensus on women's health aspects of polycystic ovary syndrome (PCOS): The Amsterdam ESHRE/ASRM-Sponsored 3rd PCOS Consensus Workshop Group. *Fertility and Sterility, 97*(1), 28–38 e25.

Ford, E. S., Giles, W. H., & Dietz, W. H. (2002). Prevalence of the metabolic syndrome among US adults: Findings from the third National Health and Nutrition Examination Survey. *Journal of the American Medical Association, 287*(3), 356–359. doi:10.1001/jama.287.3.356

Franik, S., Kremer, J. A., Nelen, W. L., & Farquhar, C. (2014). Aromatase inhibitors for subfertile women with polycystic ovary syndrome. *The Cochrane Database of Systematic Reviews, 2*, CD010287. doi:10.1002/14651858.CD010287.pub2

Franks, S. (1995). Polycystic ovary syndrome. *The New England Journal of Medicine, 333*(13), 853–861. doi:10.1056/NEJM199509283331307

Gambineri, A., Pelusi, C., Vicennati, V., Pagotto, U., & Pasquali, R. (2002). Obesity and the polycystic ovary syndrome. *International Journal of Obesity and Related Metabolic Disorders: Journal of the International Association for the Study of Obesity, 26*(7), 883–896. doi:10.1038/sj.ijo.0801994

Ghazeeri, G. S., Nassar, A. H., Younes, Z., & Awwad, J. T. (2012). Pregnancy outcomes and the effect of metformin treatment in women with polycystic ovary syndrome: An overview. *Acta Obstetricia Et Gynecologica Scandinavica, 91*(6), 658–678. doi:10.1111/j.1600-0412.2012.01385.x

Goodarzi, M. O., & Azziz, R. (2006). Diagnosis, epidemiology, and genetics of the polycystic ovary syndrome. *Best Practice & Research. Clinical Endocrinology & Metabolism, 20*(2), 193–205. doi:10.1016/j.beem.2006.02.005

Goodarzi, M. O., Dumesic, D. A., Chazenbalk, G., & Azziz, R. (2011). Polycystic ovary syndrome: Etiology, pathogenesis and diagnosis. *Nature Reviews. Endocrinology, 7*(4), 219–231. doi:10.1038/nrendo.2010.217

Hämmerli, K., Znoj, H., & Barth, J. (2009). The efficacy of psychological interventions for infertile patients: A meta-analysis examining mental health and pregnancy rate. *Human Reproduction Update, 15*(3), 279–295. doi:10.1093/humupd/dmp002

Homburg, R., & Howles, C. M. (1999). Low-dose FSH therapy for anovulatory infertility associated with polycystic ovary syndrome: Rationale, results, reflections and refinements. *Human Reproduction Update, 5*(5), 493–499. doi:10.1093/humupd/5.5.493

Hurd, W. W., Abdel-Rahman, M. Y., Ismail, S. A., Abdellah, M. A., Schmotzer, C. L., & Sood, A. (2011). Comparison of diabetes mellitus and insulin resistance screening methods for women with polycystic ovary syndrome. *Fertility and Sterility, 96*(4), 1043–1047. doi:10.1016/j.fertnstert.2011.07.002

Imani, B., Eijkemans, M. J., Faessen, G. H., Bouchard, P., Giudice, L. C., & Fauser, B. C. J. M. (2002). Prediction of the individual follicle-stimulating hormone threshold for gonadotropin induction of ovulation in normogonadotropic anovulatory infertility: An approach to increase safety and efficiency. *Fertility and Sterility, 77*, 83–90. doi:10.1016/S0015-0282(01)02928-4

Jamil, A. S., Alalaf, S. K., Al-Tawil, N. G., & Al-Shawaf, T. (2015). A case-control observational study of insulin resistance and metabolic syndrome among the four phenotypes of polycystic ovary syndrome based on Rotterdam criteria. *Reproductive Health, 12* , 7. doi:10.1186/1742-4755-12-7

Joham, A. E., Ranasinha, S., Zoungas, S., Moran, L., & Teede, H. J. (2014). Gestational diabetes and type 2 diabetes in reproductive-aged women with polycystic ovary syndrome. *The Journal of Clinical Endocrinology and Metabolism, 99*(3), E447–E452. doi:10.1210/jc.2013-2007

Kao, Y. H., Chiu, W. C., Hsu, M. I., & Chen, Y. J. (2013). Endothelial progenitor cell dysfunction in polycystic ovary syndrome: Implications for the genesis of cardiovascular diseases. *International Journal of Fertility & Sterility, 6*(4), 208–213.

Kiddy, D. S., Hamilton-Fairley, D., Bush, A., Short, F., Anyaoku, V., Reed, M. J., & Franks, S. (1992). Improvement in endocrine and ovarian function during dietary treatment of obese women with polycystic ovary syndrome. *Clinical Endocrinology, 36*(1), 105–111.

Knowler, W. C., Barrett-Connor, E., Fowler, S. E., Hamman, R. F., Lachin, J. M., Walker, E. A., & Nathan, D. M.; Diabetes Prevention Program Research Group. (2002). Reduction in the incidence of type 2 diabetes with lifestyle intervention or metformin. *The New England Journal of Medicine, 346*(6), 393–403.

Lauritsen, M. P., Bentzen, J. G., Pinborg, A., Loft, A., Forman, J. L., Thuesen, L. L., . . . Nyboe Andersen, A. (2014). The prevalence of polycystic ovary syndrome in a normal population according to the Rotterdam criteria versus revised criteria including anti-Mullerian hormone. *Human Reproduction, 29*(4), 791–801. doi:10.1093/humrep/det469

Legro, R. S., Brzyski, R. G., Diamond, M. P., Coutifaris, C., Schlaff, W. D., Casson, P., . . . & Zhang, H.; NICHD Reproductive Medicine Network. (2014). Letrozole versus clomiphene for infertility in the polycystic ovary syndrome. *The New England Journal of Medicine, 371*(2), 119–129. doi:10.1056/NEJMoa1313517

Legro, R. S., Kunselman, A. R., Dodson, W. C., & Dunaif, A. (1999). Prevalence and predictors of risk for type 2 diabetes mellitus and impaired glucose tolerance in polycystic ovary syndrome: A prospective, controlled study in 254 affected women. *The Journal of Clinical Endocrinology and Metabolism, 84*(1), 165–169. doi:10.1210/jcem.84.1.5393

Lily, M., Lilly, M., & Godwin, M. (2009). Treating prediabetes with metformin: Systematic review and meta-analysis. *Canadian Family Physician Médecin de Famille Canadien, 55*(4), 363–369.

Lim, S. S., Davies, M. J., Norman, R. J., & Moran, L. J. (2012). Overweight, obesity and central obesity in women with polycystic ovary syndrome: A systematic review and meta-analysis. *Human Reproduction Update, 18*(6), 618–637. doi:10.1093/humupd/dms030

Messinis, I. E., Messini, C. I., Anifandis, G., & Dafopoulos, K. (2015). Polycystic ovaries and obesity. *Best Practice & Research. Clinical Obstetrics & Gynaecology, 29*(4), 479–488. doi:10.1016/j.bpobgyn.2014.11.001

Mitra, S., Nayak, P. K., & Agrawal, S. (2015). Laparoscopic ovarian drilling: An alternative but not the ultimate in the management of polycystic ovary syndrome. *Journal of Natural Science, Biology, and Medicine, 6*(1), 40–48. doi:10.4103/0976–9668.149076

Murphy, M. K., Hall, J. E., Adams, J. M., Lee, H., & Welt, C. K. (2006). Polycystic ovarian morphology in normal women does not predict the development of polycystic ovary syndrome. *The Journal of Clinical Endocrinology and Metabolism, 91*(10), 3878–3884. doi:10.1210/jc.2006–1085

National Center for Health Statistics. (1994). *Plan and operation of the Third National Health and Nutrition Examination Survey, 1988–94. Series 1: Programs and collection procedures.* (No. 32, PHS 94–1308). Retrieved from http://www.cdc.gov/nchs/data/series/sr_01/sr01_032.pdf

Nieuwenhuis-Ruifrok, A. E., Kuchenbecker, W. K., Hoek, A., Middleton, P., & Norman, R. J. (2009). Insulin sensitizing drugs for weight loss in women of reproductive age who are overweight or obese: Systematic review and meta-analysis. *Human Reproduction Update, 15*(1), 57–68. doi:10.1093/humupd/dmn043

Norman, R. J., Dewailly, D., Legro, R. S., & Hickey, T. E. (2007). Polycystic ovary syndrome. *Lancet, 370*(9588), 685–697. doi:10.1016/S0140–6736(07)61345–2

Okoroh, E. M., Hooper, W. C., Atrash, H. K., Yusuf, H. R., & Boulet, S. L. (2012). Is polycystic ovary syndrome another risk factor for venous thromboembolism? United States, 2003–2008. *American Journal of Obstetrics and Gynecology, 207*(5), 377.e1–377.e8. doi:10.1016/j.ajog.2012.07.023

Pasquali, R., Casimirri, F., & Vicennati, V. (1997). Weight control and its beneficial effect on fertility in women with obesity and polycystic ovary syndrome. *Human Reproduction, 12 Suppl 1*, 82–87.

Pelletier, L., & Baillargeon, J. P. (2010). Clinically significant and sustained weight loss is achievable in obese women with polycystic ovary syndrome followed in a regular medical practice. *Fertility and Sterility, 94*(7), 2665–2669. doi:10.1016/j.fertnstert.2010.02.047

Rasgon, N. L., Rao, R. C., Hwang, S., Altshuler, L. L., Elman, S., Zuckerbrow-Miller, J., & Korenman, S. G. (2003). Depression in women with polycystic ovary syndrome: Clinical and biochemical correlates. *Journal of Affective Disorders, 74*(3), 299–304. doi:10.1016/S0165–0327(02)00117–9

Refuerzo, J. S., Viteri, O. A., Hutchinson, M., Pedroza, C., Blackwell, S. C., Tyson, J. E., & Ramin, S. M. (2015). The effects of metformin on weight loss in women with gestational diabetes: A pilot randomized, placebo-controlled trial. *American Journal of Obstetrics and Gynecology, 212*(3), e381–e389. doi:10.1016/j.ajog.2014.12.019

Rotterdam ESHRE/ASRM-Sponsored PCOS Consensus Workshop Group. (2004). Revised 2003 consensus on diagnostic criteria and long-term health risks related to polycystic ovary syndrome. *Fertility and Sterility, 81*, 19–25. doi:10.1016/j.fertnstert.2003.10.004

Setji, T. L., & Brown, A. J. (2014). Polycystic ovary syndrome: Update on diagnosis and treatment. *The American Journal of Medicine, 127*(10), 912–919. doi:10.1016/j.amjmed.2014.04.017

Stabile, G., Borrielli, I., Artenisio, A. C., Bruno, L. M., Benvenga, S., Giunta, L., . . . Pizzo, A. (2014). Effects of the insulin sensitizer pioglitazone on menstrual irregularity, insulin resistance and hyperandrogenism in young women with polycystic ovary syndrome. *Journal of Pediatric and Adolescent Gynecology, 27*(3), 177–182. doi:10.1016/j.jpag.2013.09.015

Thatcher, S. S., & Jackson, E. M. (2006). Pregnancy outcome in infertile patients with polycystic ovary syndrome who were treated with metformin. *Fertility and Sterility*, *85*(4), 1002–1009. doi:10.1016/j.fertnstert.2005.09.047

Turkmen, S., Andreen, L., & Cengiz, Y. (2015). Effects of Roux-en-Y gastric bypass surgery on eating behaviour and allopregnanolone levels in obese women with polycystic ovary syndrome. *Gynecological Endocrinology: The Official Journal of the International Society of Gynecological Endocrinology*, *31*(4), 301–305. doi:10.3109/09513590.2014.994600

Ujvari, D., Hulchiy, M., Calaby, A., Nybacka, Å., Byström, B., & Hirschberg, A. L. (2014). Lifestyle intervention up-regulates gene and protein levels of molecules involved in insulin signaling in the endometrium of overweight/obese women with polycystic ovary syndrome. *Human Reproduction*, *29*(7), 1526–1535. doi:10.1093/humrep/deu114

Vandermolen, D. T., Ratts, V. S., Evans, W. S., Stovall, D. W., Kauma, S. W., & Nestler, J. E. (2001). Metformin increases the ovulatory rate and pregnancy rate from clomiphene citrate in patients with polycystic ovary syndrome who are resistant to clomiphene citrate alone. *Fertility and Sterility*, *75*(2), 310–315. doi:10.1016/S0015-0282(00)01675-7

Vitek, W., & Hoeger, K. M. (2014). Treatment of polycystic ovary syndrome in adolescence. *Seminars in Reproductive Medicine*, *32*(3), 214–221. doi:10.1055/s-0034-1371093

Vosnakis, C., Georgopoulos, N. A., Rousso, D., Mavromatidis, G., Katsikis, I., Roupas, N. D.,...Panidis, D. (2013). Diet, physical exercise and Orlistat administration increase serum anti-Müllerian hormone (AMH) levels in women with polycystic ovary syndrome (PCOS). *Gynecological Endocrinology: The Official Journal of the International Society of Gynecological Endocrinology*, *29*(3), 242–245. doi:10.3109/09513590.2012.736557

Zimmerman, Y., Foidart, J. M., Pintiaux, A., Minon, J. M., Fauser, B. C., Cobey, K., & Coelingh Bennink, H. J. (2015). Restoring testosterone levels by adding dehydroepiandrosterone to a drospirenone containing combined oral contraceptive: I. Endocrine effects. *Contraception*, *91*(2), 127–133. doi:10.1016/j.contraception.2014.11.002

# CHAPTER 23

# TEAM COMMUNICATION: CRITICAL IN THE CARE OF THE COUPLE WITH FERTILITY CHALLENGES

*Jamie Leonard and Eleanor L. Stevenson*

Parenthood, for most couples, is an important life milestone; however, for 9% to 15% of the population becoming parents is disrupted by infertility (Phillips, Elander, & Montague, 2014). Couples have reported that infertility can be the most challenging experience faced by a couple (Phillips et al., 2014). The goal of infertility treatment is to provide appropriate care that maximizes the chance of a live birth as well as ensure that patients are satisfied with the care they receive.

Fertility providers must employ various tools to achieve the goal of helping couples to conceive including state-of-the-art knowledge; sensitivity to ethical, moral, religious, emotional, and financial issues; and well-coordinated teamwork. Central to the care that is delivered is teamwork. This chapter explores the complexity of modern reproductive care in the United States that requires all members of the team, including the patient, to work together to achieve a desirable outcome.

## TEAMWORK AND COLLABORATION

Infertility is a multidisciplinary field that requires individuals with a variety of educational and occupational training to work together to achieve successful outcomes. Effective communication and teamwork are essential in the delivery of safe high-quality patient care, particularly in a specialty as complex as infertility. Increased emphasis has been placed on teamwork in health care, primarily as a result from the Institute of Medicine's (IOM) report, *To Err Is Human: Building a Safer Health Care System* (1999). The report stated that the majority of errors were attributable to systematic failures, rather than poor performance of individuals (Clancy & Tornberg, 2007). Although other professions have acknowledged that a team approach in high stakes, high intensity environments, such as the aviation industry, generated fewer mistakes than individuals working alone, health care professionals have been slow to embrace the use of teams in practice, though this is improving (Charney, 2011). As a result of the IOM's report, teamwork has received increased attention for many health care organizations and private practices in an attempt to improve patient safety outcomes.

The idea that teamwork was a successful method to mitigate risk is not a new concept and was substantiated by the aviation industry. An investigation was opened in the 1970s when air travel fatalities were at an all-time high and accidents were correlated with failure of flight crews to use problem-solving resources during flight (Charney, 2011). Mishaps and accidents were rarely caused by lack of individual aptitude or pilot miscalculations; instead, mishaps were directly related to inadequate leadership, communication, and team coordination (Charney, 2011). The aviation industry implemented crew resource management (CRM) training to improve teamwork. CRM helped to alert the aviation industry that human interactions play an integral role in any team performance. CRM has proved to be a powerful tool that improves teamwork by providing skills that optimize both flight and crew performance. CRM skills help to alleviate the effects of distractions and interruptions, provide a benchmark for timely intervention, and provide a safety net for effectively mitigating errors (Flight Safety Foundation, 2009). Although air travel has increased over the years, the number of accidents have decreased by about one third since 1987 (Musson, 2009). It is challenging to ascertain the direct impact CRM has on the reduction of accidents as technology has also improved over the years, but what we do know is that CRM improves safety through increasing operational and team functionality and behaviors, and reducing the risk of an accident occurring.

The health care industry historically experienced similar challenges to the aviation industry because the majority of care being delivered is by individual providers in a decentralized system lacking true organization. Since the release of the IOM's (1999) report, the advantageous nature of teamwork has begun to be acknowledged in health care. "Effective teamwork and communication prevent inevitable mistakes from becoming consequential and harming patient and providers" (Leonard, Graham, & Bomacum, 2004).

Another circumstance, amplifying the importance of teamwork was The Joint Commission on Accreditation in Healthcare Organizations (2004) finding that communication breakdown and ineffective teamwork contributed to the majority of poor patient outcomes. Health care providers must strive to create a culture that focuses on safety, collaboration, and mutual respect to achieve the best possible patient outcomes (Charney, 2011).

The foundation of leadership culture, in health care, was traditionally based on establishing personal independences and control; focused on seniority of individuals, which further contributed to the resistance of seeing the benefit of group interactions (Charney, 2011). Simply gathering a group of professionals in one place does not inevitably result in optimal teamwork. Efforts must be made in health care for providers to understand the benefits of a team by sharing an understanding of common goals to promote both productivity and high-quality care.

With this understanding, the Department of Health and Human Services Agency for Healthcare Research and Quality (AHRQ) and the Department of Defense established the Team Strategies and Tools to Enhance Performance and Patient Safety (TeamSTEPPS), a teamwork and communication initiative (see Figure 23.1) designed specifically for health care providers as well as support staff to decrease

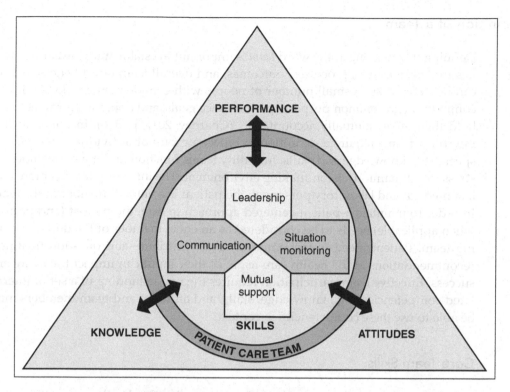

**FIGURE 23.1** TeamSTEPPS instructional framework.
*Source:* TeamSTEPPS Instructional Framework used with permission from King et al. (2008). Copyright 2008 by the Agency for Healthcare Research and Quality.

errors, improve patient outcomes, and promote patient and staff satisfaction. The TeamSTEPPS program offers tools and tactics to increase team cognizance using a shared mental model (King et al., 2008). A shared mental model involves clinical decision making between both the health care provider and the patient. They work together to make these decisions with the focus of what is best for the patient (Agency for Healthcare Research and Quality [AHRQ], 2014).

Gillespie, Chaboyer, and Murray (2010) performed a systematic review that found 70% of adverse events in the operating room can be attributed to failures in communication and that team training interventions, such as TeamSTEPPS and the use of a shared mental model, enhanced team communication, collaboration, and cohesiveness. Team training interventions offer team members the opportunity to learn and refine skills and receive feedback, which ultimately improves teamwork and patient outcomes (Salas, DiazGranados, Weaver, & King, 2008). A multisite prospective study by Haynes et al. (2009) demonstrated a significant decline in patient mortality rates after initiating team training. It is important to remember that, "In complex health care environments, teams do not exist in isolation and, as such, the effectiveness of any team training intervention must be evaluated in the context of the larger system within which the team operates" (Gillespie et al., 2010, p. 654). It is therefore logical that in the context of the complex care involved in caring for those with fertility challenges that this approach to communication would be most relevant and effective.

## Definition of a Team

Defining the meaning of the word *team* is important in establishing measurable values to describe roles, processes, outcomes, and overall team effectiveness. A team can be defined as "a small number of people with complementary skills who are committed to a common purpose, performance goals, and approach for which they hold themselves mutually accountable" (Charney, 2011, p. 336). In the context of infertility, teams require a definition to reflect a group of individuals that possess specialized knowledge and skills. Infertility teams function under a high amount of stress in a dynamic decision-making environment. The infertility team is more than just medical and laboratory personnel; the patient is a valued member of the team. In order to maintain a patient-centered approach to care, the patient (and partner, when applicable) needs to be considered as an equal member of the decision-making team. Patients need to feel empowered to contribute and question treatment recommendations of the health care team, as their input can impact their care and success. Effective team participation requires the understanding of a set of interrelated competencies (e.g., knowledge, skills, and attitude) and team members must be able to use these competencies in context.

## Core Team Skills

In order to understand the complex team structure involved in the care of the patient with infertility challenges, it is important to understand the various components of effective team communication as described by TeamSTEPPS that recognize leadership, situation monitoring, mutual support, and communication.

*Leadership*
Effective leadership is essential in the successful coordination of team efforts. "Leadership is the glue connecting all the TeamSTEPPS elements" (Clapper & Kong, 2012, p. e370). Leaders must be able to coordinate the activities of the team members by ensuring that tasks are understood, assignments are appropriate, changes in information are communicated, and team members have access to all necessary resources. Leaders are responsible for planning to ensure that the team is able to function at the highest level. Planning includes staffing, taking into consideration patient acuity and load, and making sure that each team member understands his or her role. All infertility centers are set up differently, but nurses are typically assigned a schedule of patients that they will see and work with that day. The center's manager, or leader, must ensure that the nurse's assignments are evenly distributed, so that each patient receives the highest quality care. Many times the nurse is the patient's first point of contact and someone the patient can directly relate to (Parrett, 2011). If the nurse is scheduled to see too many patients this can directly impact patient satisfaction and overall quality of care as the care is no longer patient centered. High-quality fertility care involves more than just the overall effectiveness of care or the center's statistics and live birth rates (den Breejen, Nelen, Schol, Kremer, & Hermens, 2013). Patient centeredness is also said to be an important indicator of the quality of care that a patient receives (den Breejen et al., 2013).

To ensure that the patient is receiving the highest possible quality of care, the nurse manager could have a short meeting with the nursing staff at the beginning of the day to discuss assignments for each nurse. Ad hoc meetings could be held to share information and adjust the plan for the day if patient acuity or patient load was higher than originally anticipated. Adjustments would allow for the nurse to provide care that is respectful and responsive to individual patient needs (den Breejen et al., 2013). Ensuring that the patient's values are taken into consideration to help guide the patient's treatment plan improves the patient's overall satisfaction with his or her care (den Breejen et al., 2013). The key feature here is that all members of the team are involved through the process of care delivery, and everyone has an equal voice. It is the responsibility of the leader to ensure this inclusion.

## Situation Monitoring

Infertility care is complex and often involves multiple disciplines working together to achieve a positive patient outcome. Situation monitoring is imperative, especially in care that requires collaboration, as it helps to foster mutual respect and team accountability, while providing a safeguard for not only the team but the patient as well (Ferguson, 2008). Examples of situation monitoring in the infertility setting would be a nurse or nurse manager offering to help another nurse with her patient load. Closely monitoring one another's workload helps to reduce the risk of mistakes being made and allows the patient to receive the highest quality care. This is truly a way to "watch each other's back" and ensure that any mistakes or potential mistakes are caught in a timely manner and do not negatively impact the patient (Ferguson, 2008, p. 123).

## Mutual Support

Effective teamwork depends on the ability of team members to support their coworkers and foster a culture where assistance with assignments is actively sought after and an offer is always extended to help (Charney, 2011). To be able to work in a productive environment, mutual respect is of upmost importance and should be a main focus for all team members (Charney, 2011). A team member should be able to speak up if something is not being done appropriately, regardless of his or her position. Mutual support and respect are extremely important in an infertility clinical setting where many disciplines are working together to ensure the best outcome for the patient. The patient plays an active role in infertility care and it is important that the patient feels his or her voice is heard when decisions are being made about the treatment cycle. Oftentimes, the nurse is the patient's advocate; he or she communicates the patient's wishes to the physicians and questions the treatment plan to ensure that the patient's best interests are being taken into consideration. Mutual support is the essence of teamwork and patient-centered care (AHRQ, 2014).

## Communication

Although a simplistic, universal, patient-centered approach to infertility treatment sounds appealing, infertility treatment is not straightforward, as it is individualized to meet each patient's needs. Communication must be explicit and concise and must involve consultation with other members of the team including the patient. Clear communication will ensure that the patient's values, opinions, and decisions related to his or her treatment are openly communicated with team members so that everyone is on the same page (Gameiro, Boivin, & Domar, 2013). Patients have many complex decisions to make regarding their treatment options and oftentimes they perceive a lack of clear guidance from the fertility team (Gameiro et al., 2013). Training team members in communication skills will help to diminish negative patient and staff interactions and help to increase overall patient satisfaction with care. One example is a decision aid that was developed to help the infertility team communicate with the patient on the number of embryos to transfer during an IVF cycle. The decision aid helped to improve the patient's overall knowledge and communication with the infertility team, allowing for discussions regarding the subject to occur (Gameiro et al., 2013). TeamSTEPPS provides an evidence-based model that can be applied to every team-oriented situation and aims to improve leadership, situational awareness, mutual respect, and communication to improve overall patient safety and satisfaction. TeamSTEPPS training and teamwork is a process that takes time to learn and requires reinforcement to become sustainable. Infertility care is complex and multidisciplinary and requires sound teamwork. Research has demonstrated that effective teamwork is a key factor in achieving total quality management (Mortimer & Mortimer, 2015). Teams are effective in maximizing the quality of care patients receive because they allow for skills from all of the team members to be incorporated into the care, maximizing the strengths and minimizing the weaknesses (Mortimer & Mortimer, 2015).

## Team Members

The best interests of the infertility patient will be served when a multidisciplinary approach is used involving the physician, nurses, laboratory technicians, mental health workers, clergy, and financial consultants, as well as other specialists (e.g., perinatologists, geneticists, and urologists). There is a great variation in the design of each fertility clinic; and while it is difficult to ascertain the exact members of the infertility team, the basic concepts apply to any design. In general, each fertility practice is composed of, at minimum, the physician, nurses, and laboratory technicians.

### Physicians and Advanced Practice Nurses (APNs)
Physicians and APNs will typically establish a relationship with the patient at the initial consultation. The patient is typically seeking a consultation because of an inability to conceive or maintain a pregnancy, or a known need for fertility preservation—either elective or due to a cancer diagnosis. The initial consultation usually consists of a comprehensive medical, reproductive, family history, as well as a thorough physical examination. The physician/APN may also counsel the patients concerning preconception care as well as screening for applicable genetic conditions (American Society for Reproductive Medicine, 2015). Before fertility issues can be treated, the physician/APN must identify the underlying problem. Physicians must be logical and considerate when evaluating and treating for infertility. The goal for

physicians is to maximize the fertility potential of each infertile couple or patient by providing a diagnosis, if possible, and relevant evidence-based treatments. The care provider, along with the patient and partner, will discuss the best treatment options that balance the desires of the patient with what is reasonable and achievable. Physicians/APNs help the patients understand the risks, benefits, and alternatives of all suggested treatment options so there is fully informed consent for a treatment plan. If assisted reproductive technology (ART) is the appropriate treatment plan, the physician/APN will determine the initial dosage of medication and will initiate future adjustments to the cycle, as often as required with ART cycles.

### Nurses

Infertility nurses work carefully alongside other members of the interdisciplinary team to facilitate the patient's treatment plans. Nurses also play an important role of supporting patients throughout their infertility journey. Infertility nurses are essential in patient care as they help to bridge the gap between the technical and logistical aspects of the infertility process and the patient's ability to understand the prescribed treatment regimen (Atri, 2011). The infertility nurse helps to execute the treatment plans that are established by the physician/APN at the initial consultation, including ovarian reserve testing, hysterosalpingogram (HSG), baseline ultrasounds, follow-up ultrasounds, mid-cycle ultrasounds, and semen analysis, among others, as well as provide results after testing is completed.

These tests can be difficult for patients to schedule as they often require specific timing that is centered around the patient's menstrual cycle. Not every patient's menstrual cycle is the same; some are unpredictable, which can make the timing of these tests difficult for patients to manage. In addition to timing challenges, nurses must also help patients navigate to psychosocial challenges. Patients experiencing infertility have "lost one of the most fundamental functions of life, the ability to procreate" (Lesser, 2014, p. 3). Many times patients have decreased self-esteem, feel a loss of control, and are overwhelmed with all of the complexities involved in the plan of care and infertility treatment. Infertility nurses help to empower patients, help them understand test results, and help them navigate their way through the treatment process. Nurses are frequently the patient's "go-to" person for any and all questions that they have and serve as the first line of communication for the patient.

Infertility nurses provide teaching on administration of fertility medications, including subcutaneous and intramuscular injections. Injections for fertility treatments are many times the first injections that a patient has had to self-administer, creating a lot of anxiety for the patient and/or the spouse or partner. Anxiety related to the prescribed self-injection regimen was cited as the second most common reason that infertility treatment is delayed (Domar et al., 2012). Intertility nurses help to mitigate the fears and anxiety of having to give injections by walking each patient through the process step by step and customizing teaching strategies to support the level of learning individually necessary.

The stress associated with both the diagnosis and treatment of infertility is heightened and can impact many aspects of a patient's life. Infertility is considered a "devastating life crisis"; coupled with the emotional and physical burdens of infertility, financial implications can also play a significant role (RESOLVE, n.d.). Infertility treatments are often very costly and not covered by health insurance in most states in the United States, adding to the stress and pressure patients feel throughout their fertility journey. There are resources available to patients that may help to decrease the financial burden. RESOLVE is an excellent nonprofit patient resource advocacy group that provides comprehensive information on insurance benefits as well as alternative options to help make infertility treatments a more affordable option for patients. Infertility is a very intimate journey, sometimes making it difficult for others to share in the struggles and difficulties associated with going through infertility treatments. Nurses listen, understand, and are empathetic. They provide compassionate care that patients need to feel as though they are not alone and empowers patients throughout their infertility journey (Atri, 2011).

### Laboratory Technicians/Andrologists

Laboratory technicians play an integral role on the fertility team. Laboratory technicians are responsible for running and testing lab specimens. Timely serum blood level results are critical in fertility treatment cycles as they help the physician/APN with clinical decision making such as titration of the patient's medication to safely control the simulation, to determine the optimal time to "trigger" for intrauterine insemination (IUI) or IVF (medicated controlled ovulation), and to decide if the patient requires progesterone supplementation, among others. The andrology team performs semen analyses that can be used to determine the need for waiting, IUI, IVF, or intracytoplasmic sperm injection (ICSI). The andrologist looks carefully at the semen specimen to determine the count, motility, and morphology, all critical components that help the physician/APN make treatment recommendations.

### Embryologists

Another part of the laboratory team is the embryologist who is responsible in making sure that the conditions in the embryology lab are ideal for IVF including temperature, air quality, and humidity. During an IVF procedure, embryologists look through the fluid received from the egg retrieval to identify the eggs. The embryologist will then fertilize the eggs with ICSI or conventional IVF insemination. Embryologists monitor the embryos and provide feedback to the physicians so a determination on when to transfer the embryos to the patient can be made.

It is imperative that the laboratory technicians, andrologists, and embryologists stay up to date on the latest technologies available as the field of infertility is evolving at a rapid pace. The laboratory technicians work together with both the physicians and the nurses to ensure the best possible outcomes for the patients.

### Financial Support Staff

Infertility treatment is associated with high costs, with IVF in the United States averaging over US$12,000 (RESOLVE, n.d.). Very often cost is a primary barrier to seeking or proceeding with infertility treatment. When couples do not have insurance to cover the cost of treatment, financial aid may be available for patients as there are financing options, grants, and nonprofit organizations that can help to alleviate some of the financial barriers. RESOLVE is an excellent resource that can be used to determine whether insurance covers infertility treatments, advocate for expanded coverage, and provide other avenues to pursue to help decrease the financial burden. Many states have infertility insurance laws that require health insurance to provide coverage for the diagnosis and/or treatment of infertility, but the extent of the coverage varies from state to state and in some cases employer to employer (Johnston, 2012). It is critical to include those with this knowledge in the decision making about treatment because the cost implications may drive the couple's ability to use appropriate treatments (RESOLVE, n.d.).

### Patients/Partners

Patient-centered care models stress the important role that patients play in clinical decision making and focus on care that is respectful and responsive to patient preferences and values. A patient's values are used to help direct and guide all the clinical decisions that are made. Patient involvement in infertility treatments improves the patient's overall satisfaction with care and decreases the likelihood that he or she will drop out of the fertility treatment cycle (den Breejen et al., 2013). Because the treatment ultimately is crafted for individual couples, it is logical that they should be the center of the decision making, and their involvement as a member of the health care team maximizes safety and satisfaction with care.

## Maximizing Communication With Patients

Including the patient in the discussions about treatments, risks, benefits, and alternatives is essential. Effective communication significantly improves patient satisfaction (den Breejen et al., 2013). The goal of infertility treatment is to ensure that all is being done to help achieve a live birth and patient satisfaction is a key component to achieve the overall goal.

Because of the complexity of the technology involved in fertility care, clinic staffs often speak to patients at a higher technical level than necessary, which can impact informed decision making (Knapp, Raynor, Silcock, & Parkinson, 2009). Additionally, the care team members have the potential to begin to perceive the care as routine, when in fact for that patient, it is a unique and potentially anxiety-provoking experience. Box 23.1 provides a succinct case study.

In order to maximize the communication with the patients about their care, ensure safe outcomes, and increase in patient satisfaction, some suggestions would include:

1. Answer patient questions in a nonjudgmental manner.
2. Ascertain the patient's baseline knowledge and that all members of the team, including the patient, share equality in the planning of care.
3. Provide patients written material or online references to support the specific aspects of the care plan for the patient because patients will likely not retain all the discussed information.
4. Provide patients with sufficient time to address their own concerns with the process. Staff must be available to answer follow-up questions and understand that this is not a routine process for the patient. Communication is essential in making sure that the patient understands the process. When teams are operating

efficiently, each team member feels accountable to other members on the team as well as the patient that he or she is serving. Each infertility patient is different and complex, making fertility patient care even more difficult.

5. Plan regularly scheduled (weekly) interdisciplinary team meetings in which specific patient cases are discussed. Communication and well-coordinated teamwork are critical in ensuring that the fertility process is the most successful it can be for a patient. The interdisciplinary meeting provides an opportunity to clearly communicate details about each patient and prevent miscommunications from occurring. Every team member brings a unique perspective with varying degrees of expertise and experience. Each team member must listen to others' opinions and suggestions as infertility is a complex process that takes many individuals from various fields working together to achieve the best outcomes for the patients.

## BOX 23.1 CASE STUDY FOR TEAM COMMUNICATION

TeamSTEPPS is a model that can be applied to every team-oriented situation and can help to improve patient safety by mitigating the risk for errors and improve patient satisfaction with care.

Hillary Clinton once said, "It takes a village to raise a child," but, as an infertility nurse, Parrett (2011) believes that it often takes a well-organized team to create a child. In IVF, teamwork is essential to make sure that all the moving parts are working together to ensure optimal outcomes for the patient. Sarah comes into the fertility center for consultation to discuss why she and her husband, Kevin, are not having any success in achieving pregnancy. They have been married for a little over a year, have been having unprotected intercourse for 6 months, and she just turned 34 years of age. Sarah visits with the physician and it is recommended that she has some blood work done to check her ovarian reserve and a HSG to evaluate her tubal patency and uterine cavity; in addition, her husband will have a semen analysis done. After meeting with the physician, she seems overwhelmed with all of the recommended testing and so her fertility nurse meets with her to walk her through the process and what to expect. The nurse also provides Sarah with her personal contact information, so that the patient can connect with her anytime she has questions or concerns.

As the results of each test come in, the physician reviews them and communicates with the nurse, who then calls the patient to discuss the results. Sarah's ovarian reserve testing is completely normal and her HSG reveals that her tubes are patent and no uterine abnormalities are detected. Kevin's semen analysis results reveal that no sperm are present in his semen, a condition called azoospermia. After talking with the doctor and obtaining the recommended plan, the nurse makes a follow-up call to the couple to explain the findings to Kevin and share that the doctor recommends following up with a urologist to gather more information about potential underlying conditions and potential treatment options. The nurse is responsible for calling the urologist's office to set up the appointment, sending the records, and keeping the line of communication open. The nurse asks the urologist to contact her after the consultation and sends the office notes so that everyone has all the same information and can be part of a future decision making.

(continued)

## BOX 23.1 CASE STUDY FOR TEAM COMMUNICATION (*continued*)

After a comprehensive evaluation, the urologist forwards the office notes, with the recommendation of ICSI with MESA/TESA (microepididymal and testicular sperm aspiration) to extract sperm or testicular tissue to allow for fertilization to occur. He states that he has gone over the potential success rates, risks, benefits, and alternatives with the couple and told them to contact the reproductive endocrinology office when ready to proceed.

Sarah calls the nurse and they are ready to proceed with IVF treatment. She and Kevin are scheduled for IVF orientation. At IVF orientation, a nurse, physician, and embryologist are present to explain the IVF process in detail to give the patient and her husband a much better understanding of what the IVF cycle looks like and what to expect. Sarah will call with her cycle on day 1 of her period to start the IVF cycle.

When Sarah calls to report her first day of her menstrual cycle, the IVF schedule is then planned. Coordination and collaboration with the urologist office is imperative to ensure that the urologist is available for the MESA/TESA procedure on the day of the egg retrieval. She is started on oral contraceptive pills, the IVF cycle plan is reviewed, and the numerous appointments necessary for IVF are scheduled.

At Sarah's first IVF appointment, uterine mapping is performed, in which careful measurements are made by the physician to determine exactly where the embryo(s) will be placed at embryo transfer. The nurse explains to her that this is a "trial run" so that once embryo transfer is performed, the physician is familiar with where the embryo(s) need to be placed. Sarah visits the nurse after the mapping, who will review with her the IVF plan and calendar and order the necessary medications. The nurse explains that they come from a mail-order specialty pharmacy and that the pharmacy would contact her to set up delivery and payment. The nurse then communicates with the specialty pharmacy via fax to order the medications so that they arrive in time for the start of the IVF cycle.

Next, Sarah comes in for an ultrasound before beginning to take medication to suppress natural ovulation injections to make sure she has no cysts present. The nurse explains how to inject the medication. Many patients are anxious about self-injecting and the nurse takes his or her time to walk the patient through the process. The nurse tells her that once the first injection is given, she will feel much better as the anxiety of actually giving the injection is worse than the actual injection.

Sarah will come in for another ultrasound to ensure that her ovaries are sufficiently suppressed before beginning the stimulation portion of the IVF cycle. At this visit, consents are signed for the procedure by both Sarah and Kevin. These consents can be extensive and cover not only the IVF/ICSI procedure, but also cryopreservation of nontransferred embryos, and difficult decisions regarding the disposition of cryopreserved embryos in the case of death or divorce. Because of the technical nature, both the nurse and physician ensure all information is adequately discussed and all questions are answered before the couples provide informed consent. Although the odds of finding sperm at the MESA/TESA were predicted to be good by the urologist, it is always important to make sure that the couple was asked if they wanted to have donor sperm for back-up, in the event that no sperm was found. The nurse cannot assume that the physician or the urologist already discussed this important

(*continued*)

## BOX 23.1 CASE STUDY FOR TEAM COMMUNICATION (*continued*)

information. Although it may be a difficult conversation to initiate, it is extremely important to ensure that all options are covered even if this may have been previously discussed. It is also equally important to discuss oocyte cryopreservation if no sperm is found through MESA/TESA as an alternative, so that the oocytes could be used in the future if the couple is unsure about donor sperm for backup. In this center, a communication sheet is used to ensure that all options have been explored with the patient. For example, a MESA/TESA communication sheet is useful to ensure that no steps were missed and that the couple was fully informed about their options. It is not uncommon during these complex treatment plans that couples are cared for by multiple members of the team and will see more than one nurse. It is imperative that communication between providers is clear and that protocols are in place to ensure that nothing gets overlooked, especially when multiple disciplines are involved.

Throughout the IVF stimulation, Sarah is monitored frequently using both ultrasound and serum hormone levels. The results of the ultrasound and serum tests are communicated by the nurse to the physician. The physician gives orders about medication doses and these instructions are passed onto the patient by the nurse. The nurse can help the patient to determine whether she needs to order additional medications and help to provide insight on when oocyte retrieval will occur.

When it is time for egg retrieval, the nurse reviews specific instructions on what time the patient is to take her "trigger" injection. This time is precisely calculated so that oocyte retrieval occurs 35 to 36 hours after administration of the trigger injection. The nurse also educates the patient about arrival instructions, and how to prepare for the oocyte retrieval, as well as care afterward. Because timing of the oocyte retrieval is specifically coordinated with the "trigger" injection, in order to reduce the potential for human error, the trigger time is verified with another nurse. Sarah is given an instruction sheet with all of the timing information, made aware that they will need someone to drive her home (because Kevin is having surgery as well), and a copy is made and put in the chart. Because Kevin is planning a MESA/TESA for sperm extraction, timing must also be coordinated with the urologist's office. Sarah and Kevin desire oocyte cryopreservation in the event that sperm are not found; therefore, the MESA/TESA must be scheduled before the oocyte retrieval as timing for freezing the oocytes is critical and must be done within a specified amount of time. Coordination must also occur with the embryologists to ensure that the procedures are scheduled at the appropriate times.

Kevin's MESA is performed and sperm are found in the right epididymis. Several vials are collected and what is not used for the procedure will be frozen for future use. Sarah's oocyte retrieval is performed and the couple are informed of the number of oocytes that were retrieved. The nurse reviews the importance of progesterone supplementation and what is expected after retrieval and for embryo transfer.

Each day following her oocyte retrieval, Sarah and Kevin are called by the embryologists with information about the development of their embryos. The embryologists also update the physicians and nurses regarding the patient's embryo development. Sarah is notified whether she will have embryos transferred on day 3 or day 5 following retrieval, with specific discussion about the rationale for the decision. The embryologist and the physician discuss with the couple on the day of transfer to ensure that they are active participants in the decision making.

(continued)

## BOX 23.1 CASE STUDY FOR TEAM COMMUNICATION (continued)

After embryo transfer, Sarah and Kevin must plan to receive their results on the day of the pregnancy test. Sarah comes into the center and gets her blood drawn on the day of her pregnancy test and she and Kevin anxiously await their results. The nurse calls Sarah with her test results and tells her that she and Kevin are pregnant! The nurse informs Sarah to stay on her progesterone and return to the clinic in 1 week to repeat her lab work, so that they can ensure that the pregnancy hormone is rising appropriately. Sarah and Kevin return to the clinic for Sarah's repeat lab work; the pregnancy hormone is continuing to rise as expected and her progesterone levels are within normal range. Sarah and Kevin are instructed to schedule an obstetrical ultrasound with their physician 4 weeks from the date of their embryo transfer.

Sarah and Kevin arrive for the obstetrical ultrasound and learn that they have a healthy singleton pregnancy and they are overjoyed with the news. They will have one more ultrasound with their fertility doctor in 2 weeks to ensure that the pregnancy is continuing to develop appropriately, at which time another positive report is received that everything with the pregnancy is developing as expected. Sarah is now ready to be transferred back to her OB/GYN to resume care for the remainder of her pregnancy. The fertility center will continue to monitor Sarah's progesterone, by drawing blood, until her body starts making enough progesterone on its own and progesterone supplementation can be safely stopped. The fertility center will also send a letter to Sarah and Kevin's OB/GYN so that the transfer of care goes smoothly.

Infertility and IVF treatment cycles are complex and multidisciplinary, requiring clear communication and teamwork to provide the highest quality care to patients.

## CONCLUSION

Teamwork is critical in achieving the goal of providing the patient with the best possible chance of achieving a successful outcome. However, there will be nuances between different fertility center structures; the commonality is that teamwork must be well-coordinated and interdisciplinary to provide the highest quality care. Finally, it is imperative to understand that the patient plays an integral role on the team when developing the patient's plan of care.

## REFERENCES

Agency for Healthcare Research and Quality. (n.d.). *The SHARE approach*. Retrieved from http://www.ahrq.gov/professionals/education/curriculum-tools/shareddecision-making/index.html

Agency for Healthcare Research and Quality. (2014). *TeamSTEPPS fundamentals course: Module 6. Mutual support*. Retrieved from http://www.ahrq.gov/professionals/education/curriculum-tools/teamstepps/instructor/fundamentals/module6/igmutualsupp.pdf

American Society for Reproductive Medicine. (2015). Diagnostic evaluation of the infertility female: A committee opinion. *Fertility & Sterility*, 103, e44–e50. doi:10.1016/j.fertnstert.2015.03.019

Atri, S. (2011). Role of the nurse in in vitro fertilization. *The Nursing Journal of India, C11*(4). Retrieved from http://www.tnaionline.org/Apr-11/12.htm

Charney, C. (2011). Making a team of experts into an expert team. *Advances in Neonatal Care, 11*(5), 334–339. doi:10.1097/ANC.0b013e318229b4e8

Clancy, C. M., & Tornberg, D. N. (2007). TeamSTEPPS: Assuring optimal teamwork in clinical settings. *American Journal of Medical Quality, 22*(3), 214–217. doi:10.1177/1062860607300616

Clapper, T. C., & Kong, M. (2012). TeamSTEPPS: The patient safety tool that needs to be implemented. *Clinical Simulation in Nursing, 8*, e367–e373. doi:10.1016/j.ecns.2011.03.002

den Breejen, E. M. E., Nelen, W. L. D. M., Schol, S. F. E., Kremer, J. A. M., & Hermens, R. P. M. G. (2013). Development of guideline-based indicators for patient-centredness in fertility care: What patients add. *Human Reproduction, 28*, 987–996. doi:10.1093/humrep/det010

Domar, A., Gordon, K., Garcia-Velasco, J., La Marca, A., Barriere, P., & Berligotti, F. (2012). Understanding the perceptions of and emotional barriers to infertility treatment: A survey in four European countries. *Human Reproduction, 27*, 1073–1079. doi:10.1093/humrep/des016

Ferguson, S. L. (2008). TeamSTEPPS: Integrating teamwork principles into adult health/medical-surgical practice. *Medsurg Nursing, 17*(2), 122–125.

Flight Safety Foundation. (2009). *FSF ALAR briefing note 2.2: Crew resource management.* Flight Safety Foundation ALAR Toolkit. Retrieved from http://www.skybrary.aero/bookshelf/books/851.pdf

Gameiro, S., Boivin, J., & Domar, A. (2013). Optimal in vitro fertilization in 2020 should reduce treatment burden and enhance care delivery for patients and staff. *Fertility and Sterility, 100*(2), 302–309. doi:10.1016/j.fertnstert.2013.06.015

Gillespie, B. M., Chaboyer, W., & Murray, P. (2010). Enhancing communication in surgery through team training interventions: A systematic literature review. *AORN Journal, 92*(6), 642–657. doi:10.1016/j.aorn.2010.02.015

Haynes, A. B., Weiser, T. G., Berry, W. R., Lipsitz, S. R., Breizat, A. S., Dellinger, E. P., … Guwande, A. A. (2009). A surgical safety checklist to reduce morbidity and mortality in a global population [Special Article]. *The New England Journal of Medicine, 360*(5), 491–499. Retrieved from http://www.who.int/patientsafety/safesurgery/Surgical_Safety_Checklist.pdf

Institute of Medicine. (1999). *To err is human: Building a safer health care system.* Retrieved from http://iom.nationalacademies.org/~/media/Files/Report%20Files/1999/To-Err-is-Human/To%20Err%20is%20Human%201999%20%20report%20brief.pdf

Johnston, S. (2012). *Can you afford fertility treatments?* Retrieved from http://money.usnews.com/money/personal-finance/articles/2012/08/20/can-you-afford-fertility-treatments

Joint Commission on Accreditation in Healthcare Organizations. (2004). *Sentinel event issue 30: Preventing infant death and injury during delivery.* Retrieved from http://www.jointcommission.org/sentinel_event_alert_issue_30_preventing_infant_death_and_injury_during_delivery

King, H. B., Battles, J., Baker, D. P., Alonso, A., Salas, E., Webster, J., … Salisbury, M. (2008). "TeamSTEPPS™: Team strategies and tools to enhance performance and patient safety. In K. Henriksen, J. B. Battles, M. A. Keyes, & M. L. Grady (Eds.), *Advances in patient safety: New directions and alternative approaches* (Vol. 3: Performance and Tools). Rockville, MD: Agency for Healthcare Research and Quality.

Knapp, P., Raynor, D. K., Silcock, J., & Parkinson, B. (2009). Performance-based readability testing of participant information for a Phase 3 IVF trial. *Trials, 10*, 79. doi:10.1186/1745-6215-10-79

Leonard, M., Graham, S., & Bomacum, D. (2004). The human factor: The critical importance of effective team communication in providing safe care. *Quality and Safety in Health Care, 13*, 85–90. Retrieved from http://www.ncbi.nlm.nih.gov/pmc/articles/PMC1765783/pdf/v013p00i85.pdf

Lesser, C. B. (2014). The IVF nurse: An untapped resource for recruiting and retaining patients. [Supplement: Best Practices in IVF Nursing, Newsletter Series]. *OBG Management, 26,* 1–4. Retrieved from http://cdn4.imng.com/fileadmin/qhi/obg/pdfs/1014_PDFs/Actavis_1014_V2.pdf

Mortimer, S. T., & Mortimer, D. (2015). *Quality and risk management in the IVF laboratory* (2nd ed.). Cambridge, UK: Cambridge University Press.

Musson, D. (2009). Teamwork in medicine: Crew resource management and lessons from aviation. In Croskerry, P., Cosby, K. S., Schenkel, S. M., & Wears, R. L. (Eds.), *Patient safety in emergency medicine* (pp. 188–194). Philadelphia, PA: Lippincott Williams & Wilkins.

Parrett, S. T. (2011). *The role of the nurse in your fertility treatment team.* Retrieved from http://www.resolve.org/about-infertility/medical-conditions/the-role-of-the-nurse-in-your-fertility-treatment-team.html

Phillips, E., Elander, J., & Montague, J. (2014). Managing multiple goals during fertility treatment: An interpretative phenomenological analysis. *Journal of Health Psychology, 19*(4), 531–543. doi:10.1177/1359105312474915

RESOLVE. (n.d.). *Making treatment affordable.* Retrieved from http://www.resolve.org/family-building-options/making-treatment-affordable

Salas, E., DiazGranados, D., Weaver, S. J., & King, H. (2008). Does team training work? Principles for healthcare. *Academic Emergency Medicine, 15*(11), 1002–1009. Retrieved from http://onlinelibrary.wiley.com/doi/10.1111/j.1553-2712.2008.00254.x/pdf

# CHAPTER 24

# FOCUSING ON NURSING: EMERGING SPECIALTY PRACTICE IN THE UNITED KINGDOM

*Eilis Moody*

Meeting the physical and emotional demands of infertility patients seeking assisted reproduction treatments requires a complex care structure in which nursing care is pivotal. In 2011, the Royal College of Nursing[1] (RCN) defined the role of a fertility nurse as "to provide a holistic approach to fertility investigation, treatment and early pregnancy, through compassionate, informed and evidence based practice" and recognized that fertility nursing is a highly specialized field (RCN, 2011). This broad definition of fertility nursing reflects the wide range of activities that fertility nurses perform and is in keeping with the diverse nature of the role.

As fertility nursing has evolved, nurses have reviewed their roles and sought out new ways of working for the benefit of their patients and the development of clinical services. As regulations and opinions regarding the nursing role changed, fertility nurses have gradually expanded their roles and developed areas of practice that traditionally were considered far beyond the scope of nursing practice. Roles have progressed and transformed from the early days of fertility services in which nurses had limited responsibilities to modern day services in which nurses are leading many aspects of care and taking charge of several areas previously dominated by physicians.

In this chapter, the development of specialist fertility nursing is examined, focusing on how fertility nursing has advanced across the United Kingdom. A discussion about what is needed to develop and maintain specialist fertility nursing practice and the opportunities for nurses to acquire and validate their specialist nursing skills are also addressed.

## SPECIALIST FERTILITY NURSING PRACTICE IN THE UNITED KINGDOM

The development of specialist fertility nursing practice across the United Kingdom came about for a number of reasons. Throughout the 1990s, plans by government agencies for a modern, cost-effective health care system led to changes in attitudes toward nursing roles. UK nursing guidelines reflected the changing times and allowed nurses to consider previously unexplored areas of practice. In 1992, the UK nursing regulatory body, the United Kingdom Central Council for Nurses, Midwives and Health Visiting (UKCC), resolved that the scope of nursing practice should not be limited by a set list of tasks and responsibilities but that nursing practice should be determined by knowledge and skills, thus allowing nurses to expand their roles as long as they felt competent to do so and remained accountable for their practice (UKCC, 1992). New European regulations around this time caused a reduction in junior physicians' working hours (National Health Service Management Executive, 1991) and this led to fears about meeting service needs while maintaining patient safety. Nurses were seen as a vital resource in addressing this need and they were encouraged to examine their practice and take the opportunity to extend the range of their skills.

Throughout this time, fertility services across the United Kingdom were also evolving. The number of patients undergoing fertility treatment significantly increased throughout the 1990s (Human Fertilisation and Embryology Authority [HFEA], 2008) and new clinics emerged to meet the demand. The science continued to evolve at a rapid pace, resulting in new diagnostic guidelines and appropriate treatments. Changes in societal attitudes about family structure allowed more single women and same-sex couples to consider seeking treatment. Increased activity was met with new legislation in the form of the Human Fertilisation and Embryology Act of 1990 and the formation of a new regulatory body, the HFEA[2], in 1991. Clinics offering in vitro fertilization (IVF) or donor gamete (i.e., eggs, sperm) treatments were required to be licensed by the HFEA and undergo an annual inspection to maintain their license. The HFEA Code of Practice (HFEA, 1991) set out guidelines for clinics to follow to maintain their practices within the Human Fertilisation and Embryology Act and to ensure patient safety and establish public trust in the emerging assisted reproduction field. Clinics were required to submit data on IVF procedures and the use of donated gametes. The HFEA has continued to gather data on IVF and donor gamete treatments since the establishment of the authority. The Code of Practice has been revised several times since 1991 to reflect the changing nature of assisted reproduction and it still provides comprehensive guidance for UK clinics to follow.

As the demands of fertility services increased and the importance of meeting the new regulations was understood, fertility nurses throughout the United Kingdom began to identify areas where they could develop clinical skills to support meeting the demand and to ensure that high-quality, safe, and effective care was delivered. Buoyed by changes in attitudes and seizing their opportunity, nurses stepped forward to play decisive roles in the development of fertility services across the United Kingdom.

In 1996, nurses began performing successful embryo transfers in the Oxford Fertility Unit (Barber, Egan, Ross, Evans, & Barlow, 1996), a service previously delivered by physicians only. Pregnancy rates remained unaffected and the transition into this role was seen as a huge step forward for fertility nurses. Having successfully pushed beyond the previously conceived notion of fertility nursing, the profession began considering other ways nurses could contribute to overall care in the fertility setting. In 1997, I was part of the nursing team led by Sara Frost at King's College Hospital, London, to become among the first nurses in the world performing oocyte retrievals, a change that was enjoyed by patients and the clinic staff, again without any adverse effect on outcomes. Following this, the expansion of fertility nursing continued when the nurses at Midland Fertility Services began to perform surgical sperm retrievals, again demonstrating success rates equal to their medical colleagues (Birch, 2001).

In my current clinical fertility setting, nurses enjoy a range of specialist fertility nursing activities. The nursing role began in the mid-1990s with experienced women's health nurses assisting with the development of a specialist fertility unit. Since then, the nursing team has continued to widen and develop their role to become one of the most advanced fertility nursing teams in the United Kingdom. The unit employs nurses in different capacities, ranging from senior fertility nurse specialists to junior nurses beginning their careers within infertility care. The experienced members of the nursing team play pivotal roles in all aspects of fertility care including the assessment of new patients, ultrasound scanning, consent for treatment, treatment procedures (e.g., intrauterine insemination [IUI], oocyte retrieval, embryo transfer), conscious sedation for procedures, screening and counseling of gamete donors and recipients, and research. Junior members of the team have supporting roles in the provision of services and will all be undergoing training and assessment in preparation for more senior roles as their careers progress. All members of the nursing team are trained and assessed against set competences, relevant to the roles and tasks they undertake, and work within agreed protocols that follow local and national guidelines.

Variations in clinic activities and treatments and regulations regarding nursing scope of practice will dictate the nature of the role and the extent to which it can develop. Although the development of the nursing team as described may not be within the reach of all fertility settings, it is beneficial to all settings to evaluate patient experience and to consider if any development or advanced skills of the nursing team will enhance it. Even if there is no "one size fits all" approach to developing specialist nursing practice, an assessment of patients' needs, and an evaluation of how nursing roles can help meet these, will help determine the need for specialist nursing care and any advancement of nursing practice.

## DEVELOPING SPECIALIST PRACTICE

A recent debate has called for caution regarding specialist roles and the need for specialist nurses to be adequately educated, skilled, and assessed to carry the title of specialist nurse. Although the assignment of specialist practice status is heavily influenced by national and local policies, there is a general consensus to match patients' high expectations of specialist roles to the skills and knowledge of specialist nurses. Fertility nurses cannot be considered a specialist nurse simply because they work in a specialist area; it is essential that they should have sufficient education, training, experience, and assessed competence to deliver the expert level of care the role dictates. A robust training and assessment program will help fertility nurses develop the right tools for specialist practice and ensure that they reach and maintain competence.

When beginning the journey to specialist practice, it is essential to evaluate the intended role and the specific training needs of the nurse wishing to take it on. The scope of nursing practice varies internationally; what may be common practice for one nursing nationality may be considered beyond the boundaries of nursing care by another. Indeed, this is not only limited to differences in international nursing regulations. Clinical settings vary, too, and the scope of the nursing role will be influenced by the needs of service and the desire to see nurses acting beyond traditional nursing boundaries. This variety of international nursing regulations and the diversity of clinic ethos make it difficult to define the exact nature of specialist fertility nursing; specialist practice exists in many aspects of fertility nursing and is not just limited to advanced technical skills but encompasses a range of counseling, treatment planning and coordination, and procedures. Historically, the crossing of nursing boundaries into medical aspects of care has been viewed as expanded or specialist practice. Certainly, fertility nurses who carry out embryo transfer, ultrasound scanning, and other expanded roles are generally seen as specialists in their field but there are also plenty of other less procedural aspects of fertility nursing that require specialist knowledge and skilled provision of care. Though it is difficult to be too prescriptive of the precise tasks and responsibilities each role dictates, the overall focus of training should be the development of a skilled, knowledgeable nurse who is equipped with the necessary abilities and information to confidently deliver expert care within agreed local and national guidelines.

A variety of teaching methods can be used including experiential learning, practice and supervision, attendance at external learning events and workshops, and assessment and ongoing evaluation relevant to the roles and tasks for which the individual nurse will eventually take responsibility (HFEA, 2015). Although much of specialist fertility nurse training often takes place in-house, it is useful for nurses to attend conferences and workshops relevant to their role. For expanded roles like inseminations, embryo transfer, and ultrasound scanning, it is particularly helpful to attend external events, such as the British Fertility Society[3] (BFS) embryo transfer and IUI study day or pelvic ultrasound study days, as this will help the nurse learn the background knowledge and basics of the procedures. The BFS also offers members the opportunity to complete a log book of their procedures and submit it to the BFS for accreditation of their skills. This offers nurses formal recognition of their newly acquired skills and provides evidence of a robust training program and assessment of competence.

Academic achievement for specialist nurses and those performing advanced skills has been heavily discussed in recent years, with the International Council for Nurses (ICN) recommending that specialist or advanced nurses are educated to master's level (ICN, 2009). In 2010, the RCN fertility nurses group, investigating the views of UK fertility nurses, recognized the need to protect the role extension of fertility nurses through higher education accreditation and found that many fertility nurses would welcome a clear educational pathway (Peddie, Denton, & Barnett, 2011). This led to the publication of the RCN's training and education framework for fertility nurses, which suggests academic pathways for fertility nurses to complement the training and education they receive in their practice setting (RCN, 2013). As yet there is only a recommended level of academic achievement for specialist nurses in the United Kingdom and there are wide variations between practitioners. There is, however, an increasing awareness of the need for specialist nurses to arm themselves with the appropriate academic qualifications. The recent addition of a master's-level program in advanced fertility practice at Edge Hill University will offer UK fertility nurses the opportunity to enhance their academic development.

Aside from academic achievements, proving knowledge and competence has become an important aspect of maintaining public trust in specialist nursing and validating the achievements and skills of specialist nurses. Ultimately, although it is necessary to acknowledge the specialist skills that fertility nurses possess, it is of upmost importance to protect patients. Local or nationally agreed competences are a useful tool for developing and evaluating nursing practice as they provide a benchmark for nurses to train and evaluate themselves. UK fertility nurses working in HFEA-licensed clinics are required to show evidence of competence (or working toward competence) for the roles and tasks for which they are involved (HFEA, 2015). To help with this, the RCN fertility nurses group developed specialist competences for fertility nurses that provide excellent guidance for developing competence across a wide range of fertility nursing activities. Although intended for UK nurses, the competences will assist any fertility nurse wishing to develop or evaluate his or her role (RCN, 2011). The RCN also publish several guidelines for expanded roles such as embryo transfer, oocyte retrieval, and ultrasound scanning that help guide nurses to the specific knowledge and training needed to fulfill these roles. When considering developing nursing practice into these areas, a common training program can be developed for all staff disciplines, as all staff should be expected to meet the same standard of competence before being allowed to practice independently.

Accreditation adds value to training and provides the nurse with a solid evaluation of his or her knowledge and skills. Depending on local requirements for specialist nurse training, it may also provide the necessary evidence for nurses wishing to acquire specialist nurse status. The recent addition of a nurse certification program by the European Society of Human Reproduction and Embryology[4] (ESHRE) assists specialist fertility nurses with this and follows acknowledgment of increased specialist activity in fertility nursing across Europe. The society anticipates that the certification will formally recognize fertility nurses' specialist skills and lead to an increase in the quality of care by setting high standards of knowledge and achievement. For nurses who aspire to have their specialist skills acknowledged or for those who wish to validate their skills, ESHRE certification offers an important opportunity for nurses to establish their status (ESHRE, n.d.).

To gain ESHRE certification, participants are required to have ESHRE membership, have 3 years' clinical experience in fertility practice, complete a log book, and pass an examination at the annual ESHRE conference. ESHRE has set out a detailed curriculum and reading list covering all aspects of infertility investigation, causes, and treatments. Participants are expected to work through the log book by observing, assisting, or performing tasks listed within it. Areas covered include:

- Diagnosis and diagnostic tests
- Consultation pre- and posttreatment
- Information giving
- Treatment procedures (e.g., IUI)
- Treatment coordination
- Laboratory procedures

- Psychological aspects of care
- Ethics

One of the benefits of the ESHRE program is that it does not require nurses to perform all of the tasks listed but accepts that some nurses may assist or observe certain procedures instead. ESHRE also acknowledges that local regulations may restrict direct participation in certain treatments—for example, preimplantation genetic diagnosis—and allows nurses to present alternative evidence to prove their competence.

Although adequate education and training are essential components of any path toward specialist practice, the need for ongoing evaluation at regular intervals is also a crucial factor. Developing standard operating protocols for processes such as implications counseling, as well as critical elements such as oocyte retrieval and embryo transfer, provides a solid benchmark not only to aid a consistent standard of care but also as a useful tool for staff assessment. Several different methods of assessment can be used. Peer review by another member of staff skilled in that role or procedure is very useful as it not only provides the opportunity to evaluate individual performance but also to learn from each other and discuss together the best approach to practice. Evaluation of key performance indicators is valuable in assessing procedures and can be used to look for variation between operators, identifying any areas of concern and possible need for closer inspection or further training. An audit of patient experience is always an important way of evaluating service; individual staff as fertility patients are informed consumers and are usually very happy to give honest evaluations of the care they receive. Patient audits also allow nurses and other providers to evaluate care from a more holistic approach rather than just focus on oocyte retrieval rates or pregnancy rates. Not all patients will be successful in achieving a pregnancy and it is very important not to focus all our attention on this outcome alone but to look at all aspects of care to ensure that patients have a good experience even if they do not achieve a pregnancy.

The development of specialist nursing practice takes time and the pathway will depend on the clinical setting, the role description, and the motivation and experience of the nurses involved. Providing an absolute definition of specialist fertility nursing is not without its difficulties and the answer will differ from clinic to clinic. Although responsibilities may vary, the aim of specialist fertility nursing is consistent; to provide expert, high-quality, evidence-based care while listening and responding to the needs of our patients.

## BENEFITS OF SPECIALIST NURSING PRACTICE

Although boundaries of traditional nursing care may have been expanded in part due to health care financial pressures and the need to reevaluate service provision, this does not mean that expanding the roles of nurses toward specialist care has been of little benefit to nurses and their patients.

By the start of the 21st century, the benefits of specialist fertility nursing practice had become evident, and this is well supported in the literature. Although cost-effectiveness is frequently cited as a benefit of specialist nursing, saving money cannot be the only driving force for developing fertility nursing. The advancement of our practice should not detract from patient care, it should only enhance it. Patients look to fertility nurses for support throughout their care and I have witnessed how a close relationship with the nursing staff gives patients the freedom to honestly express their concerns and feelings. Nurses often have a keen awareness of patient needs and value their position as the carer, seeing themselves as the human face of treatment (Payne & Goedeke, 2007). Qualitative research suggests that our patients enjoy specialist fertility nursing practice benefiting from continuity and consistency of care with the involvement of nurses in many stages of their treatment (Ashcroft, 2000; Harris, 2000). Hershberger and Kavanaugh (2008) found that women valued their time spent with nurses, viewing their interactions as caring and compassionate and appreciating the competence of experienced fertility nurses. Continuity of care is frequently rated by fertility patients as important throughout their care (Dancet et al., 2010) and the benefits of developing a good relationship between patient and nurse cannot be underestimated. By involving nurses in all aspects of care and letting specialist nurses lead clinics and perform procedures, it strengthens the trusting relationship between nurse and patient and allows more opportunities for patients to open up and speak freely. Although this does not undermine the excellent care given by fertility physicians, patients recognize that nurses often have a different approach to care and they value the caring environment that nurses create (Allan & Barber, 2004).

Specialist nursing care has positive effects on nurses too. Specialist practice is connected to role evaluation, acquiring new skills and knowledge, and establishing the nurses as an expert. While all of these can add confidence and improve the self-esteem of nurses, they also assist the nurse to establish their position and adds weight to their views and opinions within the multidisciplinary team. Traditionally, nurses have been accomplices rather than protagonists. Although there is concern that the cost-effectiveness of specialist nurses acting in expanded capacities and providing cheaper labor than our medical colleagues may be viewed as exploitation of nurses, the development of specialist and expanded nursing practice gives dynamic fertility nurses the opportunity to promote fertility nursing as a highly skilled, valued discipline worthy of its place among the clinical hierarchy.

The positive effects on service providers should not be ignored. Modern health care operates under increasing financial pressures and nurses have a key role in achieving cost improvements with nurse specialists proven to be clinically and financially effective (RCN, 2010). Having skilled, knowledgeable nurses capable of performing specialist procedures frees up considerable physician time, allowing appointment waiting times to remain low and increasing the flow of patients through the clinic. As nurses have been proven to be as successful as physicians at embryo transfer and oocyte retrieval, they provide a safe, effective, and cheaper option. In the United Kingdom, nursing staff also tend to be a less transient workforce than medical staff, reducing the demand for new staff training and maintaining consistency and stability of care. Having several nurses trained in expanded roles also allows greater flexibility in the clinic, allowing nursing staff to rotate through different areas and follow patients right through their treatment, offering continuity of care and thus improving patient experience and evaluation. However, above all, the benefit of specialist nurses trained in all aspects of fertility care contributes hugely to the success of a unit not simply by improving immediate patient care and reducing costs but by adding to the number of well-informed voices contributing to service evaluation and progression, working with other staff disciplines to review and improve service delivery.

## DISCUSSION

There is no doubt that specialist fertility nurses have a valuable role to play in the modern fertility service. Roles and responsibilities are diverse and reflect the changing attitudes toward fertility nursing and the great steps forward that fertility nurses have made in evaluating their care and responding to the needs and demands of their patients. But despite the proven benefits of specialist nursing and expanding the nursing role, the existence of specialist fertility nurses and particularly those performing expanded tasks is not commonplace. Although local or national regulations may limit a nurse's opportunity to take on certain roles, it is possible that there are other factors preventing nurses from considering these roles.

Corrigan (1996) and Barber (2002) explain how senior medical colleagues have been instrumental in the advancement of the nursing service in their units, viewing the nurses as equal members of the multidisciplinary team and supporting the nursing team to expand and develop their roles. I also have been fortunate to work alongside medical colleagues who understood the value of nursing care and how redefining the fertility nurses' role could benefit patients. Undeniably, support from the wider multidisciplinary team is vital to the development of nursing roles, particularly in tasks previously only performed by physicians and the support needed is not only limited to educational and training needs. To successfully implement change in the nursing role, there needs to be acceptance from all team members that nurses are knowledgeable, skilled, and experienced enough to take on these critical roles. Evaluation of performance is an important aspect of maintaining quality and offers reassurance that practitioners are fit for the roles they undertake, but it is important to evaluate all practitioners and not just limit it to nursing staff.

Nearly 20 years on from the first nurse embryo transfer and with published and local evidence that proves nurses' effectiveness in this role, the practice is not all that widespread, particularly beyond the United Kingdom. Even more so, very few nurses perform oocyte or sperm retrieval, even within the United Kingdom. I have occasionally encountered nurses who seem alarmed by the expansion of the fertility nursing role. Their argument often relates to the principles of nursing care and whether roles such as embryo transfer or oocyte retrieval fit within the remit of nursing. Clearly, nurses should be concerned with the legal and accountability implications for expanded practice. Barber (2002) warns fertility nurses of the need to remain accountable for their practice. Before considering any expansion of practice it is vital to investigate the local regulations regarding scope of practice and accountability to ensure that nurses have the appropriate support, which includes adequate insurance from their employer or practice organization.

Patient concerns are occasionally mentioned as an argument against nurses expanding their roles. Undoubtedly, fertility patients have high expectations and come to fertility clinics with the clear goal of pregnancy in their mind, wanting the best treatment available and the best person to deliver care. But who is the best person? In my experience, patients are more concerned with the knowledge, skill, and attitude of the practitioner than their job title and recognize that nurses are equally as skilled as physicians when educated and trained to perform clinical roles. Patient interviews support this notion and indicate that patients understand that the same task can be delivered in different ways. Patients also spoke of the caring environment nurses provide and their preferences for nurses to deliver their care (Allan & Barber, 2004).

In the midst of rapidly changing nursing roles Castledine (1995) opened the debate about expanding nursing roles. Nurses were cautioned not to forget their core nursing skills in pursuit of advanced nursing practice. The nursing literature voiced concerns that nurses would become "mini doctors" at the detriment of nursing care, simply stepping in to perform medical tasks without consideration of the consequences for nursing and patients. For fertility patients Allan (2002) was concerned that expanding the fertility nurse's role would adversely affect the relationship between nurse and patient, reducing the nurse's ability to care.

Although it is certain that tasks such as embryo transfer and oocyte retrieval are seen as clinical procedures, they demand much more from practitioners than just advanced technical expertise. Fertility patients are often at their most vulnerable at these points, physically and emotionally laid bare, waiting for news that will hugely impact their chance of a pregnancy. In defense of expanded nursing roles and concerns about loss of our caring role, I would argue that experienced specialist fertility nurses performing these roles are acutely aware of the emotional background to clinical procedures. They approach these tasks from a holistic point of view, understanding that care for patients at these points requires not only technical skill but also a complete understanding of the emotional aspects of the procedures and how to support patients. Specialist fertility nurses as experienced, knowledgeable practitioners are well placed to offer this type of care, fitting with the principles of nursing, at these pivotal moments.

## CONCLUSION

Since the arrival of the first IVF baby in 1978 there has been an explosion of fertility services worldwide and the demand for services continues to rise. Now more than ever nurses have the opportunity to be the forefront of service delivery and influence the nature of care. Fertility nurses are a highly educated and skilled workforce and equipping them with advanced skills for specialist practice can vastly improve patient experience and service delivery; however, the pressures on modern fertility nurse specialists are high. Fertility nurse specialists should be knowledgeable, skilled practitioners, a technical expert, while not forgoing the basics of nursing care: delivering compassionate, holistic care, listening while responding to the needs of their patients.

A transition into the role demands caution, both to protect the nurse and the patient. Nurses wishing to take on the role need time to learn; to witness the full spectrum of assisted reproduction and the effects on patients and to expand their knowledge, develop their skills, both practical and emotional, in order to meet the expectations of patients and to promote the benefits of specialist nursing.

## NOTES

1. The RCN is a UK membership organization that aims to represent nurses and nursing, promote excellence in practice, and shape health policy.
2. The HFEA is the United Kingdom's independent regulator overseeing the use of gametes and embryos in fertility treatment and research.
3. The BFS is a national multidisciplinary organization representing individuals practicing in the field of reproductive medicine. The society delivers a range of training events for nurses and physicians who wish to undertake roles such as ultrasound scanning, embryo transfer, and IUI.
4. The ESHRE was founded in 1985 and aims to promote interest in and understanding of reproductive biology and medicine.

## REFERENCES

Allan, H., & Barber, D. (2004). Nothing out of the ordinary: Advanced fertility nursing practice. *Human Fertility*, 7(4), 277–284. doi:10.1046/j.1365–2648.2002.02149.x

Allan, H. T. (2002). Nursing the clinic, being there and hovering: Ways of caring in a British fertility unit. *Journal of Advanced Nursing*, 38(1), 86–93. doi:10.1080/1464727002000199101

Ashcroft, S. (2000). Developing the clinical nurse specialist's role in fertility: Do patients benefit? *Human Fertility*, 3(4), 265–267. doi:10.1080/1464727002000199101

Barber, D. (2002). The extended role of the nurse: Practical realities. *Human Fertility*, 5(1), 13–16. doi:10.1080/1464727992000199701

Barber, D., Egan, D., Ross, C., Evans, B., & Barlow, D. (1996). Nurses performing embryo transfer: Successful outcome of in-vitro fertilization. *Human Reproduction*, 11(1), 105–108. doi:10.1093/oxfordjournals.humrep.a018999

Birch, H. (2001). The extended role of the nurse–opportunity or threat? *Human Fertility*, 4(3), 138–144. doi:10.1080/1464727012000199202

Castledine, G. (1995). Will the nurse practitioner be a mini doctor or a maxi nurse? *British Journal of Nursing*, 4(16), 938–939. doi:10.12968/bjon.1995.4.16.938

Corrigan, E. (1996). The roles and expectations of the infertility nurse practitioner and the scope for extended practice. *Journal of the British Fertility Society*, 1(1), 61–64.

Dancet, E. A. F., Nelen, W. L. D. M., Sermeus, W., De Leeuw, L., Kremer, J. A. M., & D'Hooghe, T. M. (2010). The patients' perspective on fertility care: A systematic review. *Human Reproduction Update*, 16, 467–487. doi:10.1093/humupd/dmq004

European Society of Human Reproduction and Embryology. (n.d). *Certification for ART nurses and midwives*. Retrieved from http://www.eshre.eu/Accreditation-and-Certification/Nurses-Midwives-Certification.aspx

Harris, S. M. (2000). Establishing an intrauterine insemination programme from a nursing perspective. *Human Fertility*, 3(2), 121–123. doi:10.1080/1464727002000198821

Hershberger, P. E., & Kavanaugh, K. (2008). Enhancing pregnant, donor oocyte recipient women's health in the infertility clinic and beyond: A phenomenological investigation of caring behaviour. *Journal of Clinical Nursing*, 17(21), 2820–2828. doi:10.1111/j.1365–2702.2007.02211.x

Human Fertilisation and Embryology Authority. (1991). *Code of practice*. London, UK: Human Fertilisation and Embryology Authority.

Human Fertilisation and Embryology Authority. (2008). *A long term analysis of the HFEA Register data (1991–2006)*. Retrieved from http://www.hfea.gov.uk/docs/Latest_long_term_data_analysis_report_91-06.pdf.pdf

Human Fertilisation and Embryology Authority. (2015). *Code of practice* (8th ed.). London, UK: Human Fertilisation and Embryology Authority.

International Council of Nurses. (2009). *Nursing matters fact sheet. Nurse practitioner/Advanced practice nurse: Definitions and characteristics*. Retrieved from http://www.icn.ch/images/stories/documents/publications/fact_sheets/1b_FS-NP_APN.pdf

National Health Service Management Executive. (1991). *Junior doctors. The new deal*. London, UK: Department of Health.

Payne, D., & Goedeke, S. (2007). Holding together: Caring for clients undergoing assisted reproductive technologies. *Journal of Advanced Nursing, 60*(6), 645–653. doi:10.1111/j.1365–2648.2007.04451.x

Peddie, V. L., Denton, J., & Barnett, V. (2011). Toward developing a training pathway for fertility nurses: Report of the 2010 training and educational survey. *Human Fertility (Cambridge, England), 14*(3), 167–178. doi:10.3109/14647273.2011.596893

Royal College of Nursing. (2010). *Specialist nurses. Changing lives, saving money*. Retrieved from www.rcn.org.uk/__data/assets/pdf_file/0008/302489/003581.pdf

Royal College of Nursing. (2011). *Competences: Specialist competences for fertility* nurses (2nd ed.). Retrieved from www.rcn.org.uk/__data/assets/pdf_file/0008/78740/003135.pdf

Royal College of Nursing. (2013). *An RCN training and education framework for fertility nurses*. Retrieved from www.rcn.org.uk/__data/assets/pdf_file/0003/509106/004322.pdf

United Kingdom Central Council for Nurses, Midwives and Health Visiting (1992). *The scope of professional practice*. London, UK: United Kingdom Central Council for Nurses, Midwives and Health Visiting.

# CHAPTER 25

# MEN AND INFERTILITY: THEIR EXPERIENCE WITH CHALLENGES IN FAMILY FORMATION

*Kevin McEleny*

Few life goals are as central to the human experience as are reproduction and childbirth (Purewal & van den Akker, 2007). For nearly 15% of couples, however, achieving this goal presents challenges due to infertility. Although the female partner generally receives the majority of attention in the scientific community, men are often overlooked as being an equal partner in the process. Infertile men have a lower quality of life after diagnosis (Johansson et al., 2010; Shindel, Nelson, Naughton, Ohebshalom, & Mulhall, 2008) because their childlessness is seen as central in life. Men living without children after unsuccessful treatment have a lower quality of life, years after treatment discontinuation, compared with those living with children. Fortunately, there has been a recent push for addressing male reproductive health issues, which has sparked a call for increased research (Macaluso et al., 2010). The focus of this chapter is to present an overview of what is known about male factor infertility from both clinical and psychosocial perspectives and to suggest critical areas for the future research.

## INCIDENCE OF MALE FERTILITY CHALLENGES

### Are Male Fertility Challenges Common?

Male fertility problems are the most common cause of couple infertility. They are an issue in almost 50% of cases, and the sole reason identified in 20% of cases (Thonneau et al., 1991). The severity of the defined problem can vary greatly from a small reduction in semen parameters, when compared with the normal reference ranges, to a complete absence of sperm (azoospermia) in the ejaculate.

There is evidence from some sources that the quality of semen may be declining in certain countries worldwide. The current leading theory is that testicular dysgenesis syndrome is the underlying cause of this temporal decline. This syndrome links the apparent decline in semen quality with the observed rise in the incidence of testicular cancer in some countries and the rise in certain abnormalities in male fetal development reported in some studies, such as undescended testes and hypospadias (Giwercman & Peterson, 2000). Proponents of the theory of testicular dysgenesis syndrome attribute it to a rise in the level of particular environmental pollutants that could adversely interfere with the process of masculinization in the male fetus (Skakkebæk, Rajpert-De Meyts, & Main, 2001). Such pollutants include a variety of natural and synthetic chemicals that have been shown in animal studies to possess estrogenic or antiandrogenic properties and are described as endocrine disruptors (Juul et al., 2014). Those who argue against this theory state that changes in the way semen is analyzed make it difficult to confirm a genuine deterioration, and that some of the studies at least, which reported a decline, contain significant methodological errors (Fisch, 2008). Nevertheless, interest in male fertility is currently on the rise, albeit from a low starting point.

Changes in society, such as the rise in age of first-time mothers, may expose male factor subfertility as an issue, as a young fertile female can potentially compensate for male factor infertility (Office for National Statistics, 2014). Also, there has been a rise in recent decades in the incidence of sexually transmitted infections (STIs) like chlamydia and gonorrhoea, which can adversely affect both female and male fertility by causing genital tract obstruction (Mladovsky et al., 2009). It remains to be seen if the large-scale public health interventions introduced in many countries to screen for diseases like chlamydia will ultimately reduce the number of couples who present with infertility related to sexually transmitted infections (Public Health England, 2013).

## CONTRIBUTORS TO MALE FERTILITY CHALLENGES

### Are Male Fertility Challenges a Lifestyle Problem?

Although the data for the adverse consequences of anabolic steroid abuse on semen quality (Bagatell & Bremner, 1996) and the use of certain prescribed and recreational drugs are clear cut, the evidence linking other lifestyle factors to male fertility has been conflicting. For example, some studies have shown that cigarette smoking, obesity (Eisenberg, Kim, et al., 2014), and heavy alcohol consumption can adversely affect male fertility, while other studies have shown no consistent link (Pacey et al., 2014). Other studies have implicated the role of occupation, exercise levels, and type of underwear worn to male factor infertility. Although the data are conflicting, it remains a matter of great scientific interest as well as of concern to couples with fertility issues. Despite the absence of strong evidence to link a lifestyle with fertility, the physician, nurse, counselor, or other health care professionals can use the consultation to discuss the general health benefits of a healthy diet and participating in exercise to treat obesity, to offer support in smoking cessation, and to advise on moderating alcohol consumption and the avoidance of recreational drugs. In addition to direct benefit for the men themselves, there may be additional benefit for their children. For example, it has previously been demonstrated that boys born to cigarette smokers have an increased risk of developing childhood leukemia (Chang et al., 2006). One of the issues related to the relative lack of clear scientific consensus in this area is that couples find this area confusing, due to the conflicting evidence, and are often therefore keen to seek advice about lifestyle factors during the consultation.

## Are Male Fertility Problems Related to Other Aspects of Male Health?

It is well known that some men with fertility problems are at an increased risk of testicular cancer (Doria-Rose, Biggs, & Weiss, 2005); furthermore, semen quality has been linked to male life expectancy and is described as a biomarker of male health (Eisenberg, Li, et al., 2014). This could imply that a national or regional decline in semen quality, as reported in some studies (Rolland, Le Moal, Wagner, Royère, & De Mouzon, 2013), could have wider implications for male health. Whether this reflects an environmental cause or some other common reason, such as obesity, that could potentially affect health and fertility is not clear, but work is ongoing in this important area (Sharpe, 2012).

Overall, there are clearly a number of reasons why male factor infertility should be taken seriously by couples with fertility issues along with the team that treats them. Male factor infertility can be associated with other health problems that also need to be addressed, such as obesity and diabetes. Couples presenting to fertility services provide a timely opportunity for practitioners to engage in general health promotion.

## THE EVALUATION OF MALE FERTILITY CHALLENGES

Semen analysis remains the key diagnostic test used to confirm a male factor fertility problem, which should be collected and analyzed according to World Health Organization (WHO) standards (Cooper et al., 2010). Factors assessed on semen analysis include volume, pH, sperm concentration, total sperm count, sperm motility (percentages of progressively motile sperm, nonprogressively motile sperm, and immotile sperm), and sperm morphology (sperm appearances). Any of these factors can be suboptimal when compared with the normal reference ranges (Cooper et al., 2010), but frequently men with fertility issues have impairment of all semen parameters (concentration, motility, and morphology) on testing. This is called oligoasthenoteratozoospermia (OAT). As there can be a great variation in semen quality examined from an individual, it is usual to repeat the test in men with poor sperm quality to ensure that it is a consistent finding (Keel, 2006).

One of the challenges in proper diagnosis is potential inconsistencies among those performing the analyses. It is therefore critical to establish consistency within the practice and laboratory staff performing semen analysis; these individuals should complete a formal training program. To provide oversight, laboratories performing semen analysis should be enrolled in quality assurance programs to ensure consistency of their results, such as the United Kingdom's National External Quality Assessment Service Labs. Labs and staff that consistently underperform against standard test samples are offered retraining to ensure that a high standard of assessment is maintained by participating laboratories. In the future, automated computer-aided sperm analysis systems may replace manual laboratory assessments, promoting less human error in analysis, which, in turn, may improve the diagnosis process (Mehta & Woodward, 2014)

On thorough investigation, some couples can be found to have correctable problems. A full assessment may identify male patients with reversible factors like steroid abuse, pituitary failure, and problems with sperm production and delivery that are amenable to surgical correction, such as varicocele or obstructive azoospermia caused by epididymitis. There is an association between male factor subfertility and problems with the male sexual function, like erectile dysfunction, that are distressing to the couple and can be treated if identified. Male sexual problems are more common in subfertile couples; these can reflect psychological causes linked to childlessness as well as, in some cases, a common underlying disorder such as diabetes. A careful study of sexual history can identify problems like anorgasmia that may be amenable to specific psychological treatments. Hypogonadism can cause a range of distressing symptoms that are amenable to treatment. Simple screening questions can pick out those patients who may be affected and so that appropriate treatment may commence. Furthermore, health screening can be combined with physical examination to ensure that relevant pathology is not missed.

## Why Examination of Male Patients Is Necessary

Unfortunately, many men with fertility problems are never assessed beyond abnormal semen analysis, particularly if intracytoplasmic sperm injection (ICSI) is determined to be an appropriate clinical option. Very often, the semen analysis and subsequent ICSI are coordinated by the female's care team, because the sperm required for ICSI can be procured by masturbation. This means that men are missing an opportunity to be examined to determine a potential underlying cause. Simple physical examination can provide useful information on the reason for male factor problems without the requirement for invasive or expensive tests. Important findings such as absent vas deferens, varicocele, or small volume testes can provide useful information for patients by identifying the reason for their fertility problems and enabling them to make informed choices about their treatment options. Testes cancer is the most common solid malignancy in young men (Hayes-Lattin & Nichols, 2009), and, as mentioned earlier, testes cancer is more common in subfertile men; occasionally, a tumor may be detected in clinic at examination. Furthermore, examination facilitates teaching men how to self-examine their testes, so that if in the future suspicious lumps are detected they can then be investigated at the earliest possible time.

As well as a careful genital examination, an assessment of the general body habitus can suggest an underlying cause. Men with hypogonadism, for example, may have a paucity of body hair and enlargement of the breast tissue (gynecomastia), findings that can indicate an underlying hormonal or genetic problem.

## Are Genetic Investigations Needed?

A full assessment where indicated allows for the identification of other factors that could affect a man's general health. Genetic studies are generally indicated if the sperm count is consistently less than 5 million/mL (Jungwirth et al., 2012) and abnormalities on testing are most likely in azoospermic men, that is, the chance of an identifiable genetic abnormality is proportional to the severity of the problem. Genetic studies like karyotype can pick up relatively common problems like Klinefelter syndrome that can affect other aspects of male health, like mood, bone density, and sexual function (Kamischke, Baumgardt, Horst, & Nieschlag, 2003). Klinefelter syndrome is a meiotic nondisjunction disorder, resulting in the affected person having an extra "X" chromosome, resulting in the XXY genotype. Although some males with Klinefelter syndrome are diagnosed in childhood, or even antenatally following amniocentesis or chorionic villous biopsy, many are only diagnosed when they attend for infertility investigations. Younger men with Klinefelter syndrome, particularly mosaics with a mixed genotype, can sometimes have sperm in their ejaculate (Selice et al., 2010), but the progressive deterioration in testicular function seen in this condition means that virtually all such patients are azoospermic by the time they reach their 20s. In some instances, however, surgical sperm retrieval can be successful, giving men with this genetic condition a potential chance of biological fatherhood (Aksglaede & Juul, 2013). Overall, fertility preservation strategies such as cryopreservation of ejaculated sperm where possible should be considered in young men with Klinefelter syndrome.

Cystic fibrosis is a common autosomal recessive disorder that usually presents in infancy with a failure to thrive, due to chronic respiratory problems and pancreatic insufficiency. A cystic fibrosis gene mutation is carried by one in 25 people of Northern European heritage. Men who are cystic fibrosis carriers often present via fertility services with azoospermia, as do on occasions men with homozygous mutations, due to a congenital absence of the vas deferens. While sperm can be recovered from them in the vast majority of cases, it is imperative that the female partner's cystic fibrosis status be checked to exclude that she does not also have carrier status. If both partners are cystic fibrosis carriers, then there will be a one in four chance that any children that they have together will have cystic fibrosis. Preimplantation genetic diagnosis can enable some couples to avoid having a child that is homozygous for the disorder. Because of the significance that being a cystic fibrosis carrier has on decision making about parenting, patients who have vasal abnormalities on examination or a family history of cystic fibrosis should be screened.

The genes that are responsible for making sperm are located on the long arm of the Y chromosome and small deletions of parts of these genes (microdeletions) are one of the commoner identifiable genetic causes of male infertility. Men who have the microdeletion patterns known as AZFa and AZFb are not believed to have any chance of becoming biological parents, but identifying this problem can contribute to providing the patients with closure on the issue, by giving a precise reason for their infertility and enabling them to avoid procedures like testicular biopsy that may prove costly and carry the risk of adverse side effects like scrotal infections and painful hematomas.

Another more common microdeletion pattern (AZFc) is different in that some men with this problem will have sperm that can be recovered surgically from their testes, or even small numbers of sperm in their ejaculate, and in these cases there is some potential for biological parenthood. However, it is imperative that the couple receive appropriate education as any male offspring conceived using this sperm would grow up to have the same fertility problems as their fathers, as they would inherit their father's Y chromosome.

## What Other Tests Are Useful?

It is apparent that conventional semen analysis may not be the final arbitrator of male fertility. There is a growing body of evidence that reactive free oxygen species, caused by a variety of problems including infection, obstruction, and varicocele, can damage sperm DNA and contribute to couple infertility. Some experts believe that the identification of sperm DNA damage, which can be picked up by laboratories using a number of commercially available kits, can explain some cases of recurrent miscarriage and identify couples for whom certain types of treatment (e.g., ICSI rather than IVF) may be more appropriate because they can potentially improve fertility outcomes (Lewis et al., 2013).

Ideally, the method of sperm selection for treatment would allow the lab team the ability to detect and use the best available sperms present in the sample for treatment. Improved methods of sperm selection based on tests of sperm functionality, like the ability of normally functioning sperm to bind hyaluronic acid, may also ultimately provide a better solution when used in conjunction with current methods of assessment, although definitive clinical evidence is awaited (McDowell et al., 2014).

A full assessment is essential in determining how best to treat a couple with male factor infertility; while this will enable the mechanism of subfertility to be explained (e.g., a sperm production issue), it is disappointing that relatively few men complete the process with a clear explanation of the precise reason for their problem. Many couples at this point will just be treated with ICSI, but there is a clear requirement to improve male fertility diagnostics. It is unusual in specialty areas of medicine for treatment to be commenced without a clear understanding of the reason for the problem in the first place. This is very different to medical specialities that have sophisticated diagnostics but limited treatment options such as perhaps neurology. It is important that the ability to proceed directly to treatment does not mean that an attempt to find a remediable cause, or even an explanation, for the problem should be overlooked.

## Why Evaluate Male Patients When ICSI Is Available?

The development of ICSI has revolutionized the treatment of couples with male factor subfertility, allowing couples where male partners have the poorest quality of ejaculated sperm the chance to become biological parents. However, there is a desire for men to find out what the cause of their problem is and this may not always be satisfactorily answered. Indeed, some experts believe that one consequence of the success of ICSI has been a decline in the role traditionally played by male fertility assessment and the attempt to find out the cause of the male problem.

It must be borne in mind that many couples who pursue assisted reproductive technology (ART) never become pregnant, meaning that they are left to deal with the long-term consequences of childlessness. In the longer term, emotional support may not always be available and this, combined with the uncertainty caused by the lack of a clear explanation of what caused the male fertility problem, can have implications for a couple's well-being.

A question to consider is that if a couple can proceed to treatment using ICSI without a clear understanding of what the problem is, does it matter? To answer this question, the potential risks of treatment must be considered. The risks associated with ICSI are low but not zero. Studies have shown that children born through the use of ICSI have an increased risk of certain developmental problems including abnormalities of the genitourinary system (Seggers et al., 2015) and disorders of imprinting, a situation in which gene expression is modified by processes like methylation (Lazaraviciute, Kauser, Bhattacharya, Haggarty, & Bhattacharya, 2014). The latter includes conditions like Beckwith-Wiedemann syndrome, an imprinting disorder characterized by macrosomia, macroglossia, abdominal wall defects, and a propensity to certain tumors (Soejima & Higashimoto, 2013). According to some, Angelman syndrome, which is associated with intellectual impairment, may be more common in children conceived by ICSI (Ludwig et al., 2005; Vermeiden & Bernardus, 2013). Not all epidemiological studies have confirmed a clear increase in the incidence of these rare disorders; overall, the absolute risk to the fetus remains very low (Alukal & Lamb, 2008) and any confirmed risk may not be due to the technique of ICSI itself but rather to risks from the parents'genetics (Fauser et al., 2014; Palermo, Neri, & Rosenwaks, 2015). Although the absolute risk of congenital problems is unclear, much more is known about the well-recognized risks of ART themselves including ovarian hyperstimulation and the risks associated with multiple pregnancies (both of these topics are covered in other chapters). Allowing couples to conceive without the need for ART is beneficial from a medical, aesthetic, and financial standpoint. Where possible, this should be discussed, while bearing in mind that female factors and couple choice may ultimately determine the best way for the couple to achieve their aims.

Another important point to consider is that ICSI can only be performed if sperm is available. The 1% of men who are azoospermic require specific consideration. In many cases, such men undergo procedures in an attempt to recover sperm from their testicles for use in ICSI. If the reason for the lack of sperm is due to a production-type problem rather than a genital tract blockage, the procedure has a much higher chance of failure. Surgical sperm retrieval itself is not without potential complications; while the risks are low, problems such as scrotal hematoma, infection, and even hypogonadism can occur.

## TREATMENT OPTIONS FOR MALE FERTILITY CHALLENGES

### What About Azoospermic Men?

Although ICSI requires the presence of at least a small number of ejaculated sperms to be successful, this procedure is not possible for the 1% of men with azoospermia who will require special consideration. Although some of them have problems that are correctable, like vasectomised men, the majority will require some form of surgical sperm retrieval in order that they may become biological parents. Although successful sperm recovery, by biopsy or aspiration techniques, is very likely in cases of obstructive azoospermia, men with nonobstructive azoospermia have a much less certain outcome. The development of the MicroTESE technique by Schlegel et al. at Cornell has greatly improved their prognosis, but many men still will be left at the end of their treatment pathway, childless and without a clear explanation of what precisely has caused the problem. There is an urgent requirement that male fertility researchers continue to investigate the causes of this most perplexing of issues as it is clear that many patients deserve a more comprehensive explanation than we are currently able to provide.

## If There Is No Sperm Available From the Male Partner, Couldn't the Couple Just Use Donor Sperm?

The use of donor sperm has enabled many couples to become parents and the evidence supports that children born in this way grow up as well adjusted as children born to both their biological parents. The use of donor sperm can enable treatment options like intrauterine insemination (IUI), which are less invasive, less expensive, and carry less risk than ICSI using surgically recovered sperm. However, the use of donor gametes is not acceptable to all couples at a personal level or because of cultural or religious considerations. Sometimes couples can have a discordant attitude toward the use of donor sperm when it is raised as a treatment choice, which can lead to tensions in the relationship. Every effort should be taken to ensure that couples considering the use of donor gametes are appropriately counseled to reduce the chance that a couple passes through fertility assessment and treatment with donor sperm without a full understanding of the implications of what they have chosen to do.

In many countries, the disclosure of the identities of gamete donors is mandated by law. This can mean that children who are born by the use of donor sperm, in for example the United Kingdom, have the legal right to find out the identity of the donor when they reach a defined age. The implications of what has been a change in national legislation have led, in some countries, to a reported decline in the numbers of men who wish to become sperm donors (Gudipati et al., 2013). This has had a number of consequences, including a reduction in patient choice due to a reduction in the number of available donors, a rise in the amount of sperm that is imported from other countries where attitudes to sperm donation are different, a rise in cross border fertility treatment (where couples travel abroad to countries with different regulations on the use of donor sperm), and also to a rise in the use of donors who are known to the couple being treated (often a family member). Known donors tend to provide sperm for only one family and therefore contribute less to addressing the rising demand for donor sperm, seen in many countries. Due to the difficulties in some countries in accessing sperm from registered and screened donors, there have been cases where couples have sought the use of sperm sourced from unregistered private donors that has not been properly screened and could therefore be potentially unsafe (BBC News, 2010).

## PSYCHOSOCIAL CONSIDERATIONS FOR MEN WITH FERTILITY CHALLENGES

### How Do Men Feel About Fertility Assessment?

Unfortunately, the issue of how men feel about their own fertility has not been extensively researched and most work in this area has concentrated on the female experience (Purewal & van den Akker, 2007). For many younger men, this will be their first reason for involvement with health services and the anxiety pertaining to the consultation alone can be significant. Many men find genital examination and production of a semen sample for analysis very stressful (Karalovos, Haimes, Quinton, & McEleny, 2014).

The knowledge level pertaining to fertility is often a challenge once men liaise with the health care team. In general terms, many men do not have a full understanding of basic fertility concepts and frequently the female partner takes the lead in arranging assessment and investigation. Cultural stereotyping and ineffective health education mean that some men do not even realize that there could ever be a problem with their own fertility, assuming that if there is a problem, it can only ever be with their female partner and never themselves. Many men react with shock and disbelief to finding out that they have a male factor fertility problem, with some in fact proceeding through a grieving process, before coming to terms with the situation, as they realize that the family life they had assumed that they would have with their partner may not be the one that they end up with. For many cultures it is expected that a couple will have children and men report that the additional family pressure can make things even less tolerable. As mentioned earlier, men find the lack of a clear reason for the problem frustrating and often attribute it to a lifestyle event or choice, such as using a recreational drug, that may have happened many years before and will clearly be unrelated to the current episode (Karalovos et al., 2014).

## How Do Men Cope With Fertility Treatment?

Little is known about how men cope with the diagnosis of male factor infertility; it is an important area for future research. However, inferences can be made by examining male attitudes in other contexts. Many cultures demonstrate a traditional masculine identity (Barnett, Raudenbush, Brennan, Pleck, & Marshall, 1995), which comprises a number of defined characteristics including emotional repression and self-reliance. In such cultures, the defined gender roles for men can be more strongly defined than for women (Wentworth & Chell, 2001). This could potentially explain why men are less likely to seek help, including medical opinions, than women (Addis & Mahalik, 2003).

Some men state that being labeled subfertile makes them feel less masculine, as they cannot dissociate their fertility from their masculine identity. The lack of disclosure seen often outside the immediate family reflects the fact that male factor infertility in many cultures remains a taboo subject. Many men are reluctant to seek support from colleagues and friends for fear of receiving insensitive remarks, instead preferring to seek support from their partner and close family only. Men are perhaps less likely than women to seek psychological support with childlessness.

## How Do Fertility Challenges Impact Relationships?

Most men tell us that they deal with the fertility problems they have encountered as a couple and therefore do not feel isolated within their relationship. However, some aspects of their relationship can be harmed; for example, some couples report a negative aspect of fertility problems on physical intimacy. Whether this is due to the perceived loss of masculine identity, stress of being labeled infertile, or replacement of "recreational" sex with "reproductive" sex is not clear. Although some men have stated that they felt a need to "release" their female partner from the relationship to enable her to find another partner who may be able to allow her to achieve her goal of motherhood, most couples state that the problem has brought them closer together.

## CONCLUSION

Male fertility problems are common and may be becoming more common. They can be associated with other significant health issues and in some cases lifestyle issues; therefore, a full assessment of the male partner, including psychosocial requirements, is important to enable the couple to make an informed choice about their fertility options. Modern medical developments can allow even men with profound sperm production problems the chance of becoming biological parents, but male fertility assessment requires a high-quality laboratory service and access to genetic testing.

It is distressing that so little research has been conducted on the impact of fertility problems on the emotional well-being of men diagnosed with male factor infertility. Although much of the focus of fertility assessment and treatment has been on the female, as most fertility assessment and treatment is carried out on the female partner, there is a clear requirement to find out more about the male perspective to ensure that we as fertility practitioners have the right systems of support in place for our male patients.

There is a view that male patients do not feel a part of the process and are just there to provide sperm (where available) for ICSI treatment. Nowadays men rightly expect more from fertility services and we owe them a responsibility to provide it. Male assessment is about so much more than just a means to an end; an explanation of the underlying cause can be extremely helpful, particularly when it is borne in mind that many couples will not become biological parents together. As well as attempting to find out the reason for the male factor problem, assessment enables an environment where broader male health issues can be discussed.

## REFERENCES

Addis, M. E., & Mahalik, J. R. (2003). Men, masculinity, and the contexts of help seeking. *The American Psychologist, 58*(1), 5–14. doi:10.1037/0003–066X.58.1.5

Aksglaede, L., & Juul, A. (2013). Testicular function and fertility in men with Klinefelter syndrome: A review. *European Journal of Endocrinology/European Federation of Endocrine Societies, 168*(4), R67–R76. doi:10.1530/eje-12–0934

Alukal, J. P., & Lamb, D. J. (2008). Intracytoplasmic sperm injection (ICSI)—What are the risks? *The Urologic Clinics of North America, 35*(2), 277–288, ix. doi:10.1016/j.ucl.2008.01.004

Bagatell, C. J., & Bremner, W. J. (1996). Androgens in men—Uses and abuses. *The New England Journal of Medicine, 334*(11), 707–714. doi:10.1056/nejm199603143341107

Barnett, R. C., Raudenbush, S. W., Brennan, R. T., Pleck, J. H., & Marshall, N. L. (1995). Change in job and marital experiences and change in psychological distress: A longitudinal study of dual-earner couples. *Journal of Personality and Social Psychology, 69*(5), 839–850. doi: 10.1037/0022–3514.69.5.839

BBC News. (2010, October 12). *Suspended jail term for illegal sperm website pair BBC News.* Retrieved from http://www.bbc.co.uk/news/uk-england-berkshire-11521464

Chang, J. S., Selvin, S., Metayer, C., Crouse, V., Golembesky, A., & Buffler, P. A. (2006). Parental smoking and the risk of childhood leukemia. *American Journal of Epidemiology, 163*(12), 1091–1100. doi:10.1093/aje/kwj143

Cooper, T. G., Noonan, E., von Eckardstein, S., Auger, J., Baker, H. W., Behre, H. M., . . . Vogelsong, K. M. (2010). World Health Organization reference values for human semen characteristics. *Human Reproduction Update, 16*(3), 231–245. doi:10.1093/humupd/dmp048

Doria-Rose, V. P., Biggs, M. L., & Weiss, N. S. (2005). Subfertility and the risk of testicular germ cell tumors (United States). *Cancer Causes & Control: CCC, 16*(6), 651–656. doi:10.1007/s10552–005-0169-x

Eisenberg, M. L., Kim, S., Chen, Z., Sundaram, R., Schisterman, E. F., & Buck Louis, G. M. (2014). The relationship between male BMI and waist circumference on semen quality: Data from the LIFE study. *Human Reproduction (Oxford, England), 29*(2), 193–200. doi:10.1093/humrep/det428

Eisenberg, M. L., Li, S., Behr, B., Cullen, M. R., Galusha, D., Lamb, D. J., & Lipshultz, L. I. (2014). Semen quality, infertility and mortality in the USA. *Human Reproduction (Oxford, England), 29*(7), 1567–1574. doi:10.1093/humrep/deu106

Fauser, B. C., Devroey, P., Diedrich, K., Balaban, B., Bonduelle, M., Delemarre-van de Waal, H. A., . . . Wells, D.; Evian Annual Reproduction (EVAR) Workshop Group 2011. (2014). Health outcomes of children born after IVF/ICSI: A review of current expert opinion and literature. *Reproductive Biomedicine Online, 28*(2), 162–182. doi:10.1016/j.rbmo.2013.10.013

Fisch, H. (2008). Declining worldwide sperm counts: Disproving a myth. *The Urologic Clinics of North America, 35*(2), 137–146, vii. doi:10.1016/j.ucl.2008.01.001

Giwercman, A., & Petersen, P. M. (2000). Cancer and male infertility. *Baillière's Best Practice & Research. Clinical Endocrinology & Metabolism, 14*(3), 453–471.

Gudipati, M., Pearce, K., Prakash, A., Redhead, G., Hemingway, V., McEleny, K., & Stewart, J. (2013). The sperm donor programme over 11 years at Newcastle Fertility Centre. *Human Fertility (Cambridge, England), 16*(4), 258–265. doi:10.3109/14647273.2013.815370

Hayes-Lattin, B., & Nichols, C. R. (2009). Testicular cancer: A prototypic tumor of young adults. *Seminars in Oncology, 36*(5), 432–438. doi:10.1053/j.seminoncol.2009.07.006

Johansson, M., Adolfsson, A., Berg, M., Francis, J., Hogström, L., Janson, P. O., . . . Hellström, A. L. (2010). Gender perspective on quality of life, comparisons between groups 4–5.5 years after unsuccessful or successful IVF treatment. *Acta Obstetricia Et Gynecologica Scandinavica, 89*(5), 683–691. doi:10.3109/00016341003657892

Jungwirth, A., Giwercman, A., Tournaye, H., Diemer, T., Kopa, Z., Dohle, G., & Krausz, C.; European Association of Urology Working Group on Male Infertility. (2012). European Association of Urology guidelines on male infertility: The 2012 update. *European Urology, 62*(2), 324–332. doi:10.1016/j.eururo.2012.04.048

Juul, A., Almstrup, K., Andersson, A. M., Jensen, T. K., Jørgensen, N., Main, K. M., . . . Skakkebæk, N. E. (2014). Possible fetal determinants of male infertility. *Nature Reviews. Endocrinology, 10*(9), 553–562. doi:10.1038/nrendo.2014.97

Kamischke, A., Baumgardt, A., Horst, J., & Nieschlag, E. (2003). Clinical and diagnostic features of patients with suspected Klinefelter syndrome. *Journal of Andrology, 24*(1), 41–48. doi:10.1002/j.1939–4640.2003.tb02638

Karalovos, S., Haimes, E., Quinton, R., & McEleny, K. (2014). *"There is not a day goes by that I don't think about it": The experience and meaning of male factor infertility to men.* Poster presented at the European Society of Human Reproduction and Embryology (ESHRE) Annual Congress 2014. Retrieved from http://eshre2014.congressplanner.eu/showabstract.php?congress=ESHRE2014&id=362

Keel, B. A. (2006). Within- and between-subject variation in semen parameters in infertile men and normal semen donors. *Fertility and Sterility, 85*(1), 128–134. doi:10.1016/j .fertnstert.2005.06.048

Lazaraviciute, G., Kauser, M., Bhattacharya, S., Haggarty, P., & Bhattacharya, S. (2014). A systematic review and meta-analysis of DNA methylation levels and imprinting disorders in children conceived by IVF/ICSI compared with children conceived spontaneously. *Human Reproduction Update, 20*(6), 840–852. doi:10.1093/humupd/dmu033

Lewis, S. E. M., Aitken, R. J., Conner, S. J., De Iuliis, G., Evenson, D. P., Henkel, R.,...Gharagozloo, P. (2013). The impact of sperm DNA damage in assisted conception and beyond: Recent advances in diagnosis and treatment. *Reproductive Biomedicine Online, 27*, 325–337. doi:10.1016/j.rbmo.2013.06.014

Ludwig, M., Katalinic, A., Gross, S., Sutcliffe, A., Varon, R., & Horsthemke, B. (2005). Increased prevalence of imprinting defects in patients with Angelman syndrome born to subfertile couples. *Journal of Medical Genetics, 42*(4), 289–291.

Macaluso, M., Wright-Schnapp, T. J., Chandra, A., Johnson, R., Satterwhite, C. L., Pulver, A.,...Pollack, L. A. (2010). A public health focus on infertility prevention, detection, and management. *Fertility and Sterility, 93*(1), 16.e1–16.10. doi:10.1136/jmg.2004.026930

McDowell, S., Kroon, B., Ford, E., Hook, Y., Glujovsky, D., & Yazdani, A. (2014). Advanced sperm selection techniques for assisted reproduction. *The Cochrane Database of Systematic Reviews, 10*, CD010461. doi:10.1002/14651858.CD010461.pub2

Mehta, J., & Woodward, B. (2014). *Male infertility: Sperm diagnosis, management and delivery.* London, UK: JP Medical.

Mladovsky, P., Allin, S., Masseria, C., Hernandez-Quevedo, C., McDaid, D., & Mossialos, E. (2009). *Health in the European Union: Trends and analysis.* Retrieved from http://www .euro.who.int/__data/assets/pdf_file/0003/98391/E93348.pdf

Office for National Statistics. (2014). *Births in England and Wales, 2013.* Retrieved from http:// www.ons.gov.uk/ons/dcp171778_371129.pdf

Pacey, A. A., Povey, A. C., Clyma, J. A., McNamee, R., Moore, H. D., Baillie, H., & Cherry, N. M.; Participating Centres of Chaps-UK. (2014). Modifiable and non-modifiable risk factors for poor sperm morphology. *Human Reproduction, 29*(8), 1629–1636. doi:10.1093/ humrep/deu116

Palermo, G. D., Neri, Q. V., & Rosenwaks, Z. (2015). To ICSI or not to ICSI. *Seminars in Reproductive Medicine, 33*(2), 92–102. doi:10.1055/s-0035-1546825

Public Health England. (2013). *The National Chlamydia Screening Programme: An overview.* Retrieved from http://www.chlamydiascreening.nhs.uk/ps/overview.asp

Purewal, S., & van den Akker, O. (2007). The socio-cultural and biological meaning of parenthood. *Journal of Psychosomatic Obstetrics and Gynaecology, 28*(2), 79–86. doi:10.1080/01674820701409918

Rolland, M., Le Moal, J., Wagner, V., Royère, D., & De Mouzon, J. (2013). Decline in semen concentration and morphology in a sample of 26,609 men close to general population between 1989 and 2005 in France. *Human Reproduction, 28*(2), 462–470. doi:10.1093/ humrep/des415

Seggers, J., de Walle, H. E., Bergman, J. E., Groen, H., Hadders-Algra, M., Bos, M. E.,...Haadsma, M. L. (2015). Congenital anomalies in offspring of subfertile couples: A registry-based study in the northern Netherlands. *Fertility and Sterility, 103*(4), 1001–1010.e3. doi:10.1016/j.fertnstert.2014.12.113

Selice, R., Di Mambro, A., Garolla, A., Ficarra, V., Iafrate, M., Ferlin, A., & Foresta, C. (2010). Spermatogenesis in Klinefelter syndrome. *Journal of Endocrinological Investigation, 33*(11), 789–793. doi:10.1007/BF03350343

Sharpe, R. M. (2012). Sperm counts and fertility in men: A rocky road ahead. Science & Society Series on Sex and Science. *EMBO Reports, 13*(5), 398–403. doi:10.1038/embor.2012.50

Shindel, A. W., Nelson, C. J., Naughton, C. K., Ohebshalom, M., & Mulhall, J. P. (2008). Sexual function and quality of life in the male partner of infertile couples: Prevalence and correlates of dysfunction. *The Journal of Urology, 179*(3), 1056–1059. doi:10.1016/j.juro.2007.10.069

Skakkebaek, N. E., Rajpert-De Meyts, E., & Main, K. M. (2001). Testicular dysgenesis syndrome: An increasingly common developmental disorder with environmental aspects. *Human Reproduction (Oxford, England), 16*(5), 972–978. doi:10.1093/humrep/16.5.972

Soejima, H., & Higashimoto, K. (2013). Epigenetic and genetic alterations of the imprinting disorder Beckwith-Wiedemann syndrome and related disorders. *Journal of Human Genetics, 58*(7), 402–409. doi:10.1038/jhg.2013.51

Thonneau, P., Marchand, S., Tallec, A., Ferial, M. L., Ducot, B., Lansac, J.,...Spira, A. (1991). Incidence and main causes of infertility in a resident population (1,850,000) of three French regions (1988–1989). *Human Reproduction, 6*(6), 811–816.

Vermeiden, J. P., & Bernardus, R. E. (2013). Are imprinting disorders more prevalent after human in vitro fertilization or intracytoplasmic sperm injection? *Fertility and Sterility, 99*(3), 642–651. doi:10.1016/j.fertnstert.2013.01.125

Wentworth, D. K., & Chell, R. M. (2001). The role of house husband and housewife as perceived by a college population. *The Journal of Psychology, 135*(6), 639–650. doi:10.1080/00223980109603725

# CHAPTER 26

# Exemplar: AN ADOLESCENT SEEKING FERTILITY TREATMENT

*Anne Derouin*

Reproductive health for teens has primarily focused on preventing or delaying pregnancies (and sexually transmitted infections [STIs]) rather than treating infertility issues, even though these concerns exist. There continues to be millions of teen pregnancies per year (Martin, Hamilton, Osterman, Curtin, & Mathews, 2015), many *intended* by females and/or her partner, especially in developing countries where adolescent parenting is commonplace to the cultural norms (Haimov-Kochman, Imbar, Farchat, Bdolah, & Hurwitz, 2008). There is evidence in media reports (e.g., "Massachusetts Pregnancy Pact" [Kingsbury, 2008]; reality TV program *Teen Mom*) and in the medical literature that some adolescents consider pregnancy desirable. Crosby et al.(2001) found that 21% of their nonpregnant adolescent subjects wanted to become pregnant. Young women who perceived that their partners favored pregnancy were three times more likely to stop using contraception and expressed concerns about fertility. Crump et al. (1999) found that adolescents in focus groups believed that pregnancy was a desirable but unachievable goal. Early- and middle-stage adolescents typically seek independence from authorities and their adult caregivers. They possess intense self-focus, desire for romantic relationships with peers, a sense of "immediacy," and a limited ability to calculate long-term consequences of their actions (Feigelman, 2015). They often have sought health information about sexual health and fertility from media sources or one another rather than a health care professional (Lundsberg et al., 2014). The following case is an exemplar for considerations related to adolescent infertility.

## CASE STUDY

J.G. is a 16-year-old Hispanic female who presents at the adolescent clinic with two female peers requesting a pregnancy test. During the health history J.G. states that her last menstrual period (LMP) was about 5 weeks ago and that she is having nausea and mild abdominal cramping. She denies emesis, headaches, fever, dysuria, flank pain, vaginal discharge, or trauma. She has no allergies and takes no medications. She cannot recall her last medical visit but believes her immunizations are up to date. She has an unremarkable past medical or surgical history. Her diet and activity is normal; she is passing all her classes except math at school and works on the weekends for a cleaning service. She denies using tobacco, alcohol, or recreational drugs. She reports having unprotected intercourse with the same male partner for the past 9 months; they do not use any form of contraception. Her parents are aware of the relationship and approve of it. She lives with her parents and four younger siblings in a small single-family home.

The physical examination reveals a well-groomed, alert teen who appears anxious. Estimated weight is 130 pounds, height is 63 inches, and body mass index (BMI) is 23 (normal). All vital signs are normal, the blood pressure is 102/60; she is afebrile. She appears well hydrated with clear skin and normal heart and lung sounds. Her abdomen is soft and rounded with active bowel sounds in all quadrants. There are no masses, tenderness to palpation, rebound tenderness, or suprapubic or flank pain. She is cooperative, and moves all extremities with equal strength and full range of movement. Her gait is steady and even.

Clinical lab testing includes a urinalysis and urine pregnancy test. The urinalysis reveals positive (trace) protein and positive (trace) leukocytes. All other indicators are negative (–). The urine pregnancy test is negative (–). When the lab findings are reported to the patient, she begins to cry and asks, "Why can't I get pregnant, this is the fifth negative test!" J.G. further explains that she has been trying to get pregnant over the past 5 months because her partner is active in a neighborhood street gang and if she became pregnant, it would save his life by "getting him off the streets." She reports that the gang "rules" would disallow him from committing violent or criminal activities typically engaged in, if he was an expectant father and that they both desire starting a family.

As she continues to cry, she explains that after the last negative pregnancy test, completed at home about 6 weeks ago, he was angry and said, "something must be wrong with her." She believes that he will be angry again on learning about today's negative test result. She states that she is afraid to share test results with him and is certain that she will "never" become pregnant. She brought friends with her to the clinic visit for support and consolation.

## DISCUSSION

This case illustrates reasons adolescents may intentionally try to become pregnant—either as a cultural or societal norm, attention-seeking behavior or peer pressure, or as a goal a couple has mutually agreed on. Over the past decade, teens in my clinical setting have sought health care information about fertility and shared various rationales for desiring pregnancy including "wanting to be loved and needed by someone unconditionally," having a baby to "show off" like other girls in their community (a contagion factor), being the "Mama they never had," having a reason to avoid an undesirable school setting through a maternity leave or home–school arrangement, wanting to keep their male partner from "leaving them," and like J.G., wanting to start a family and provide a seemingly legitimate reason for avoiding further violence or danger to the partner. Other teens have sought to become pregnant after intentionally terminating a pregnancy, experiencing a miscarriage, or following the death of a family member. My clinical team has generally considered this a "blessing" rather than a concern for infertility when adolescents do not subsequently become pregnant following consultation. In those cases, extensive fertility workup has not been performed. Instead, we have ensured recommended preventative care, routine SIT screening, and counseling prior to their transition to adult health care services.

Not surprisingly, there are limited reports of infertility treatment recommendations or rates of infertility among teens and young adults—the focus among fertility has been on prevention of adolescent pregnancies globally and in the United States. Because of higher morbidity and mortality rates among pregnant teens and unfavorable (and costly) risks for preterm births, considerable efforts among health care providers, educators, and government agencies have aimed to reduce adolescent pregnancy rates through education interventions and promotion of contraception. Only one case study, found in a literature search on PubMed, documented infertility treatment for a teen who was not undergoing gonotoxic therapies. This case was presented from Israel, where fertility treatment technology is more readily available than in other developed countries, including the United States (Haimov-Kochman et al., 2008). The scarcity of reports suggest a lack of concern for infertility among health care providers who care for teens. Instead, the primary focus for adolescent health care has been to promote safety (including abstinence and/or contraception) and continue routine preventative health visits among adolescents to reduce the injury or illness (American Academy of Pediatrics Committee on Adolescents, 2014; Centers for Disease Control and Prevention [CDC], n.d. a).

Research on family planning and promoting adolescent fertility options among adolescents with chronic illness such as sickle cell disease, immunotherapy, and oncology conditions that use gonadotoxic treatments has increased in recent years, but there is limited evidence on the infertility rates among teens and clinical management guidelines for healthy adolescents with infertility concerns. Fallat and Hutter (2008) report difficult ethical issues surrounding the management of children and teens undergoing cancer therapies who are at risk for sterility, infertility, or subfertility. The American Society of Clinical Oncology recommends addressing the possibility of infertility to all patients treated during their reproductive years and referring patients to reproductive specialists as indicated, there is no consensus on what age would be appropriate to initiate the discussion and if the fertility treatment recommendations would apply to patients with cancer who are younger than 18 years (Hutter & Klosky, 2009). Even with clear guidelines, there is often a failure to communicate the infertility risks and treatment options to the teens undergoing chemotherapy or radiation treatments; rather, the discussion is held with the patients' adult caregivers, if at all.

Teens have questions and concerns about their ability to conceive yet often lack knowledge on even basic information about ovulatory cycles, as well as the effects of diet, weight (obesity or low weight), stress, exercise, toxins, and STIs on fertility. Lundsberg et al. (2014) reported younger women (18–24 years) believed more readily in common myths and misconceptions about fertility and demonstrated less knowledge about reproductive health than women 25 to 40 years of age. In this study, younger women cited websites as top sources of health-related information and discussion with health care providers about specific factors affecting fertility was sparse (Lundsberg et al., 2014). Rainey, Stevens-Simon, and Kaplan (1993) found nearly a quarter of teen females in an urban setting, aged 14 to 18 years, were concerned about their fertility. When further considering adolescent females' understanding about conception, Wimberly, Kahn, Kollar, and Slap (2003) found that most were able to define fertility as an ability to become pregnant but had an extensive range of misconceptions and beliefs about the causes of infertility—many of them inaccurate or unrealistic.

## CONCLUSION

The case example and the adolescent infertility research findings indicate the ongoing need for effective education and communication with adolescents about all aspects of reproductive health, not just contraception and STI prevention as recommended by the American College of Obstetricians and Gynecologists Committee on Gynecologic Practice (2005). Although concerted health care and regulatory efforts should continue to focus on preventing unwanted pregnancies among teens, it is critical that efforts include dispelling false beliefs about fertility and providing accurate information about menstrual cycles and conception. Health care providers need to consider the possibility of infertility among adolescents attempting to conceive as well as treatment options for teens at risk for infertility. Listening with sincerity to the fertility concerns and accurately answering the questions of an adolescent are among the initial steps in establishing trust, providing meaningful education, and initiating reproductive health care. Often, the attentive assessment of teens also leads to insight and awareness of trends and risks to adolescents in the community, as well as relevant social, cultural, and individual beliefs of the patient, his or her peer group, and the family system. The frank discussion of an adolescent's concerns about infertility, even if unwarranted, offers the health care provider an opportunity to correct misconceptions and positively impacts health care behaviors.

Finally, this exemplar points to the need for improved understanding of current adolescent infertility rates—how many women are *actually* affected but not evaluated carefully by health care providers. Current rates of infertility are speculated to be less than 8% among women younger than 19 years (CDC, n.d. b) but these may be underreported. The data are especially important as we consider the impact of rising childhood obesity rates (and comorbidities including diabetes and polycystic ovarian syndrome) on infertility in the United States. The obesity epidemic ultimately may have a tremendous impact on fertility of adolescents and adults in the future, requiring refined infertility recommendations and management strategies.

## SAMPLE DISCUSSION QUESTIONS

1. Considering this case, what additional risk factors might the health care provider screen this patient for besides infertility?
2. How does infertility testing, planning, and patient education differ among adolescents as compared with older women and/or couples?
3. How do cultural, environmental, and socioeconomic statuses affect adolescent fertility considerations?

# REFERENCES

American Academy of Pediatrics Committee on Adolescents. (2014). Policy statement: Contraception for adolescents. *Pediatrics, 134*, e1244–e1256. doi:10.1542/peds.2014–2299

American College of Obstetricians and Gynecologists Committee on Gynecologic Practice. (2005). ACOG committee opinion #313: The importance of preconception care in the continuum of women's health care. *Obstetrics & Gynecology, 106*, 665–666. doi:10.1097/00006250-200509000-00052

Centers for Disease Control and Prevention. (n.d. a). *About teen pregnancy: CDC priority: Reducing teen pregnancy and promoting health equity among youth*. Retrieved from http://www.cdc.gov/teenpregnancy/about/index.htm

Centers for Disease Control and Prevention. (n.d. b). *Fast stats: Infertility*. Retrieved from http://www.cdc.gov/nchs/fastats/infertility.htm

Crosby, R. A., DiClemente, R. J., Wingood, G. M., Sionean, C., Cobb, B. K., Harrington, K.,...Oh, M. K. (2001). Correlates of adolescent females' worry about undesired pregnancy. The importance of partner desire for pregnancy. *Journal of Pediatric and Adolescent Gynecology, 14*(3), 123–127.

Crump, A. D., Haynie, D. L., Aarons, S. J., Adair, E., Woodward, K., & Simons-Morton, B. G. (1999). Pregnancy among urban African-American teens: Ambivalence about prevention. *American Journal Health Behavior, 23*, 32–42. doi:10.5993/AJHB.23.1.4

Fallat, M. E., & Hutter, J.; American Academy of Pediatrics Committee on Bioethics; American Academy of Pediatrics Section on Hematology/Oncology; American Academy of Pediatrics Section on Surgery. (2008). Preservation of fertility in pediatric and adolescent patients with cancer. *Pediatrics, 121*(5), e1461–e1469.

Feigelman, S. (2015). Overview and assessment of variability. In R. M. Kliegman, B. F. Stanton, J. W. St. Geme, & N. F. Schor (Eds.), *Nelson textbook of pediatrics* (20th ed.). Philadelphia, PA: Elsevier, Inc.

Haimov-Kochman, R., Imbar, T., Farchat, M., Bdolah, Y., & Hurwitz, A. (2008). Adolescent infertility—To treat or not to treat. *Fertility and Sterility, 90*(5), 2009.e1–2009.e4.

Hutter, J., & Klosky, J. L. (2009). Communicating risk of infertility to adolescents prior to chemotherapy. *The Virtual Mentor: VM, 11*(8), 589–597.

Kingsbury, K. (2008, June). Gloucester pregnancy plot thickens. *Time*. Retrieved from http://content.time.com/time/nation/article/0,8599,1817272,00.html

Lundsberg, L. S., Pal, L., Gariepy, A. M., Xu, X., Chu, M. C., & Illuzzi, J. L. (2014). Knowledge, attitudes, and practices regarding conception and fertility: A population-based survey among reproductive-age United States women. *Fertility and Sterility, 101*(3), 767–774.

Martin, J. A., Hamilton, B. E., Osterman, M. J. K., Curtin, S. C., & Mathews, T. J. (2015). *Births: Final data for 2013* (National Vital Statistics Report Vol. 64, No. 1). Retrieved from http://www.cdc.gov/nchs/data/nvsr/nvsr64/nvsr64_01.pdf

Rainey, D. Y., Stevens-Simon, C., & Kaplan, D. W. (1993). Self-perception of infertility among female adolescents. *American Journal of Diseases of Children (1960), 147*(10), 1053–1056.

Wimberly, Y. H., Kahn, J. A., Kollar, L. M., & Slap, G. B. (2003). Adolescent beliefs about infertility. *Contraception, 68*, 385–391. doi:10.1016/j.contraception.2003.07.006

# EPILOGUE: FAMILY FORMATION— WHAT IS AHEAD?

*Eleanor L. Stevenson and Patricia E. Hershberger*

The science that led to significant advances in assisted reproductive technology (ART) and fertility treatment began just a few decades ago. With Drs. Robert Edwards and Patrick Steptoe's research leading to the first in vitro fertilization (IVF) baby in 1978, Louise Brown became synonymous with what was possible for those who previously had little to no hope of a biological child. Since that significant event, scientists and clinicians have strived to understand the complex phenomenon of the human body as it relates to conception and the development of a healthy baby. The curiosity and dedication that scientists, clinicians, and other scholars have put forth toward helping those with fertility challenges have resulted in a wondrous amount of knowledge. This knowledge has further led to highly technical approaches to fertility challenges, including ARTs.

Although there seemed to be limitless topics to include in this book, we decided to present information in four different sections: "Theory: Engaging Theories and Conceptual Concepts in ART"; "Research and Reviews: Delineating the State of the Science in ART"; "Policy: Exploring Access and Challenges in ART"; and "Practice: Improving the Delivery of Care in the ART Setting." We felt that each of these four areas represented the necessary components of fertility care worldwide and are all inextricably linked. Although the topics covered are by no means comprehensive, our goal was to start a discussion about what we felt were important topics in each area.

## THEORY: ENGAGING THEORIES AND CONCEPTUAL CONCEPTS IN ART

We began this book by addressing theoretical components of ART as the scientific process. In assisted reproduction and fertility care, theory is an important component of inquiry, thus guiding and shaping so many impressive discoveries that have advanced modern fertility care across the world. Yet, much of the theoretical underpinning in ART, beyond the physiological sciences, has not been articulated well. The "Theory: Engaging Theories and Conceptual Concepts in ART" section of this book provided a snapshot of how some theories are applicable in this clinical area. Jacqueline Fawcett, an expert on conceptual models and theories, particularly in nursing science, was able to apply the Roy Adaptation Model (RAM) to create a comprehensive theory of infertility. Investigators and clinicians can now implement Fawcett's theory about "adaptation" into their clinical practice or test her theory in future research. It is this creative approach that will continue to push scientists to expand our understanding of the phenomenon and improve care delivery systems. As Fawcett indicated, application of the RAM can be replicated using other conceptual models to allow for frameworks for understanding concepts that can be empirically tested. Because few new theoretical concepts have emerged in fertility research that address practice delivery over the past years despite the rapidity of physiological scientific growth, never is it so important to consider with more scrutiny the underlying theoretical underpinnings that support fertility research that touches on the quality of care, in particular to ART settings.

In the subsequent chapters discussing theory and theoretical conceptions, Wagner examined the changing family structure via a theoretical perspective about how family structure is shifting globally, in part because of fertility care. She posited that because family structure is fluid, it is critical that clinicians achieve a greater level of cultural competency in caring for those in the fertility setting. Clinicians must be flexible in practice by addressing the cultural needs of individuals and couples, thus allowing for comprehensive and appropriate care. This knowledge will help those working with individuals who are in the process of building families to frame their care from a culturally appropriate framework. Stevenson and Cobb examined the current literature to ascertain approaches to stress during pregnancies conceived via IVF. Because of the challenge in adequately defining psychological stress, this review considered the current research examining this concept from a multidimensional theoretical framework, which has its basis in Lazarus and Folkman's transactional model of stress and coping (Lazarus, 1966; Lazarus & Folkman, 1984; Lazarus & Launier, 1978) and was extended by Lobel et al. (Lobel, 1994; Lobel, Dunkel-Schetter, & Scrimshaw, 1992). This review provided a comprehensive approach to evaluation of stress, particularly when considering the impact stress may have on pregnancy outcomes. Because clinicians in the ART setting manage the early pregnancy care of individuals and couples who achieve a pregnancy via IVF, awareness of the effects of psychological stress can provide a basis for modifying care early in the pregnancy and allow for implementation of appropriate stress-reduction strategies. Finally, Hershberger and Yeom took a novel approach by exploring the unit of analysis used in ART research that addresses education and counseling. The authors articulated benefits and challenges to conceptualizing research designs around the individual, couple, or family. Future research might consider focusing on the family versus the individual when appropriate. Taken together with Wagner's discussion of the fluidity of family structure, investigators can more appropriately consider research designs that expand our understanding beyond the individual level.

## RESEARCH AND REVIEWS: DELINEATING THE STATE OF THE SCIENCE IN ART

In the "Research and Reviews: Delineating the State of the Science in ART" section, the contributing authors of this book offered a deeper look into many of the research areas that support fertility care, including psychological stress of fertility treatments, the experience that follows successful oocyte donation as well as older parenthood, critical factors in decision making about fertility preservation for young women with cancer, important aspects of adhering to rabbinic law for Jewish couples seeking fertility care, and how patients and clinicians diverge in their opinion of multiple gestation pregnancies. Although we consider each of these topics important, it is a sampling of the research that has been—and needs to be—conducted.

There are critical needs for fertility research and its application in order to move practice forward. Our collaborators have specifically indicated that existing research must be better incorporated into clinical care. Lawson stated that because of the associated stress, it is important that those receiving fertility treatment receive emotional support during fertility treatment, which is currently not consistently provided. Lawson also offered that anecdotal stories of a relationship between stress and success with fertility treatment often result in women placing blame on themselves for not conceiving. This review illuminated that clinicians are in an optimal position to reassure women and couples that stress is both common and not necessarily deleterious to them or their ability to achieve pregnancy.

Despite the increased prevalence of oocyte donation, there is limited understanding about the experience of pregnancy, birth, and breastfeeding of oocyte-recipient women. Indekeu and Daniels provided new qualitative data to help better understand the specific psychological processes that occur during the pre-, peri-, and postnatal periods for women who are recipients of donor oocytes. Based on these data, the authors posited that there is a special care pathway for pregnancies after oocyte donation that can foster the support and development of a confident maternal identity. What is needed is a greater awareness and understanding of the distinctive psychological qualities of oocyte-recipient pregnancies. Additionally, this chapter illustrated that more research is needed to help understand cultural expectations about the oocyte treatment process and resulting postnatal care. This information has the potential to provide appropriate and sensitive care to those seeking to expand their families with donated oocytes.

With all the advances in technology that have provided the opportunity for parenthood to many, we now have additional important questions to consider. Woodward and MacDuffie presented a review of the literature on parenting during later life, as this technology has allowed older individuals to become parents. They found a mix of both positive and negative outcomes. Although there are better outcomes for both older parents and their children, waiting until middle age to become parents when one's personal, social, and financial circumstances are more ideal is associated with significant risks for both later-life parents and their children. In the future, a more comprehensive study is necessary to determine the optimal window for parenthood and increase our understanding of the advantages and disadvantages of later-life parenthood. Additionally, as older individuals seek parenthood, we are better positioned to counsel comprehensively and provide appropriate anticipatory guidance about what to expect in the years ahead, should they be successful in their ART pursuits.

It is essential that we have a broad understanding of the impact of ART on the lives of those whom we are treating. To extend our understanding of older parenthood, Romain and Nachtigall presented data about the potential impact of delayed parenting on paid work and work–family strategies. The investigators found that because of current cultural and workplace beliefs that do not support working parents, many women are delaying parenthood and thereby potentially missing their optimal fertility window. This often leads to the necessity for ART treatment to achieve parenthood. The authors also stressed the need for modifications to policy in the workplace as well as more broadly in U.S. culture. Specifically, there is a need to modify policy around parenthood for those who work outside the home, thereby providing women and men the opportunity to simultaneously build their careers and establish their lives as well as their families in the modern world. Much work is still needed for increased public awareness about age-related infertility, and the findings discussed in their chapter support the need for changes to the structures of the American workplace to include the following: reducing the American workweek across professions; providing stimulating and protected part-time jobs; providing benefits to those in part-time positions; providing high-quality, affordable childcare and on-site childcare; protecting maternity as well as paternity leave; and ceasing to discriminate against those who have gaps in their résumés due to childrearing. Because of differences in workplace expectations following parenthood among countries, it is imperative to have increased discussions about changes to societal structures in a global setting; although the medical care surrounding ART is relatively similar among countries, how individuals are able to parent and maintain careers following their care is not.

Hershberger provided an analysis of literature spanning the past 20 years about what is known regarding the reasons that drive young women's decisions about whether to undergo fertility preservation treatment. She concluded that reasons for women's decisions about whether to undergo fertility preservation treatment are complex and preference based. There are direct practice applications from this information for clinicians and others who assist young women with cancer in their decision-making processes about fertility preservation treatment. Going forward, critical understanding of this process can help other areas of fertility preservation treatment that include young women who are diagnosed with autoimmune disorders (e.g., systemic lupus erythematosus and rheumatoid arthritis) and those affected by sickle cell disease. These are important areas in need of expanded research attention so that we may better care for this growing and often vulnerable population. Additionally, these data have direct care implications, including improving the decision-making process for fertility preservation for young women facing a cancer diagnosis, which currently is an area where many clinicians and patients struggle to exchange information and identify patient preferences.

Of interest and relevance to a population often not given enough consideration in the clinical setting are those who follow rabbinic law and are seeking fertility treatment including ART. Ivry provided a comprehensive review and insight from her research about the many considerations and nuances that pertain to caring for this population. The information is relevant to anybody who is interested in providing religiously sensitive health care. The challenge, however, is that clinicians who consider patients' or personal religious principles when providing care might compromise their professional and even ethical standards of care. Ivry suggested that going forward, we need further discussion and research about whether such compromises contribute to the health and well-being of fertility patients and what effects this can have on patients' mental health status. Religious sensitivity is a broader issue beyond those who follow rabbinic law, and this chapter gives pause about the need to appreciate the potential impact of religion on care for those seeking ART.

Cooper, Flynn, and Duthie provided a novel insight into the perception of multiple gestation following ART from the patient perspective and spoke in depth about the discord between what patients value regarding the number of embryos to transfer during IVF and what clinicians perceive as optimal for maternal and child health. They further indicated that going forward, optimal care will include the provision of accurate, evidence-based information to make informed choices about embryo transfer and the potential for twins or larger gestations. The authors discussed how this information is not yet being delivered effectively. The challenge is, however, about how clinicians mediate a situation in which they and patients disagree on the number of embryos. The authors provided substantial evidence about why additional counseling and education are needed during the ART process, but this still may not resolve with both parties satisfied. Perhaps a broader public educational effort is needed to increase understanding of the risks of multiple gestational births. One question still to be answered is about the rights of the patient versus the rights of the clinicians. This important question must continue to be considered as the science refines research questions to address the problem and more individuals and couples seek ART.

It truly is an exciting time in the fertility area; although we have learned so much about the human body's capacity for reproduction and addressed many of the deviations, there is much on the horizon. Increasingly important is our understanding of genetics and its implications in the fertility setting. The genetic cause of some infertility is gaining attention among scientists, and work is focused on elucidating potential genetic determinants of infertility so that it can have practical applications for women and men. For example, we currently do not know the cause of male-factor infertility in more than 50% of the cases. What is needed is a better understanding of the genetic components of male infertility. This would in turn help clinicians advise male patients by providing more accurate calculations about success rates in terms of fathering a child. These data may also help find ways to correct the potential genetic defects, thus giving hope to those from whom we currently have no answers.

Another critical area of inquiry is the evolving knowledge of genetics in female infertility. At present, there is no way to predict the remaining years in a woman's reproductive life span, which impacts decision making in women planning for their families. Research could in the future allow clinicians the ability to predict the remaining years of optimal fertility based on the number of ovarian follicles. There is a need for increased research attention in the coming years that will advance knowledge about female infertility including polycystic ovary syndrome, endometriosis, and certain anomalies of the female reproductive system, for which currently we do not have diagnostic genetic testing available. The genetic basis of male and female infertility has real potential to help diagnose the cause of many currently unexplained cases of infertility.

## POLICY: EXPLORING ACCESS AND CHALLENGES IN ART

Despite all the current scientific advances, not all people who have infertility or are at risk of fertility loss currently receive the care that is appropriate. In the "Policy: Exploring Access and Challenges in ART" section, contributors highlighted some key issues that surround access to fertility care. Although much of the discovery related to fertility care is performed in the United States, citizens of this country often have challenges accessing care, in part because of the current structure of health care. Collura and Stevenson discussed some of the key issues related to access in the United States and offered suggestions for improvement. Going forward, Collura and Stevenson brought to light the need for social justice regarding infertility care. As they state, there continues to be much work needed to ensure comprehensive access to needed fertility care and treatments. As we write this epilogue, the American Society for Reproductive Medicine (ASRM) is planning to launch an "Access to Care" campaign in late 2015. The intention of the campaign will be to utilize ASRM's position to enhance the ability of infertile couples to obtain affordable, successful care over the next 5 years. The initial focus of this campaign is on improving access to care for infertile couples within the United States and then eventually move globally. It is critical that there be an increased focus on the prevention of infertility, as well as increased and equitable access to necessary and appropriate fertility care.

It seems that the logical next step should be toward universal access for all Americans; however, challenges to meet this goal still exist. This is demonstrated, in part, by the fact that many Americans seek the care they need outside of their own country, where costs are often more affordable. Looking more globally, Stevenson and Kanehl examined the legal and monetary reasons why individuals and couples in other developed countries often do not receive care within their own country and seek it from others. Currently, specific countries' laws and regulations have necessitated a rise in cross-border reproductive care (CBRC), a process in which citizens will travel to other locations outside their country or state to seek the necessary care. As science continues to advance and governments grapple with the decisions to make these new technologies available, those in need will continue to seek care elsewhere; this has individual and more global ramifications. Looking forward, an example of an important ethical dilemma is the recent technological development on mitochondrial transfer. This technology gives hope to those with inherited mitochondrial disorders. Although still experimental, governments are grappling with the ethical considerations surrounding this issue. In the United States, the Food and Drug Administration is currently considering clinical trials of this controversial cutting-edge fertility procedure (Farahany, 2014). As this science moves forward, new legal, ethical, and reimbursement issues will most likely come to light. It will be imperative that those working in this area continue to ask difficult and challenging questions and ensure that the policy that underlies the science is fair and ethically sound for individuals and their future offspring, families, *and* society.

Access to fertility care is an additional challenge in resource-poor countries, such as many countries in sub-Saharan Africa, where there are multiple health care challenges. Dhont and Ombelet examined the issue that surrounded access and utilization of services and also discussed an emerging cost-effective option, the

Walking Egg. Because of economic and health care challenges faced by many countries in sub-Saharan Africa, provision of adequate fertility care is currently limited. Infertility in developing nations such as those in sub-Saharan Africa has special considerations, in part because the psychosocial burden of infertility is so substantial (Hemmerling, 2010). Access to services is particularly challenging in a health care system that is striving to meet the basic needs of individuals. The rate of infertility is comparable with other areas of the world but the need for this care is further challenged by the cultural emphasis on parenthood and the social ramifications of childlessness. The authors discussed their organization, the Walking Egg, which is a nonprofit organization that works to increase awareness about childlessness in resource-poor countries, such as those in sub-Saharan Africa. The goal of the project is to make ART available to those who otherwise would not have access. The care that is becoming available in these areas utilizes more cost-effective strategies by making available "low-cost IVF" procedures in which this technology is provided at a significantly lower cost. Although still early in their implementation, there is a potentially significant positive impact on those living in these countries. Additionally, given the previous discussion about the challenges to access in developed countries such as the United States, future care may be impacted by these lower cost options. Those working in this field must stay informed about the shift in political, legal, and monetary nuances to ART care, so that care can be appropriately available to those in need.

Although it is with the very best intention that available ART treatment is used appropriately and judiciously in all situations, Scholten and Mol challenged conventional beliefs about the time frame in which infertility treatment should be initiated. The authors suggested that perhaps not all patients require prompt or immediate care. They posited that when these services are used appropriately, there is greater access for all those who are in need. Individuals and couples from all parts of the globe struggle with policies that hinder their ability to establish or maintain pregnancies because of the perception that fertility care is not of vital importance. As future advances are made in treatment options, scientists, clinicians, and health care leaders must assess the appropriate use of these innovations, to ensure optimal, safe care on an individual level, and appropriate use of resources on a broader level.

Although research in these areas will advance the care of patients with infertility, more knowledge about emerging issues such as care of the same-sex couples, as discussed by Everett, Apatira, and McCabe, would be beneficial. Because of the changing climate in many countries around the world about same-sex relationships, their civil and reproductive rights have precipitated numerous transformations to the legal, technological, and medical fields. What is necessary in today's world are changes in social and cultural attitudes toward sexual minority persons. Despite increased access to care for same-sex couples and sexual minority families, bias and exclusion of prospective sexual minority parents still often exist during fertility care. It is imperative for clinicians and researchers to work together to better understand the unique fertility experiences of lesbian, gay, bisexual, and transgender (LGBT) populations in areas in which same-sex marriage and/or sex are legal as well as other areas where same-sex sex is a criminal offense. As societal views toward inclusion of diverse populations continue to shift (i.e., the recent Supreme Court ruling to allow same-sex marriage in the United States) and there are nearly two dozen countries that currently have national laws allowing same-sex marriage (Pew Research Center, 2015), there is hope for a more seamless integration of LGBT patients into the fertility care settings.

## PRACTICE: IMPROVING THE DELIVERY OF CARE IN THE ART SETTING

The aim of fertility care is ultimately to serve patients. All the other areas—theory that supports and guides inquiry, knowledge that emerges from that inquiry, and policy that helps shape utilization of care—are focused on the end product: health care of patients. The "Practice: Improving the Delivery of Care in the ART Setting" section of this book presented several aspects of clinical care. An overview of treatment with a focus on ART was presented by Stevenson, which allowed readers outside of direct patient care an increased understanding of the treatment options available. A more in-depth examination of the complexity of care involving those with polycystic ovary syndrome was provided by Abdalmageed, Eaton, and Hurd. Polycystic ovary syndrome is a challenging clinical condition that has specific fertility ramifications as well as broader health implications. Although these broader health conditions are discussed, particular attention is paid to those seeking a pregnancy, and both clinicians and those beyond the clinical setting have had an increased appreciation about caring for this challenging population.

Infertility care is complex with many different clinicians serving a common goal. In order for proper coordination of care to patients, effective communication among the team is necessary. For example, the principles of TeamSTEPPS, a shared mental model in the fertility setting, were presented by Leonard and Stevenson. The authors discussed how communication is essential in effective care delivery, which can be modeled in other care settings seeking to maximize efficiency of the delivery of care. In order to allow for a glimpse into another way in which care might be improved and made more efficient, Moody provided insight into the expanded role of the fertility nurse in the United Kingdom. Moody delineated nursing care that allows skilled nurses to perform procedures such as oocyte retrieval and embryo transfer that were once relegated to physicians only. The expanded role of the nurse is inconsistent globally, and the United Kingdom has demonstrated forward thinking about the potential for expansion of clinical roles that only have the potential to improve patient care and meet care needs. This expanded role may have a positive impact on the care being delivered in resource-poor countries. Additionally, although countries such as the United States have demonstrated expanded roles for nurses to meet health care needs with the role of the advanced practice nurse, much of the specific care involved in fertility settings remains within the domain of physicians. Because of access issues discussed in the policy section, it is possible that consideration of expanded roles, such as being modeled in the United Kingdom, has utility in other settings. This may prove to be an essential component of care in countries such as the United States, as nursing roles continue to evolve and as financial costs and issues of access are considered.

One promising area for nurses in the United States is the re-institution of a National Subspecialty Certification for nurses and other licensed professionals working in the reproductive endocrine and infertility (REI) setting. By obtaining this certification, the care that nurses offer to patients with fertility challenges has the potential for improvement. The certification can also serve to advance nursing practice by bringing awareness about the importance and skill requirements of fertility nurses.

Most of the focus in research and care has been on females, as females are often the individuals who receive the majority of evaluation and treatment as they ultimately carry the pregnancy after conception is established. It is, therefore, imperative that we in this field expand our vision of who is the patient with the inclusion of the male partner. In the final practice chapter, McEleny presented some key clinical issues in caring for men with male factor infertility, a complex and often overlooked area. Recently, there has been a focus on male reproductive health issues and a call for increased research (Centers for Disease Control and Prevention, 2010). This chapter provided readers a substantial overview of the clinical and psychosocial needs of men diagnosed with infertility. McEleny suggested that substantial work, in particular the impact of fertility problems on the emotional well-being of men diagnosed with male factor infertility, is ahead to improve care for this specific population.

There has been a recent increase in the research focus on family planning and promoting adolescent fertility options among adolescents with chronic illness such as sickle cell disease, immunotherapy, and oncology conditions; however, there is limited evidence on the infertility rates among teens and clinical management guidelines for healthy adolescents with infertility concerns. This provides pause about the ethical dimensions associated with adolescents who may technically be experiencing fertility challenges and desire a pregnancy. In many societies, a delay in childbearing until after adolescents have met educational goals and are in a position to build families once they are able to sustain themselves autonomously is generally desired. Derouin highlighted an area not seen in the literature but often experienced by clinicians who care for adolescents. Clearly, what is needed is an improved understanding of current adolescent infertility rates and how many adolescents are being adequately evaluated for fertility concerns by clinicians. There is no clear answer about whether and, if so, how clinicians should help adolescents in family-building efforts that require advanced fertility care. Increased evaluation could, however, impact the delivery of more comprehensive care for underlying conditions that contribute to infertility such as the rising childhood obesity rates and associated comorbidities, including diabetes and polycystic ovarian syndrome, in many developed countries.

The practice section provided a cross-section of some of the clinical issues involved in patient care. The pace of the physiological sciences in ART is moving so rapidly that it is often awe-inspiring to see the advances and options that we have available for patients, especially in westernized countries. Although several of the emerging populations that receive care in ART clinics were addressed (i.e., same-sex couples, those seeking to preserve fertility in the setting of health issues such as cancer), the future will continue to focus on other populations that will require the best practice. These include couples at genetic risk who use preimplantation genetic diagnosis and screening individuals who will use a single-embryo transfer to increase singleton gestation, those who are able to undergo low-cost

IVF, and even those individuals requiring a uterine transplant (Heinonen, 2015). Practitioners and care teams must stay abreast of these evolving clinical practice considerations when caring for those with fertility challenges that surround ART. Future work in the area of practice must align with the science that continues to evolve. As we understand more and develop new technologies to meet these complex challenges, those who care for patients will need to ensure that their practice is current and evidence based.

## CONCLUSION

When we set out to put a book together that highlighted and addressed some of the key challenges and issues surrounding ART, we lacked a full appreciation of the awe and inspiration that is occurring throughout the world. The process of putting this book together has given us both personal and professional satisfaction and taught us that truly, the world is getting smaller. The ability to connect together so many thought leaders, both those with numerous years of working in this setting who offer wisdom and experience and some who are embarking on their careers and who offer hope and passion for the future, was tremendous. With each theoretical approach to a research question, surprising scientific discovery, significant policy change, and evolution of safe and comprehensive patient care, it is critical that we keep the discussion alive in order to identify solutions to fertility care challenges that surround ART in the future.

Although open to debate, many people view parenthood as an entitled "right" (Bartlam & Birch, 1998). Some even argue that IVF, a component of ART, is also a right (Tännsjö, 2008). The reproductive technology that has developed and been made available for the past 30 years has allowed countless individuals and couples the opportunity to have a biological child. Those who are passionate about this area like us can add additional inspiration and provide a much needed and desired reservoir of hope to those who might not otherwise have had any; we believe the type of commitment and energy that has been demonstrated in this book to theoretical underpinnings, research and review discoveries, perspectives about policies, and practice delivery will be synergistic in our global society and will lead to improved fertility care.

## REFERENCES

Bartlam, B., & Birch, S. (1998). A right to parenthood. *Journal of Child Health Care, 2*, 36–40. doi:10.1177/136749359800200108

Centers for Disease Control and Prevention. (2010). *Advancing men's reproductive health in the United States: Current status and future directions*. Retrieved from http://www.cdc.gov/reproductivehealth/ProductsPubs/PDFs/Male-Reproductive-Health.pdf

Farahany, N. (2014, February 25). FDA considers controversial fertility procedure. What's at stake? *The Washington Post*. Retrieved from www.washingtonpost.com/news/volokh-conspiracy/wp/2014/02/25/fda-considers-controversial-fertility-procedure-whats-at-stake

Heinonen, P. K. (2015). Livebirth after uterus transplantation. *Lancet, 385*(9985), 2352. doi:10.1016/S0140–6736(15)61097–2

Hemmerling, A. (2010). Infertility in developing countries: Scope, psychosocial burden, and the need for action. In P. Murthy & C. L. Smith (Eds.), *Women's global health and human rights* (pp. 299–310). Sudbury, MA: Jones and Bartlett Publishers.

Lazarus, R. S. (1966). *Psychological stress and the coping process.* New York, NY: McGraw-Hill.

Lazarus, R. S., & Folkman, S. (1984). *Stress, appraisal, and coping.* New York, NY: Springer.

Lazarus, R. S., & Launier, R. (1978). Stress-related transactions between person and environment. In L. A. Pervin & M. Lewis (Eds.), *Perspectives in interactional psychology* (pp. 287–327). New York, NY: Plenum.

Lobel, M. (1994). Conceptualizations, measurement, and effects of prenatal maternal stress on birth outcomes. *Journal of Behavioral Medicine, 17,* 225–272. doi:10.1007/BF01857952

Lobel, M., Dunkel-Schetter, C., & Scrimshaw, S. C. (1992). Prenatal maternal stress and prematurity: A prospective study of socioeconomically disadvantaged women. *Health Psychology, 11,* 32–40. doi:10.1037/0278–6133.11.1.32

Pew Research Center. (2015). *Gay marriage around the world.* Retrieved from http://www.pewforum.org/2015/06/26/gay-marriage-around-the-world-2013

Tännsjö, T. (2008). Our right to in vitro fertilisation—Its scope and limits. *Journal of Medical Ethics, 34,* 802–806. doi:10.1136/jme.2008.024232

# INDEX

acupuncture, 73–74
adolescent fertility treatment, 337–340
adoption
  family building, 87, 176, 217
  heterosexuals, 247
  and relaxation, 76–77
advocacy and networking, Walking Egg
    Project, 230
Affordable Care Act (ACA), 195–198
alpha amylase, 71–72
American Society for Reproductive Medicine
    (ASRM), 106, 112, 113, 161, 168, 169, 192,
    196, 348
  Ethics Committee, 106
American Society of Clinical Oncology
    (ASCO), 144
amniocentesis, 327
andrologists, 302
andrology team, 302
aneuploidy, 104
anxiety
  country origin, ethnicity, and cultural identity
    impact, 41–42
  gestational age impact, 42
  pregnancy-specific, 31
  previous pregnancies impact, 40–41
ART. See assisted reproductive
    technologies (ART)
ASRM. See American Society for Reproductive
    Medicine (ASRM)
assisted reproductive technologies (ART).
    See also couples with fertility issues
  awareness, 49
  in CBRC. See cross-border reproductive
    care (CBRC)
  couple and family unit of analysis findings,
    53–55
  cycles, 201, 203
  donor oocytes, 87

first-time parents older than 40 years, 103
funding. See funding for ART
individual unit of analysis findings, 50–52
multifetal pregnancies, 168–170
physician/advanced practice nurse, 300–301
practice and guidelines, 168–170
pregnancy and birth rates, 87
rabbinic law
  culturally and religiously appropriate
    reproductive medicine, 153–154
  fertility and medicine according to halacha,
    155–156
  medical practitioners on trial, 157–158
  religiously observant fertility patients,
    156–157
  religiously sensitive health care, 158–159
reproductive medicine, culturally and
    religiously appropriate, 153–154
same-sex relationship, 245
sexual minority women (SMW), 246
surrogates and gestational
    carriers, 183–186
Walking Egg Project, 223–231
azoospermia
  azoospermic men, 329–330
  gamete donation, 268
  infertility investigations, 327
  male fertility challenges, 323
  obstructive, 326
  team communication, 304

Beckwith-Wiedemann syndrome, 329
biomarker
  male semen quality, 325
  stress, 66, 70–73
birth defects. See also delayed parenting
  genetic disorders risk, 104
  gestational carriers, 185
  later-life parenting, 104, 105

Blair-Loy's concept, 136–137
breast cancer
    fertility preservation, 146
    letrozole, 283
    survivors, fertility, 144
breastfeeding
    delayed parenting, 136
    donor-oocyte recipients, 97
    oocyte donation, 98
    oocyte-recipient women, 99–100, 345
    women's feeling about 88, 94–96
British Fertility Society (BFS), 314

cardiovascular disease (CVD)
    couple and individual partner concerns, 271
    and polycystic ovary syndrome, 285
CBRC. See cross-border reproductive care (CBRC)
Centers for Disease Control and Prevention
        (CDC), 20, 162
cesarean deliveries, 94, 105–106, 185
child-bearing age for women, 202–203
child-centered mothering, 137–138
children born to later-life parents, 111–112
chorionic villous biopsy, 327
chronic anovulation, 280
clinical counseling, cancer, 145–146
clinicians and care providers considerations,
        later-life parenting
    age-related fertility, 114
    conversations, 115
    elective egg freezing, 114
    patients counseling, 115
    preparedness plan, 115
    written guidelines, 115
clomiphene, 281–283
cognator coping subsystem, 4
cohabitation and family structure, 19–20, 23–24
communication. See also team communication
    core team skills, 299–300
    health care providers, 296
    leadership culture, 296
    with patients, 303–304
    safe, high-quality patient care, 295
compensation, gestational carriers, 185, 196, 268
complementary and alternative medicine (CAM)
    depressive and anxious symptomatology, 79
    infertile patient populations, 73
    yoga, 75
complications, 91–92
    expectations and, 93
    self-confidence during, 93

comprehensive theory of infertility
    adaptation theories, 11
    adjustment, 7
    couple resilience, 7–8
    nursing conceptual models and, 7
    PubMed/MEDLINE search, 5–6
    quality of life, 8
    relinquishing infertility, 7
    restitution, 8
    Roy Adaptation Model concepts, 3–4, 8–10
    subjective well-being, 8
conception
    chances, 72
    couples with failed IVF and ICSI treatment, 54
    delayed, 109, 111
    distressing, 43
    donor, 90, 96
    family planning, 20
    natural course of, 235–236
    oocyte donor, 90, 99
    primary infertility and, 68
    reproductive processes and infertility
        treatments, 163
    spontaneous, 76–78
    successful vs. unsuccessful, 76
congenital conditions of male infertility, 265
contemporary infertility treatments, 161
contextual stimuli, 4, 8
continuity of care, specialist nursing practice, 317
contraception and abortion, 122
co-parenting relationship, later-life parenting, 108
coping processes, Roy Adaptation Model (RAM), 4
core team skills
    communication, 299–300
    leadership, 298–299
    mutual support, 299
    situation monitoring, 299
cost-effective health care system, 311–312
cost-effective treatments
    Millennium Development Goal 5 (MDG5), 223
    WE Project. See Walking Egg Project
couple and family unit of analysis
    behavior, 53
    genetic risks, 54
    heterosexual couples, 55
    intentions, 53
    interviews, 54
    in vitro fertilization treatment, 53
    marital stress, 55
    psychosocial characteristics, 53–54
    quality of care, 53

couple resilience, 7–8
couples with fertility issues
    assisted reproductive technology (ART)
        gamete donation, 268
        gestational carrier, 268, 269
        intracytoplasmic sperm injection (ICSI), 267
        mitochondrial transfer, 268–269
        preimplantation genetic diagnosis, 267
        in vitro fertilization, 266–267
    couple and individual partner concerns, 271
    educational needs, 270
    etiology of infertility, 264–265
    physiological considerations, 270–271
    psychosocial needs, 270
    socioeconomic considerations, 270
crew resource management (CRM) training, 296
cross-border reproductive care (CBRC)
    baby business, 205
    gamete donation, 206
    legal restrictions, 205
    outgoing countries, 205
    patient consideration, 206–207
    preimplantation genetic diagnosis, 204–206
    rates, 205
    religious and ethical constructs, 205
    single and lesbian women, 206
cryopreservation, 113, 168, 169, 229, 305, 327
cultural competency, 24–25, 251, 344
current duration approach, infertility, 193
cystic fibrosis, infertility investigations, 206, 258, 267, 327

dehydroepiandrosterone sulfate (DHEAS), 278–279
delayed conception, 109, 111
delayed parenting
    Blair-Loy's concept, 136–137
    "career" and "parenting roles" codes, 124
    contraception and abortion, 122
    dual-earner families, 122
    expectations, parenting value and career, 126–128
    financial security and career achievement, 135
    gender impact, 131–133
    heterosexual couples, 135–136
    later-life parenting, 123
    middle-class dual-earner couples, 137
    motherhood penalty, 121–122
    Nam–Boyd Occupational Status Scale, 124
    paid work reductions and structural inequality, 131–133
    participants, demographic description, 124–126
    qualitative data analysis methods, 123
    structural inequalities in workplace, 135
    unpaid housework and caregiving, 122
    women
        fertility, 134–135
        participation in workplace, 121–122
    workplace policy, 133–134
    work-related commitments, limits for, 128–130
Demographic Health Surveys, 212
depressive symptomatology, 75, 110
diabetes
    gestational, 40, 87, 105, 162, 265, 282
    male fertility challenges, 325
    and polycystic ovary syndrome, 285
diagnostic hysteroscopy, 225
Dickey–Wicker Amendment, 198
discordant attitude, male fertility challenges, 330
distress and infertility, 68–69
domestic groups, 16
donor-conceiving couples, 87
donor oocytes
    assisted reproductive technology (ART), 87
    first-time parents older than 40 years, 103
    in vitro fertilization with, 115
    recipients, 88, 108
donor sperm, 88, 204, 206, 268, 330
Down syndrome, later-life parenting, 104–105
dual-earner families, 122, 137

educational needs for couples with fertility issues, 270
egg donation, 59, 60, 88–89, 106, 158, 206
egg donor, 60
    donor-conceived children, 59
    genetic lineage, 59–60
    pregnancy in infertile women, 59
egg-freezing parties, 113
EHB plan. See Essential Health Benefits (EHB) plan
elective cesareans, later-life parenting, 105–106
elective oocyte cryopreservation, 113
embryologist, 164, 302, 305–306
embryo transfers, 87, 312–313
emotional distress, 67, 69, 73–75
emotional response component, 31, 40, 42, 43
endocrine disruptors, male fertility challenges, 324
endometrial cancer, 280, 287, 288
endometriosis, 264, 347
environmental stimuli, 4
Essential Health Benefits (EHB) plan, 197

Ethics Committee of the American Society for
     Reproductive Medicine, 245
etiology of infertility
   contributors to female infertility, 264–265
   contributors to male infertility, 265
European Society of Human Reproduction and
     Embryology (ESHRE), 315–316
expectations, parenting value and career, 126–128

family formation
   planning and fertility care, 217
   policy, 348–350
   practice, 350–352
   research and reviews, 344–347
   schema, 136
   theories and conceptual concepts, 343–344
family structure
   anthropological view, 15–16
   cohabitation and, 19–20, 23–24
   fertility rates, 17–18, 23
   health care providers, implications for, 24–25
   households, 22
   in vitro fertilization/intracytoplasmic sperm
     injection treatment, 20–21
   life expectancy, 18–19
   national trends, 21–22
   sociological view, 16
   U.S. families, 22–24
FCSRCA. See Fertility Clinic Success Rate and
     Certification Act (FCSRCA)
fecundity, 193
federal research restrictions, 198
female personality characteristics, 69
fertility care
   awareness counseling, 225–226
   breast cancer survivors, 144
   medicine according to halacha
     biomedicine, 156
     halachic supervisors, 156
     Judaism, 155
     mamzer children, 155
     medico-religious expertise, 155
     PUAH, 155–156
     PUANIT, 156
   natural pregnancy post-cancer, 144
   perceptions about assessment, men's, 330–331
   programs, same-sex relationship, 245
   rates, 17–18
   stress and. See psychological stress and
     fertility
   workup and diagnoses, 236

fertility care, in developing countries (DCs)
   access of, 214–215
   controversial issue, 215
   costs, 218–219
   family planning and, 217
   HIV care, 217–218
   infertility
     causes, 212–213
     consequences of, 213
     definition, 211
     health-seeking behavior, 213–214
     HIV, 214
     magnitude of problem, 212
     primary and secondary, 211–212
   integrated reproductive health services,
     216–217
   limited resources argument, 216
   overpopulation, 216
   prevention, 215–216
   risk management, 218
Fertility Clinic Success Rate and Certification Act
     (FCSRCA), 166, 167
fertility nursing practice in the UK
   clinic activities and treatments variations, 313
   embryo transfers, 312–313
   fertility services development, 312
   HFEA Code of Practice, 312
   nursing guidelines, 311–313
   "one size fits all" approach, 313
   roles, 313
fertility preservation treatment after cancer
     diagnosis
   autoimmune disorder and, 149
   decision-making processes, 148
   natural pregnancy post-cancer, 144
   preference-sensitive decisions, 148
   young women with cancer
     clinical counseling effect, 145–146
     culture, society, and policies effect, 147
     sociodemographics effect, 146–147
financial security and career achievement,
     delayed parenting, 135
financial support staff, 302–303
first-time motherhood
   age 45 years or older, 103–104
   male fertility challenges, 324
first-time parents older than 40 years
   advanced maternal age, 103
   assisted reproductive technologies
     (ART), 103
   delayed child bearing, 103

donor oocytes, 103
later-life parenthood, 103
older motherhood, 103, 104
focal stimulus, 4, 11
follicular development, IVF, 228
funding for ART
access, 204–206
CBRC. *See* cross-border reproductive
care (CBRC)
coverage for, 203–204
eligibility and restrictions, 202–204
heterosexual relationship, 203
homosexual couples, 203
privatization of health care, 204
soft guideline for women, 202
waiting times for services, 204

gamete donation, 206, 207, 268
gamete intrafallopian transfer (GIFT), 162
genital tract blockage, male fertility
challenges, 329
gestational age, 40, 42, 238
gestational carriers
compensation, 185
couples with fertility issues, 268, 269
independent legal representation, 185
lifestyle and other habits, 185
partners, 185
gestational diabetes, 40, 87, 105, 162,
265, 282
glucose intolerance, and polycystic ovary
syndrome, 285
gonadotropin-releasing hormone (GnRH) in
women and men, 67–68, 284
gross national income (GNI), in developing
countries, 211

"halachic infertility," 158
halachic supervisors, 156
health care providers
family structure, 24–25
reproductive medicine, culturally and
religiously appropriate, 154
same-sex relationships, 251–252
team communication, 296
health-seeking behavior, infertility, 213–214
heterosexual couples, 250
couple and family unit of analysis
findings, 54
delayed parenting, 135–136
hirsutism, 278, 289

HIV
care and fertility care, 217–218
infertility, 214
hormonal biomarkers, stress and infertility
alpha amylase, 71–72
cortisol, 73
hormonal imbalances, 264–265
Human Fertilisation and Embryology Act
1990, 312
hyaluronic acid, male fertility challenges, 328
hyperandrogenism, polycystic ovary syndrome,
278–279, 286–287
hypogonadism, 326, 329
hypothalamic–pituitary–gonadal (HPG) axis,
67–68
hysterosalpingography, 224–225
hysteroscopy, 225

iatrogenic multifetal pregnancies, 162–163
idiopathic premature-ovarian failure, 89
in vitro fertilization/intracytoplasmic sperm
injection treatment, 20–21
impaired fecundity, 23, 193, 198
inability to conceive, 68, 183, 235, 300
individual unit of analysis findings
Chinese society, 52
concept of hope, 51
education, 51
esophageal atresia, IVF pregnant woman, 51
intracytoplasmic sperm injection (ICSI), 51
physiological report, 51
regret, 51
social and cultural history, 52
infertile couples, 30, 53–54, 211–214, 216, 217,
224, 230, 263
infertility
action plan, 194
barriers to access
Affordable Care Act (ACA), 196–197
complacency in states with mandates, 196
federal research restrictions, 198
insurance, 194–195
personhood and other anti-family state
bills, 196
restrictive federal benefits, 197
state mandates status, 195–196
causes, 212–213
CBRC. *See* cross-border reproductive care
(CBRC)
consequences of, 213
definition, 192–193, 211

infertility (*cont.*)
 conception, natural course of, 235–236
 fertility workup and diagnoses, 236
 implications for treatment usage, 238–239
 safety, 238
 treatment effectiveness, 236–237
 health-seeking behavior, 213–214
 HIV, 214
 incidence of, 193
 magnitude of problem of, 212
 male, 193
 primary and secondary, 211–212
 services utilization, 194
 stress
 female personality characteristics, 69
 hormonal biomarkers, 71–73
 psychogenic infertility, 69
 relaxing conditions/activities and
 fertility, 73
 survey-based assessment, 70–71
 treatment
 advocacy and networking, 230
 countries/pilot centers selection, 230
 effectiveness, 236–237
 multifetal pregnancies, 177–178
 restrictive federal benefits to, 197
 safety, 238
informal donor relationships, 247
inseminating motile count (IMC), 225
insulin resistance, and polycystic ovary
 syndrome, 285
insurance and infertility, 194–195
integrated reproductive health services,
 216–217
intensive mothering, 137–138
interactive parenting style, 108
interdependence mode, adaptation modes, 4
International Committee for Monitoring
 Assisted Reproductive Technology, 192
International Council for Nurses (ICN), 314
intracytoplasmic sperm injection (ICSI), 225
 couples with fertility issues, 267
 male fertility challenges, 326, 328–329
 pregnancies, 87
 reproductive processes and infertility
 treatments, 164
 treatment, 20–21
intrauterine insemination (IUI)
 infertility treatment and non-IVF-assisted
 reproduction, 225–227
 multifetal pregnancies, 162

study, 314
 treatment, 236–237
in vitro fertilization (IVF) pregnancies
 anxiety
 country of origin, ethnicity, and cultural
 identity impact, 41–42
 gestational age impact, 42
 pregnancy-specific, 31
 previous pregnancies impact, 40–41
 conception, natural course of, 235–236
 couples with fertility issues, 266–267
 emotional response component, 31, 40
 fertility clinic success rate and certification act,
 166–168
 fertility workup and diagnoses, 236
 findings regarding stress outcomes, 39–40
 follicular development, 228
 Human Fertilisation and Embryology
 Authority (HFEA) licensed, 312
 implications for treatment usage, 238–239
 infertile couples, 30
 low-cost. *See* Walking Egg Project
 maternal death, 238
 multifetal pregnancies, 162
 ovarian stimulation, 227–228, 238
 perceptual component, 31
 polycystic ovary syndrome, 283–284
 preimplantation genetic diagnosis, 257–259
 quantitative perspective, 30
 restrictive federal benefits to infertility
 treatments, 197
 safety, 238
 simplified laboratory procedures, 227
 stress, 29–30
 stress reduction, later parenting, 108
 studies, 32–38
 success rate, 87
 theoretical model, 30–31
 treatment effectiveness, 236–237
Israel Ministry of Health (IMOH), 153
IUI. *See* intrauterine insemination (IUI)

Joint Commission on Accreditation in Healthcare
 Organizations, 296

karyotype, male fertility, 326–327
Kleinfelter syndrome
 later-life parenting, 105
 male fertility, 326–327
knowledge and competence, specialist nursing
 practice, 315

laboratory technicians, 300, 302
later-life parenting
  aneuploidy, 104
  birth defects and genetic disorders risk, 104
  children, psychosocial implications for, 111–112
  clinicians and care providers, 114–116
  Down syndrome, 104–105
  egg quality, 104
  elective oocyte cryopreservation, 113
  female fertility declines with age, 104
  health outcomes, 106–107
  Klinefelter syndrome, 105
  pregnancy risks associated with advanced
      maternal age, 105–106
  psychosocial implications of
    co-parenting relationship, 108
    depressive symptomatology, 110
    donor oocyte recipients, 108
    interactive parenting style, 108
    maternal maturity hypothesis, 108
    negative outcomes, 109
    nonnormative birth experience, 110
    parental regret, 109
    postmenopausal parenting, 110
    respondents discomfort, 109
    satisfaction and behaviors, 108
    stressful IVF treatment, 108
  research, 113–114
leadership
  ad hoc meetings, 299
  communication, 296, 299–300
  culture, 296
  high-quality fertility care, 296
  leaders, responsibility of, 298–299
legal recognition, same-sex relationship, 245–246
legal restrictions, CBRC, 205
lesbian donor insemination, 248
lesbian gay, bisexual and transgender persons
    (LGBT), 245, 251
letrozole, 283
life expectancy, 18–19, 107, 112, 325
lifestyle problem, male fertility challenges, 324
limited resources argument, 216
low-cost ovarian stimulation protocols for IVF,
    227–228

male fertility challenges
  analysis process inconsistencies, 325
  Beckwith–Wiedemann syndrome, 329
  cope with fertility treatment, 331
  endocrine disruptors, 324

fertility assessment, 330–331
first-time mothers, 324
genetic investigations, 326–327
genital examination, 326
genital tract blockage, 329
hyaluronic acid, 328
hypogonadism, 326, 329
impact on relationships, 331–332
infertility factor, 225, 227
intra-cytoplasmic sperm injection (ICSI), 326,
    328–329
lifestyle problems, 324
male sexual function, 326
obesity and diabetes, 325
oligoasthenoteratozoospermia (OAT), 325
pollutants, 324
quality of semen, 323
semen analysis, 325, 326
sexually transmitted infections (STIs), 324
testes cancer, 326
testicular cancer and, 325
testicular dysgenesis syndrome, 323–324
tests for, 328
treatment options
  azoospermic men, 329–330
  donor sperm usage, 330
mamzer children, 155
masculine identity, 331
maternal and fetal outcomes, same-sex
    relationship, 249–250
maternal complications, 162, 284
maternal maturity hypothesis, 108
medically assisted reproduction (MAR),
    246–248
medical practitioners on trial, 157–158
"medical tourism," 204–206
men participation in parenting, 137–138
metabolic syndrome, and polycystic ovary
    syndrome, 286
metformin
  infertility treatments, 281–282
  and polycystic ovary syndrome, 288
microdeletion patterns, male infertility, 327
MicroTESE technique, 329–330
middle-class, dual-earner couples, delayed
    parenting, 137
Midland Fertility Services, 313
Military Treatment Facilities (MTF), 197
mindfulness meditation, 74–75
"mini doctors," 319
mistimed/nonnormative birth experience, 110

mitochondrial transfer, 268–269, 348
modern mothering, 137–138
motherhood, 213. *See also* first time motherhood penalty, 121–122
MTF. *See* Military Treatment Facilities (MTF)
multifetal pregnancies
  American Society for Reproductive Medicine (ASRM), 161
  assisted reproductive technologies practice and guidelines, 168–170
  Centers for Disease Control and Prevention (CDC), 162
  contemporary infertility treatments, 161
  gamete intrafallopian transfer (GIFT), 162
  iatrogenic, 162–163
  infertility treatment, 177–178
  intrauterine insemination (IUI), 162
  IVF and fertility clinic success rate and certification act, 166–168
  IVF procedures, 162
  maternal complications, 162
  multiple gestation, 162, 171, 177–178
  ovarian stimulation, 162
  patient decision making, 170–177
  practitioner's role, 177–178
  reproductive processes and infertility treatments, 163–166
  single-embryo transfer (SET), 165
  zygote intrafallopian transfer (ZIFT), 162
multiple gestation, 162, 171, 177–178
multiple healthy embryos, 164
multiple-infant births, 167
multiple pregnancies, 227
mutual support, 299

Nam–Boyd Occupational Status Scale, 124
National Infertility Association, 191, 258, 259
National Survey of Family Growth (NSFG), 192–193
National Vital Statistics Reports, 112
natural pregnancy post-cancer, 144
non-biologic child, 183
non-IVF-assisted reproduction, 225–227
nonnormative birth experience, 110
NSFG. *See* National Survey of Family Growth (NSFG)
nuclear family, 15, 19
nulliparous women, 194
nurses
  self-esteem of, 317
  team members, 301–302

nursing care
  benefits, 316–318
  fertility nursing practice in UK, 311–313
  regulations and opinions, 311
  specialist practice, 313–316
nursing practice (specialist)
  academic achievement, 314–315
  accreditation, 315
  benefits of, 316–318
  British Fertility Society (BFS) embryo transfer and IUI study, 314
  caution, 313
  clinical settings, 314
  conferences and workshops, 314
  continuity of care, 317
  European Society of Human Reproduction and Embryology (ESHRE), 315–316
  evaluation, 316
  guidelines, 315
  International Council for Nurses (ICN), 314
  knowledge and competence, 315
  local or nationally agreed competences, 315
  "mini doctors," 319
  oocyte/sperm retrieval, 318
  patient concerns, 318–319
  public trust, 315
  Royal College of Nursing fertility nurses group, 314–315
  roles and responsibilities, 318
  self-esteem of nurses, 317
  teaching methods, 314
  training and assessment program, 313

obesity
  male fertility challenges, 325
  polycystic ovary syndrome, 285
obstructive azoospermia, 326
occupational schema, 136
office mini-hysteroscopy, 225
OHSS. *See* ovarian hyperstimulation syndrome (OHSS)
oligoasthenoteratozoospermia (OAT), 325
one-stop diagnostic phase, 224–227
oocyte cryopreservation, 113
oocyte donation
  breastfeeding, 94–96
  complications, 89, 91–93
  donor-conceived nature, of pregnancy, 90
  donor gametes, 89
  donor-oocyte pregnancies, 90
  emotionless thought, 96–97

infertile women, medical and professional
  knowledge, 89
interviews, 90–91
motherhood feeling, 93–94
participants, 89
pregnancy, 88–89
professional care and oocyte recipients, 90
woman's privacy, 90
oocyte-donor conception, 99
oral contraceptives, 280, 286–289
ovarian drilling, 283
ovarian hyperstimulation syndrome (OHSS),
  238, 270–271
ovarian stimulation, 162, 163–164, 238
overpopulation in developing countries
  (DCs), 216
ovulation induction
  with injectable gonadotropins, 283
  with oral medications, 282–283
ovulatory dysfunction, 227, 278

paid work reductions and structural inequality,
  131–133
parasympathetic dominance, 75
parental regret, later-life parenting, 109
patient care, team communication, 295
patient decision making
  awareness, 176–177
  comparing treatment options, 176
  insemination, 173
  interview, 171
  multifetal pregnancies risk, 170
  multiple gestation, 171
  participant-initiated discussions, 172
  reproductive specialist (RS), 171
  treatment, multiple cycles, 170
  twins, positive and negative prospect, 172
patients/partners, team members, 303
PCOS. See polycystic ovary syndrome (PCOS)
personhood and other anti-family state
  bills, 196
PGD. See preimplantation genetic diagnosis (PGD)
physicians and advanced practice nurses
  (APNs), 300–301
placing limits, 137
pollutants, male fertility challenges, 324
polycystic ovary syndrome (PCOS)
  diagnosis, 277–279
  endocrine disorder in women, 277
  infertility, 280–284
  long-term treatment of, 287–289

medical conditions associated
  with, 285–286
menstrual irregularity, 278, 280
pregnancy, 284
psychological support, 289
psychosocial implications of, 286–287
reproductive impact, 279–280
Rotterdam criteria, 278
postmenopausal parenting, 110
pregnancy
  anxiety, 31
  complications, later-life parenting,
    105–106
  hypertension, 87
  outcome anxiety, 92
  risks associated with advanced maternal age,
    105–106
preimplantation genetic diagnosis (PGD),
  204, 327
  couples with fertility issues, 267
  cross-border reproductive care (CBRC),
    204–206
  genetically at-risk couple, 257–259
  sickle cell disease, 257–259
preterm birth, later-life parenting, 106
privatization of health care, 204
psychogenic infertility, 69
psychological stress and fertility. See also stress
  acupuncture, 73–74
  distress and, 68–69
  hormonal biomarkers of stress and, 71–73
  inability to conceive, 68
  mindfulness meditation, 74–75
  primary and secondary infertility and, 68
  psychotherapy and psychological
    intervention, 75–76
  relaxation
    adoption, 76–77
    conditions/activities and fertility, 73
    treatment stopping/starting, 77–78
  stress, 69–70
  survey-based assessment, 70–71
  woman, egg donor, 59–60
  yoga, 75
psychosocial needs, couples with fertility
  issues, 270
psychotherapy and psychological intervention,
  infertility, 75–76
PUAH, fertility and medicine, 155–159
PUANIT, for PUAH's couples, 156
public trust, specialist nursing practice, 315

rabbinic law, ART
  culturally and religiously appropriate
      reproductive medicine, 153–154
  fertility and medicine according to halacha,
      155–156
  medical practitioners on trial, 157–158
  religiously observant fertility patients, 156–157
  religiously sensitive health care, 158–159
recreational sex, 332
recurrent pregnancy loss, 192
regulator coping subsystem, 4
relaxation
  adoption, 76–77
  conditions/activities and fertility, 73
  treatment stopping/starting, 77–78
religiously observant fertility patients, 156–157
reproductive medicine, 239
  assisted reproductive technologies (ARTs) in
      Israel, 153–154
  authority and complex power relations, 154
  awareness, 153
  biomedical professionals, 153
  health care professionals, 154
  Israel Ministry of Health initiative, 153
  "kosher" reproductive medicine, 154
  patient autonomy, 153
  triadic provider–patient–rabbi relations, 154
reproductive processes and infertility treatments,
      163–166
  iatrogenic multifetal pregnancies, 162–163
  ovarian stimulation, 163–164
  take-home baby, 165
reproductive sex, 332
residual stimuli, 4, 7
role function mode, adaptation modes, 4
Roy Adaptation Model (RAM)
  adaptation level, 6
  comprehensive theory of infertility, 3–4, 8–10
  concepts and propositions, 5, 8
  physiological mode of adaptation, 7
  summary, 4
Royal College of Nursing (RCN) fertility nurses
      group, 314–315

safety, infertility, 238
same-sex relationship
  assisted reproductive technology (ART), 245
  care experiences in reproductive care settings,
      248–249
  fertility programs, 245

  health care providers and future
      recommendations, 251–252
  legal recognition, 245–246
  maternal and fetal outcomes, 249–250
  medically assisted reproduction
      (MAR), 246
  sexual minority parents, 245
  sexual minority women (SMW), 246–247
  sperm donor selection, 247–248
  surrogacy and gay men, 250
  transgender experiences in fertility care
      settings, 250–251
scaling back, 137
self-concept mode, adaptation modes, 4
self-esteem of nurses, 317
semen analysis, 225, 325, 326
SET. See single embryo transfer (SET)
sex hormone binding globulin (SHBG), 288
sexually transmitted infections (STIs), 212, 224,
      247, 264, 324
sexual minority parents, 245, 252, 349
sexual minority women (SMW)
  assisted reproductive technologies and, 246
  homophobic and discriminatory
      interactions, 246
  lesbians, 246, 247
  medically assisted reproduction methods,
      246–247
SHBG. See sex hormone binding
      globulin (SHBG)
sickle cell disease, preimplantation genetic
      diagnosis, 257–259
simplified infertility treatment, 225–227
simplified IVF laboratory procedures, 227
single and lesbian women, and CBRC, 206
single embryo transfer (SET), 165, 238
situation monitoring, 299
societal attitudes, 312
Society for Assisted Reproductive Technology
      (SART), 167
socioeconomic considerations for couples with
      fertility issues, 270
sperm donor selection
  informal relationships, 247
  lesbian donor insemination, 248
  personal preferences, 247–248
  racial/ethnic minority women, 248
  sexual minority women, 247–248
  socioeconomic status (SES), 248
spontaneous conception, 76–78

state mandates status, 195–196
stillbirth and maternal death, later-life
    parenting, 106
stress
  biological plausibility and reduced fecundity,
    68–69
  infertility
    female personality characteristics, 69
    hormonal biomarkers, 71–73
    psychogenic infertility, 69
    relaxing conditions/activities and
      fertility, 73
    survey-based assessment, 70–71
  physiology
    adrenocorticotropic hormone (ACTH), 67
    autonomic system, 66
    breed and feed system, 66
    chronic stress, 66–67
    defined, 65
    epinephrine, 66
    norepinephrine, 66
    responses, 65
    rest and digest system, 66
    sympathetic–adrenal–medullary (SAM)
      pathway, 65
    sympathetic nervous system, 66
  pregnancy and. *See in vitro* fertilization (IVF)
    pregnancies
subfertile couples, 237
surrogacy. *See also in vitro* fertilization (IVF)
    pregnancies
  gay men, 250
  surrogates and gestational carriers, 183–186
survey-based assessment, stress and infertility,
    70–71

take-home baby, 165
team communication
  Agency for Healthcare Research and Quality
    (AHRQ), 296–297
  case study, 304–307
  core team skills
    communication, 299–300
    leadership, 298–299
    mutual support, 299
    situation monitoring, 299
  crew resource management (CRM)
    training, 296
  health care industry, 296
  health care providers, 296

Joint Commission on Accreditation in
    Healthcare Organizations, 296
  leadership culture, 296
  maximizing communication with patients,
    303–304
  safe high-quality patient care, 295
  team members
    andrologists, 302
    embryologists, 302
    financial support staff, 302–303
    laboratory technicians, 302
    nurses, 301–302
    patients/partners, 303
    physicians and advanced practice nurses
      (APNs), 300–301
  TeamSTEPPS, 296–297, 304
  teamwork, 295–297, 307
  training interventions, 297
testes cancer, male fertility challenges, 326
testicular cancer, 325
testicular dysgenesis syndrome, 323–324
testosterone, and polycystic ovary
    syndrome, 278
total fertility rate (TFR), 17–18
traditional Chinese acupuncture, 73–74
transgender experiences in fertility care settings,
    250–251
tubal blockage, 264
tubal obstruction, one-stop diagnostic phase,
    224–225
tubal patency, 227

UK nursing guidelines, 311–313
unpaid housework and caregiving, 122
unprotected sexual intercourse, 23, 192, 211

vaginal bleeding, 87

Walking Egg (WE) Project
  action plan, 223–224
  advocacy and networking, 230
  countries/pilot centers selection, 230
  goal, 223
  low-cost ovarian stimulation protocols for IVF,
    227–228
  non-IVF-assisted reproduction, 225–227
  one-stop diagnostic phase, 224–227
  simplified infertility treatment, 225–227
  simplified IVF laboratory procedures, 227
  ⁺We Pilot centers implementation, 229–230

weight loss
  infertility treatments, 280–281
  and polycystic ovary syndrome,
    286–287
women's participation in workplace,
  121–122
workplace policy, delayed parenting,
  133–134

yoga, 53, 75
young women with cancer
  clinical counseling effect, 145–146
  culture, society, and policies effect, 147
  fertility preservation, 145
  sociodemographics effect, 146–147

zygote intrafallopian transfer (ZIFT), 162

Printed in the United States
By Bookmasters